DOPAMINE

Advances in Biochemical Psychopharmacology
Volume 19

Advances in Biochemical Psychopharmacology

Series Editors:

Erminio Costa, M.D.
Chief, Laboratory of Preclinical Pharmacology
National Institute of Mental Health
Washington, D.C.

Paul Greengard, Ph.D.
Professor of Pharmacology
Yale University School of Medicine
New Haven, Connecticut

Dopamine

Advances in Biochemical Psychopharmacology
Volume 19

Edited by:

Peter J. Roberts, B.Sc., Ph.D.

Department of Physiology and Pharmacology
School of Biochemical and Physiological Sciences
University of Southampton
Southampton, England

Geoffrey N. Woodruff, B.Pharm., Ph.D.

Department of Physiology and Pharmacology
School of Biochemical and Physiological Sciences
University of Southampton
Southampton, England

Leslie L. Iversen, M.A., Ph.D.

MRC Neurochemical Pharmacology Unit
Department of Pharmacology
University of Cambridge
Cambridge, England

Raven Press ▪ New York

Raven Press, 1140 Avenue of the Americas, New York, New York 10036

Made in the United States of America

(Advances in biochemical psychopharmacology, v. 19)
Papers from a symposium held in the summer of 1977 at the University of Southampton, England.
Includes bibliographical references and index.
I. Dopamine-Congresses. 2. Dopamine-Physiological effect-Congresses. I. 3. Brain chemistry-Congresses. I. Roberts, Peter J.
II. Woodruff, Geoffrey N. III. Iversen, Leslie Lars. IV. Series. (DNLM: 1. Dopamine-Congresses 2. Receptors-Dopamine-Congresses.
W1 AD437 v. I9/WLI02.8 S797d I977)
RM3I5,A4 vol. I9 (QP563.D66) 6I5'.78'08s
ISBN 0-89004-239-X   (6I6.8)   78-4355

Preface

This volume provides a comprehensive review of the anatomy, biochemistry, and pharmacology of the dopamine systems in the brain. The initial chapters are devoted to the anatomy of the dopaminergic neuron systems in the brain, the uptake and release of the transmitter from its storage sites, the nature of the dopamine receptor, and the pharmacological properties of this receptor. This is followed by a consideration of the effects of pharmacologic agents on the function of the dopamine systems and their role in neurology and psychiatry.

This volume will be of interest to neurochemists and pharmacologists, as well as to those psychiatrists and neurologists interested in the chemical basis of neural disorders.

The Editors

Acknowledgments

In conjunction with the sixth meeting of the International Society for Neurochemistry in Copenhagen, a Satellite Symposium on Dopamine was held at the University of Southampton, England. The meeting on which this volume is based provided up-to-date information on the neurochemistry and pharmacology of dopamine, ranging from molecular mechanisms, to therapeutic approaches to disorders of brain dopamine metabolism.

All who participated in the symposium will testify to its success in promoting the frank and open exchange of information and ideas, as well as in the formation of new research collaborations, and friendships. A major factor in the friendly and relaxed atmosphere was the superlative effort of our colleague, Dr. Judith Poat who dealt with each and every problem or inquiry of the participants: to her, we express our special thanks. Thanks are also due to the University and the City of Southampton for providing two receptions; the latter being in the splendid surroundings of the City's art gallery.

Finally, the meeting would not have been possible in these financially stringent times for scientists, without the extremely generous support which was accorded the symposium. It is therefore a pleasure to express our gratitude to the following organizations: The Wellcome Trust (London), Paul-Martini-Stiftung (Frankfurt, Main), Boehringer Ingelheim (Ingelheim am Rhein), The Royal Society (London), Merck Institute for Therapeutic Research (West Point, Pennsylvania), Ciba-Geigy (UK) Ltd. (Macclesfield), Roche Products Ltd. (Welwyn Garden City), H. Lundbeck & Co. A/S (Copenhagen), Eli Lilly Research Centre (Indianapolis), Smith Kline & French Laboratories (Philadelphia), Pfizer Central Research (Sandwich), Parkinson's Disease Society (London), Sandoz Ltd. (Basel), Schering A. G. (Berlin), Allen & Hanbury's Ltd. (London), Beecham Pharmaceuticals, Research Division (Harlow), Hoechst UK Ltd. (Hounslow), ICI Ltd., Pharmaceuticals Division (Macclesfield), Brocades (GB) Ltd. (Weybridge), Janssen Pharmaceutical Ltd. (Marlow), Arnold R. Horwell Ltd. (London).

Peter J. Roberts
Geoffrey N. Woodruff
Leslie L. Iversen

Contents

Short Communications

Contributors

G. M. Anlezark
Department of Neurology
Institute of Psychiatry
Denmark Hill
London SE5 8AF, England

L. Annunziato
Department of Pharmacology
Michigan State University
East Lansing, Michigan 48824

G. W. Arbuthnott
M. R. C. Brain Metabolism Unit
University Department of Pharmacology
Edinburgh EH8 9JZ, Scotland

J. Arnt
Department of Pharmacology
The Royal Danish School of
    Pharmacy
Copenhagen, Denmark

J. S. de Belleroche
Department of Biochemistry
Imperial College of Science and
    Technology
London SW7 2AZ, England

Brigitte Berger
INSERM U134
Neuropathology Laboratory
Charles Foix Hospital, Salpêtrière
75634 Paris, Cedex 13, France

W. Birkmayer
Ludwig-Boltzmann Institute of Clinical Neurobiology
Lainz Municipal Hospital
A-1130 Vienna, Austria

Anders Björklund
Department of Histology
Biskopsgatan 5
S-223 62 Lund, Sweden

G. Blanc
Groupe NB—INSERM U 114
College of France
75231 Paris Cedex 5, France

E. P. Bonetti
Pharmaceutical Research Department
F. Hoffmann-La Roche and Company, Ltd.
Basel, Switzerland

H. F. Bradford
Department of Biochemistry
Imperial College of Science and Technology
London SW7 2AZ, England

C. Braestrup
Psychopharmacological Research
    Laboratory
Department E.
Sct. Hans Hospital
4000 Roskilde, Denmark

W. P. Burkard
Pharmaceutical Research Department
F. Hoffmann-La Roche and Company, Ltd.
Basel, Switzerland

R. del Carmine
Institute of Pharmacology
Catholic University
00168 Rome, Italy

C. J. Carter
Department of Pharmacology
The Medical School
University of Bristol
Bristol BS8 1TD, England

F. Cattabeni
Institute of Pharmacology and
    Pharmacognosy
University of Milan
Milan, Italy

F. Cerrito
Institute of Pharmacology
Catholic University
00168 Rome, Italy

A. M. Cervoni
Institute of Pharmacology
Catholic University
Cellular Biology Laboratory
Rome, Italy

A. Cheramy
Groupe NB (INSERM U 114)
College of France
75231 Paris Cedex 5, France

A. V. Christensen
Department of Pharmacology
H. Lundbeck and Company, A/S
DK-2500 Copenhagen, Denmark

A. R. Cools
Department of Pharmacology
University of Nijmegen
Nijmegen, The Netherlands

G. U. Corsini
Institute of Pharmacology
University of Cagliari
09100 Cagliari, Italy

T. J. Crow
Division of Psychiatry
Clinical Research Centre
Northwick Park Hospital
Harrow, Middlesex HA1 3UJ,
   England

M. Da Prada
Pharmaceutical Research Department
F. Hoffmann-La Roche and Com-
   pany, Ltd.
Basel, Switzerland

A. Davis
Pharmacology Group
School of Biochemical and Physio-
   logical Sciences
University of Southampton
Southampton SO9 3TU, England

L. De Angelis
Institute of Pharmacology and
   Pharmacognosy
University of Milan
Milan, Italy

J. Dedek
Synthélabo, L.E.R.S.
Department of Biology
Neurochemistry Unit
92220 Bagneux, France

G. Di Chiara
Institute of Pharmacology
University of Cagliari
09100 Cagliari, Italy

P. C. Emson
M. R. C. Neurochemical Pharma-
   cology Unit
Department of Pharmacology
Medical School
Cambridge, England

Irene J. Farley
Clarke Institute of Psychiatry
Toronto M5T 1R8, Canada

G. L. Gessa
Institute of Pharmacology
University of Cagliari
09100 Cagliari, Italy

J. Glowinski
Groupe NB (INSERM U 114)
College of France
75231 Paris Cedex 5, France

Leon I. Goldberg
Committee on Clinical Pharmacology
Departments of Pharmacological and
   Physiological Sciences and Medi-
   cine of Chicago
Chicago, Illinois 60637

S. Govoni
Institute of Pharmacology and
   Pharmacognosy
University of Cagliari
Cagliari, Italy
and
Institute of Pharmacology and
   Pharmacognosy
University of Milan
Milan, Italy

A. Groppetti
Institute of Pharmacology
University of Milan
Milan, Italy

G. A. Gudelsky
Department of Pharmacology
Michigan State University
East Lansing, Michigan 48824

Midori Hiramatsu
Institute for Neurobiology
Okayama University Medical School
Okayama, 700 Japan

Alan S. Horn
Department of Pharmacy
University of Groningen
Groningen, The Netherlands

Oleh Hornykiewicz
Institute of Biochemical Pharmacology
University of Vienna
A-1090 Vienna, Austria

R. W. Horton
Department of Neurology
Institute of Psychiatry
London SE5 8AF, England

J. Hyttel
Department of Pharmacology and Toxicology
H. Lundbeck and Company, A/S
DK 2500 Copenhagen-Valby, Denmark

L. L. Iversen
M. R. C. Neurochemical Pharmacology Unit
Department of Pharmacology
Medical School
Cambridge, England

K. Jellinger
Ludwig-Boltzmann Institute of Clinical Neurobiology
Lainz Municipal Hospital
A-1130 Vienna, Austria

T. M. Jessell
M. R. C. Neurochemical Pharmacology Unit
Department of Pharmacology
Medical School
Cambridge, England

E. C. Johnstone
Division of Psychiatry
Clinical Research Center
Northwick Park Hospital
Middlesex HA1 3UJ, England

John W. Kebabian
Experimental Therapeutics Branch
National Institute of Neurological and Communicative Disorders and Stroke
National Institutes of Health
Bethesda, Maryland 20014

H. H. Keller
Pharmaceutical Research Department
F. Hoffmann-La Roche and Company, Ltd.
Basel, Switzerland

Marie Kenny
Pharmacology Department
University College
Galway, Republic of Ireland

Jin-Soo Kim
Neurobiology Division
Max-Planck-Institute
6 Frankfurt, Germany

Mutsutoshi Kohsaka
Institute for Neurobiology
Okayama University Medical School
Okayama, 700 Japan

J. Korf
Synthélabo L.E.R.S.
Department of Biology
Neurochemistry Unit
92220 Bagneux, France

B. E. Leonard
Pharmacology Department
University College
Galway, Republic of Ireland

G. Levi
Cellular Biology Laboratory
01668 Rome, Italy

Olle Lindvall
Department of Histology
Biskopsgatan 5
S-223 62 Lund, Sweden

Tomas Ljungberg
Department of Histology
Karolinska Institute
S-104 01 Stockholm, 60 Sweden

A. Longden
Division of Psychiatry
Clinical Research Center
Northwick Park Hospital
Middlesex HA1 3UJ, England

G. Magelund
Psychopharmacological Research
* Laboratory*
Department E., Sct. Hans Hospital
Roskilde, Denmark

A. Maggi
Institute of Pharmacology and
* Pharmacognosy*
University of Milan
Milan, Italy

John McDermed
Department of Chemistry
Wellcome Research Laboratories
Research Triangle Park
North Carolina 27709

B. S. Meldrum
Department of Neurology
Institute of Psychiatry
Denmark Hill
London SE5 8AF, England

G. P. Mereu
Institute of Pharmacology
University of Cagliari
09100 Cagliari, Italy

M. Monduzzi
Institute of Pharmacology and
* Pharmacognosy*
University of Milan
Milan, Italy

K. E. Moore
Department of Pharmacology
Michigan State University
East Lansing, Michigan 48824

Akitane Mori
Institute for Neurobiology
Okayama University Medical School
Okayama, 700 Japan

I. Møller Nielsen
Department of Pharmacology and
* Toxicology*
H. Lundbeck and Company, A/S
DK 2500 Copenhagen-Valby, Den-
* mark*

A. Nieoullon
Groupe NB (INSERM U 114)
College of France
75231 Paris Cedex 5, France

Neville N. Osborne
Neurochemical Research Department
Biochemical Pharmacology Division
Max-Planck-Institute
3400 Göttingen, Germany

F. Owen
Division of Psychiatry
Clinical Research Center
Northwick Park Hospital
Middlesex HA1 3UJ, England

M. Parenti
Institute of Pharmacology
University of Milan
Milan, Italy

L. Pieri
Pharmaceutical Research Department
F. Hoffmann-La Roche and Com-
* pany, Ltd.*
Basel, Switzerland

M. Pieri
Pharmaceutical Research Department
F. Hoffmann-La Roche and
* Company, Ltd.*
Basel, Switzerland

Kathleen S. Price
Department of Psychopharmacology
Clarke Institute of Psychiatry
Toronto M5T 1R8, Canada

C. J. Pycock
Department of Pharmacology
The Medical School
University of Bristol
Bristol BS8 1TD, England

G. Racagni
Institute of Pharmacology and
  Pharmacognosy
University of Milan
Milan, Italy

M. Raiteri
Institute of Pharmacology
Catholic University
00168 Rome, Italy

J. C. Reubi
M. R. C. Neurochemical Pharma-
  cology Unit
Department of Pharmacology
Medical School
Cambridge, England

M. T. Ribera
Institute of Pharmacology
Catholic University
00168 Rome, Italy

P. Riederer
Ludwig-Boltzmann Institute of
  Clinical Neurobiology
Lainz Municipal Hospital
A-1130 Vienna, Austria

P. J. Roberts
Pharmacology Group
School of Biochemical and Physio-
  logical Sciences
University of Southampton
SO9 3TU Southampton, England

B. Scatton
Synthélabo L.E.R.S.
Department of Biology
Neurochemistry Unit
92220 Bagneux, France

J. Scheel-Krüger
Psychopharmacological Research
  Laboratory
Department E., Sct. Hans Hospital
4000 Roskilde, Denmark

Michel Schorderet
Department of Pharmacology
School of Medicine
CH 1211 Geneva, 4 Switzerland

Wolfram Schultz
Department of Histology
Karolinska Institute
S-104 01 Stockholm, 60 Sweden

P. Seeman
Department of Pharmacology
University of Toronto
Toronto, Canada M5S 1A8

D. F. Sharman
Agricultural Research Council
Institute of Animal Physiology
Babraham
Cambridge CB2 4AT, England

D. Sinclair
Department of Pharmacology
University of Toronto
Toronto, Canada M5S 1A8

Karl-H. Sontag
Neurochemical Research Department
Biochemical Pharmacology Division
Max-Planck-Institute
3400 Göttingen, Germany

P. F. Spano
Institutes of Pharmacology and
  Pharmacognosy
University of Cagliari
Cagliari, Italy
and
Institute of Pharmacology and
  Pharmacognosy
University of Milan
Milan, Italy

E. Stefanini
Institutes of Pharmacology and
  Pharmacognosy
University of Cagliari
Cagliari, Italy
and
Institute of Pharmacology and
  Pharmacognosy
University of Milan
Milan, Italy

J. P. Tassin
Groupe NB-INSERM U 114
College of France
75231 Paris Cedex 5, France

J. Tedesco
Department of Pharmacology
University of Toronto
Toronto, Canada M5S 1A8

M. Titeler
Department of Pharmacology
University of Toronto
Toronto, Canada M5S 1A8

A. M. Thierry
Groupe NB-INSERM U 114
College of France
75231 Paris Cedex 5, France

M. Trabucchi
Institute of Pharmacology and
Pharmacognosy
University of Cagliari
Cagliari, Italy
and
Institute of Pharmacology and
Pharmacognosy
University of Milan
Milan, Italy

Urban Ungerstedt
Department of Histology
Karolinska Institute
S-104 01 Stockholm, 60 Sweden

P. Weinreich
Department of Pharmacology
University of Toronto
Toronto, Canada M5S 1A8

B. H. C. Westerink
Laboratory for Pharmaceutical and
Analytical Chemistry
Department of Clinical Chemistry
Groningen University
Groningen, The Netherlands

G. N. Woodruff
Pharmacology Group
School of Biochemical and
Physiological Sciences
University of Southampton
Southampton SO9 3TU, England

M. B. H. Youdim
Ludwig-Boltzmann Institute of
Clinical Neurobiology
Lainz Municipal Hospital
A-1130 Vienna, Austria

Advances in Biochemical Psychopharmacology, Vol. 19,
edited by P. J. Roberts et al.
Raven Press, New York © 1978.

Anatomy of the Dopaminergic Neuron Systems in the Rat Brain

Olle Lindvall and Anders Björklund

Department of Histology, Biskopsgatan 5, S-223 62 Lund, Sweden

Since dopamine was found biochemically in the brain (13,24,79) and its intraneuronal localization first demonstrated histochemically (23), numerous studies on the organization of central dopaminergic neuron systems have been carried out. This work was first performed with the Falck-Hillarp formaldehyde fluorescence method in combination with mechanical or chemical lesions using 6-hydroxydopamine (3,27,28,41,102). With the introduction of the glyoxylic acid fluorescence method (70) in combination with the Vibratome sectioning procedure (54) the catecholamine systems could be studied in greater detail, and because of the higher sensitivity of this method previously unknown dopamine-containing fiber systems were discovered (16,18,68,69, 72,73). During recent years several other techniques have been found highly useful for neuroanatomical studies on central dopaminergic systems. These methods include horseradish peroxidase (HRP) tracing (see, e.g., refs. 64 and 83), Fink-Heimer staining (46,77,96–98), and determination of dopamine and the dopamine-synthesizing enzyme tyrosine hydroxylase (TH) in minute amounts of tissue (9,21,62,93). Of particular interest is the recently evolved technique of immunohistochemical visualization of TH, since TH antiserum seems to demonstrate preferentially dopamine neurons (49,52, 87,88). However Hökfelt et al. (52) have pointed out that TH can be demonstrated also in at least some norepinephrine and particularly in epinephrine nerve endings at the light microscopic level.

This chapter will summarize the presently available data on the organization of central dopaminergic neurons in the rat brain. The emphasis has been put on our own investigations using mainly the glyoxylic acid fluorescence method, but also results obtained with other techniques, such as immunohistochemistry and HRP tracing, will be referred to in the text. Table 1 summarizes the major dopaminergic projection systems. Each system will be described separately in the text.

MESOTELENCEPHALIC DOPAMINE SYSTEM

Dopamine-containing cell bodies in the mesencephalon were first demonstrated by Dahlström and Fuxe (27). In further histochemical studies in com-

TABLE 1. *Central dopaminergic projection systems*

System	Cells of origin	Projections
1. Mesostriatal system	Substantia nigra	Nucleus caudatus-putamen: probably also globus pallidus
	Ventral tegmental area	Nucleus accumbens
2. Mesocortical system	Substantia nigra and ventral tegmental area	*Allocortical subdivision:* olfactory tubercle, septum, interstitial nucleus of the stria terminalis, amygdala; probably also the piriform cortex
		Neocortical subdivision: suprarhinal cortex, pregenual and supragenual anteromedial cortex, ventral entorhinal cortex
3. Periventricular system	Mesencephalic periaqueductal gray and periventricular gray of caudal thalamus	Periaqueductal gray; medial thalamus and hypothalamus
4. Incertohypothalamic system	Zona incerta and periventricular hypothalamus	Zona incerta; anterior, medial preoptic, and periventricular hypothalamus; septum
5. Tuberohypophyseal system	Arcuate and periventricular hypothalamic nuclei	Median eminence; pars nervosa and pars intermedia of the pituitary
6. Periglomerular dopamine neurons	Olfactory bulb	Dendritic processes into olfactory glomeruli
7. Retinal dopamine system	Mainly in the inner nuclear layer of the retina	Local dendritic projections

bination with lesions, Andén et al. (2) and Bertler et al. (12) provided more direct evidence for a nigrostriatal dopaminergic system, giving rise to a dense terminal network distributed throughout the nucleus caudatus-putamen (4,41). Apart from the neostriatum, Fuxe (41) demonstrated dense dopaminergic innervations in several basal forebrain areas, such as the olfactory tubercle, the central amygdaloid nucleus, the nucleus accumbens, and the interstitial nucleus of the stria terminalis. From lesion experiments, Andén et al. (3) proposed that these innervations were the terminals of dopamine neurons located in the ventromedial mesencephalic tegmentum. Their axons ascend along the medial forebrain bundle, constituting the so-called mesolimbic dopaminergic system (102).

Our knowledge of the projections of the mesencephalic dopamine neurons has subsequently been expanded through the biochemical (100,101) and histochemical (10,11,50,68,69,71,72) demonstrations of termination areas in the neocortex, septum, and probably also in the piriform cortex. The neocortical projections have been called the mesocortical dopaminergic system.

In the present account the terminology suggested by Björklund et al. (17) has been used. The mesotelencephalic system, which refers to the entire ascending forebrain projection of the mesencephalic dopamine neuron system, is divided into two major subsystems (Table 1): the *mesostriatal system* [including both the classic nigrostriatal system and the projection from the ventral tegmental area to the nucleus accumbens (which is part of the striatum)] and the *mesocortical system* which, according to this terminology, includes both the mesolimbic system as defined by Ungerstedt (102) and the more recently described mesocortical projections. Within the mesocortical dopamine system are distinguished an *allocortical projection* innervating the olfactory tubercle, septum, interstitial nucleus of the stria terminalis, amygdala, and probably also the piriform cortex, and an *iso-* or *neocortical projection* innervating the pregenual and supragenual parts of the antero-medial cortex, the suprarhinal cortex, and the ventral part of the entorhinal cortex.

MESOSTRIATAL SYSTEM

In the rat striatum the dopaminergic neurons give rise to a dense terminal network that is distributed throughout the nucleus caudatus-putamen (Fig. 1). This terminal pattern extends without interruption also into nucleus accumbens (4,41). In the rat, globus pallidus appears, in specimens processed according to the Falck-Hillarp formaldehyde method, to lack a catecholaminergic innervation (41). Globus pallidus is traversed by axons of the nigrostriatal pathway on their way to the neostriatum (69,102). It has therefore been assumed that the relatively high concentrations of dopamine that have been detected chemically (13) are located in these preterminal axons. Observations with the glyoxylic acid histofluorescence method in the rat (O. Lindvall and A. Björklund, *unpublished observations*) indicate, however, that dopamine fibers actually terminate also in globus pallidus. In the rat, axons continuing into the caudate-putamen as they pass through the globus pallidus send out long collaterals into the nucleus, making close contacts with the pallidal nerve cell bodies. These observations suggest that one and the same dopamine axon might establish contacts with neurons in both the neostriatum and the globus pallidus.

The mesostriatal dopamine pathway projecting to the nucleus caudatus-putamen originates in the substantia nigra (in the rat mainly in cells located in the pars compacta) and probably also in the A10 and A8 cell groups of the mesencephalic tegmentum. The striatal projection of the nigral neurons has been established with a large variety of techniques, including fluorescence histochemistry, immunohistochemistry, biochemistry, stains for terminal degeneration, HRP tracing, and electron microscopy (2–4,8,12,25,52,56,69, 80,83,85,90,102).

There is at least a crude topographic relation between the mesencephalic dopamine cells and the area of termination in the striatum. Thus, the lateral part of the substantia nigra projects to a lateral part of the neostriatum, the medial part of the nigra to a more medial part of the neostriatum, and the

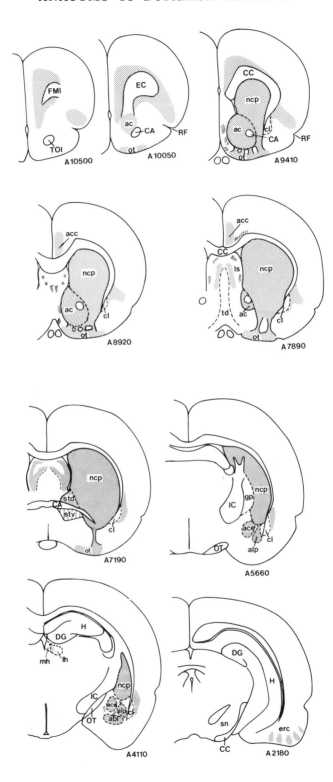

laterally situated A10 neurons to the most medial and ventral parts of the head of the nucleus caudatus-putamen (33,71,82). Moreover, Nauta (82) has suggested from HRP material that the neurons of the A8 cell group give rise to an innervation in the ventral neostriatum.

As observed in glyoxylic acid-treated material (69), the nigral axons are, in their initial course, directed medially (Fig. 2). Medial to the substantia nigra they are joined by axons from the A8 group. The axons turn sharply rostrally and assemble into a well-defined bundle that ascends in the H-field of Forel immediately dorsolateral to the median forebrain bundle (MFB) system. The most dorsal fibers in the nigrostriatal pathway leave the bundle first. At the level of the subthalamic nucleus, these dorsal fibers bend first sharply laterally, above the crus cerebri, and then rostrally to turn into the internal capsule from the caudal side toward the caudal parts of the neostriatum. The somewhat more ventrally located fibers deviate less sharply, and run in a rostrolateral direction through the subthalamic region into the internal capsule. The centrally and ventrally located fibers continue rostrally along and partly within the dorsomedial edge of the internal capsule. Along this course, the more dorsally situated fibers in the bundle deviate in a rostrolaterodorsal direction into the internal capsule, toward the central parts of the nucleus caudatus-putamen. The ventral portion of the nigrostriatal pathway continues further rostrally up to the level of the globus pallidus. Here, most of the fibers fan out in rostrodorsolateral directions to run along the myelinated fascicles through the globus pallidus into the head of the nucleus caudatus-putamen. The most ventral portion, however, continues rostrally, in a position just dorsal to the MFB, up to the anterior commissure; the axons pass ventrally to the commissure, and medially and laterally to its anterior limb they run into the ventromedial part of the nucleus caudatus-putamen and the dorsal part of the interstitial nucleus of the stria terminalis. The ventral portion of the pathway also contributes fibers to the ansa lenticularis, probably innervating the amygdala (e.g., the central amygdaloid nucleus). From this description it is evident that there is a topographic arrangement of the axons within the nigrostriatal pathway. The fibers going to the caudal regions lie more dorsally and laterally, and those going to rostral and ventral regions lie more ventrally.

←

FIG. 1. Schematic representation in 9 frontal planes of the terminals of the mesotelencephalic dopamine system. In addition, the dopaminergic innervation of the lateral habenular nucleus, probably originating in the mesencephalic cell groups, is represented. Areas of termination are indicated by hatchings. Data compiled from Berger et al. (11), Fuxe (41), Fuxe et al. (43), Lindvall (68), Lindvall et al. (71–73), and Ungerstedt (102). Abbreviations: abl, basal amygdaloid nucleus, lateral part; ac, nucleus accumbens; acc, anterior cingulate cortex (supragenual cortex); ace, central amygdaloid nucleus; alp, lateral amygdaloid nucleus, posterior part; cl, claustrum; erc, entorhinal cortex; gp, globus pallidus; lh, lateral habenular nucleus; ls, lateral septal nucleus; mh, medial habenular nucleus; ncp, nucleus caudatus-putamen; ot, olfactory tubercle; sn, substantia nigra; st, interstitial nucleus of stria terminalis, std = dorsal part, stv = ventral part; td, nucleus of diagonal band; CA, anterior commissure; CC, corpus callosum; DG, dentate gyrus; EC, external capsule; FMI, forceps minor; H, hippocampus; IC, internal capsule; OT, optic tract; RF, rhinal fissure; TOI, intermediary olfactory tract.

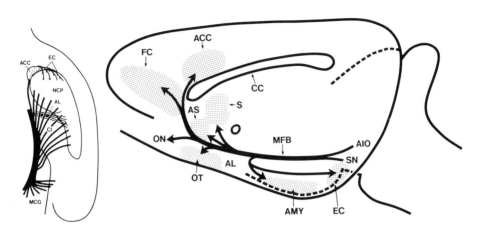

FIG. 2. Schematic representation of the mesostriatal (*left*) and the mesocortical (*right*) dopaminergic systems in horizontal and sagittal projections, respectively. Modified from Lindvall and Björklund (69) and Lindvall et al. (72). Abbreviations: ACC, anterior cingulate cortex (supragenual system) or nucleus accumbens; AL, ansa lenticularis; AMY, amygdala; AS, nucleus accumbens; CC, corpus callosum; CI, internal capsule; EC, external capsule or entorhinal cortex; FC, frontal cortex (anteromedial system); MCG, mesencephalic dopamine cell group; MFB, medial forebrain bundle; NCP nucleus caudatus-putamen; ON, olfactory nuclei; OT, olfactory tubercle; S, septum; SN, substantia nigra.

The part of the mesostriatal dopamine system projecting to nucleus accumbens originates in the ventromedial tegmental area, medial to substantia nigra (see below; 3,98,102). The axons ascend in the dorsal portion of the MFB, in a position immediately ventromedial to the nigrostriatal pathway (69,102). The axons reach nucleus accumbens along the MFB. Part of the axons pass dorsally on the rostrolateral aspects of the nucleus to fan out over the external capsule (Fig. 2A). Part of these fibers continue into the frontal cortex; others appear to project into the head of the nucleus caudatus-putamen.

Apart from the axonal processes, projecting to the basal ganglia, also the dendrites of the substantia nigra neurons have been shown to store dopamine (16). As described originally by Cajal (22) in Golgi preparations, the nigral dendrites form long branching processes that ramify both among the dopamine neurons in the pars compacta as well as into the depth of the pars reticulata. Jessell et al. (57) and Korf et al. (61) have demonstrated a release of dopamine from the pars reticulata upon electrical stimulation. This might suggest a role for dopamine at the dendritic level within the nigra itself. Whether these properties of the dendrites also are valid for other mesencephalic dopamine neurons is so far unknown.

MESOCORTICAL SYSTEM

The dopaminergic innervation of the olfactory tubercle consists of densely packed, fine varicose fibers with a morphology similar to that of the neostriatal innervation. According to Fuxe (41) the innervation is mainly confined to the medial part of the tubercle, within the lamina pyramidalis, and the islands of Calleja are devoid of innervation. In glyoxylic acid-treated material an innervation of the insula Calleja magna has, however, been demonstrated (O. Lindvall, *unpublished observations*). Furthermore, Hökfelt et al. (53) have demonstrated a significant supply of tyrosine hydroxylase-containing fibers in the islands of Calleja, although the density is lower than in other parts of the olfactory tubercle. The dopaminergic innervation of the olfactory tubercle is continuous with that of the neostriatum along the cell bridges connecting the two structures.

The mesencephalic dopamine innervation of the septal area is in the rat of morphologically two different types (68). One type is fine varicose and the other smooth with few varicosities. The latter type of axon often outlines the cell body and the proximal dendrites of septal neurons, forming pericellular basket-like arrangements (see also ref. 81). At the most rostral levels of the septum, scattered pericellular arrangements and smooth fibers are found in the lateral septal nucleus and in the area ventral to the hippocampal rudiment (Fig. 1). Further caudally, the dopamine innervation increases progressively and the highest terminal density is found medially and ventrally in the middle portion of the lateral septal nucleus. The fine-varicose dopamine fibers are aggregated in a dense band outlining the fornix in the medial part of the lateral nucleus. Pericellular arrangements and smooth fibers occur mainly in its lateral and dorsal parts, close to the lateral ventricle. The density of innervation again decreases in the caudal part of the septum (Fig. 1).

The interstitial nucleus of the stria terminalis has partly a dense dopaminergic innervation that is closely related to that of the septum, on one hand (O. Lindvall, *unpublished observations*), and the nucleus caudatus-putamen on the other (3,41,102). The dorsal part of the nucleus has the densest innervation, but also the ventral part has a definite dopaminergic nerve supply, scattered among the dense noradrenergic innervation present in this part of the nucleus (O. Lindvall, *unpublished observations;* see also ref. 53). Dopamine axons can be traced from the interstitial nucleus of the stria terminalis into the dense terminal system in the lateral septal nucleus (O. Lindvall, *unpublished observations*).

In amygdala a dopamine innervation of high density is found in the central nucleus (41,102), and rich innervations have also been reported in the lateral and basolateral nuclei and the so-called intercalated masses (Fig. 1; 39,43). The innervation in the central nucleus has been described as an extension of that in the nucleus caudatus-putamen.

The neocortical projections of the mesocortical dopaminergic system are found in the entorhinal cortex and in the frontal lobe (10,11,50,55,71,72) (Fig. 1). In the ventral entorhinal area the dopamine fibers form a series of clusters, which are principally located in the second and third layers but extend into the molecular layer (see also refs. 26,53). On the basis of fiber morphology and localization of cell bodies of origin (see below), three dopaminergic terminal systems have been distinguished in the frontal lobe (71; Fig. 1). The anteromedial system is formed by smooth axons distributed mainly in the pregenual part of the anteromedial cortex, and the highest fiber density is found in the basal cortical layers. A much more sparse, caudal extension of this system is present in the basal layers in the supragenual part of the anteromedial cortex. The suprarhinal system forms the dorsal part of the dopaminergic innervation which is found in the perirhinal cortex, surrounding the rhinal sulcus. It can be regarded as a direct lateral continuation of the anteromedial system, and can be followed from a coronal level just rostral to the nucleus accumbens to the level of the most rostral part of the nucleus caudatus-putamen. The axons are distributed mainly in the basal cortical layers. The supragenual system is formed by very fine-varicose axons distributed in a restricted area of the supragenual anteromedial cortex (anterior cingulate cortex). The axons are localized in the superficial cortical layers (I–III).

The mesocortical pathways have been shown with fluorescence histochemistry (3,43,68,71,72,102), Fink-Heimer staining (46,98), and HRP tracing (7,71) to originate in the ventromedial tegmental area, with one notable exception: the pathway innervating the outer layers of the supragenual anteromedial frontal cortex originates by all probability in the substantia nigra (71,72).

The different components of the mesocortical dopamine system originate in different parts of the mesencephalic dopamine cell system, suggesting that there is at least a crude topographical arrangement among these neurons. Figure 3 shows schematically a summary of our own observations obtained from fluorescence histochemical observations in combination with small electrolytic lesions (68,71,72) and from observations using the HRP tracing method (71,74). Other literature is generally in agreement with this picture (3,43,98,102). When comparing our HRP data obtained after injections into the anteromedial frontal cortex with those of Beckstead (7), it seems that the medially located A10 cells project to the pregenual part of the anteromedial cortex, whereas the dopamine innervation in the supragenual anteromedial cortex originates from more laterally situated cells and from medial substantia nigra neurons. Our lesions of the substantia nigra consistently remove the fine-varicose supragenual terminal system. From lesions of varying size and position we have concluded that this innervation originates in cells distributed throughout the mediolateral extent of the nigra (71,72). Despite this, localized HRP injections into this terminal area label cells only in the medial part of the substantia nigra, as well as cells in the lateral A10 area (7,71). We believe, therefore, that only part of the cells innervating the supragenual anteromedial cortex are labeled with HRP, and that some of those which become labeled are identical to those sending axons to the caudal extension of the anteromedial system in the supragenual cortex (see above). As Beckstead (7) has pointed out, the projection fields from the ventral tegmental and substantia nigra neurons thus overlap in the supragenual cortex. In the cat, Avendaño et al. (5) have reported labeling of both substantia nigra and A10 neurons after HRP injections into the frontal lobe. In contrast to the rat where the entire mesotelencephalic system appears to project only ipsilaterally, these latter authors reported labeling also in the contralateral mesencephalon in the cat.

There is thus substantial evidence that the substantia nigra dopamine neurons project not only to neostriatum but also to neocortex. Simon et al. (98) have, on the basis of anterograde degeneration staining, suggested a projection from substantia nigra also to the entorhinal cortex. In our own material (*unpublished observations*), a near total destruction of the nigra did not cause any substantial reduction in the dopaminergic innervation of the ventral entorhinal cortex, whereas a lesion involving both the nigral and ventral tegmental projections removed this system totally (see also ref. 43). This points to an origin of the entorhinal cortex innervation in the ventral tegmental area, although the exact location of the cells has not yet been clarified.

It is interesting to note that in our material the cells labeled after HRP injections in the anteromedial frontal cortex and in the lateral septal nucleus had a similar distribution in the medial A10 area (Fig. 3A and B). This would be consistent with the fact that the same dopaminergic cells project to both the frontal cortex and the septum, an arrangement that finds support in the observation that the axons running into the frontal cortex give off collaterals into the septum (69). Preliminary lesion studies and HRP injection experiments have demonstrated that the cells projecting to nucleus accumbens are distributed over the mediolateral extent of the A10 cell group. These cells thus partly overlap with those innervating the anteromedial

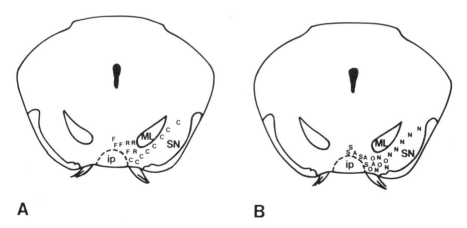

A   **B**

FIG. 3. Relative location of dopamine cell bodies in ventral mesencephalon projecting to neocortical areas (A) and to striatal and allocortical areas (B). Abbreviations: F, anteromedial dopamine system; C, supragenual dopamine system; R, suprarhinal dopamine system; S, septum; A, nucleus accumbens; O, olfactory tubercle; N, neostriatum; ip, interpeduncular nucleus; ML, medial lemniscus; SN, substantia nigra. The position of cells projecting to nucleus accumbens and the olfactory tubercle rests on preliminary observations with electrolytic lesions and the HRP method (74).

frontal cortex and the septum (Fig. 3B). Interestingly, there seems to be a crude topographic arrangement of the A10 cells in the mediolateral direction, the medial cells projecting to medial telencephalic structures (septum, accumbens, medial frontal cortex) and the lateral cells to areas situated more laterally (olfactory tubercle and neostriatum). As described above (see ref. 71) the rostral cortical areas (such as the pregenual anteromedial cortex) have their cell bodies of origin more medially (in the A10 cell group; Fig. 3A). Going caudally in the medial cortex (i.e., into the supragenual cortex), the cell bodies of origin are found more laterally (in the lateral A10 and substantia nigra), and going caudally along the rhinal sulcus, the cells of origin are again found more laterally in the ventral tegmental area. Such a topographic arrangement is also supported by the recent study of Fallon and Moore (39).

In the rat (see ref. 69) the mesocortical axons ascend along the MFB, in a position ventromedial to the mesostriatal axons. The axons continue apparently unbranched up to the retrochiasmatic region where fibers (at least partly as collaterals) leave the bundle laterally along the ansa lenticularis toward amygdala and the piriform and entorhinal cortices (see Fig. 2B). After having given off fibers ventrally into the olfactory tubercle and dorsally along the diagonal band into the septum, the remaining portion of the mesocortical pathway leaves the MFB at the level of the rostral septum in a dorsomediorostral direction to run in a position well corresponding to the septohypothalamic tract. The fibers sweep as a broad band along the medial and the medioventral aspects of the nucleus accumbens. In the region rostromedial to the nucleus accumbens, the bundle separates into four main branches: First, the branch of greatest abundance runs dorsorostrally and laterally into the deep layers of the pregenual part of the anteromedial frontal cortex. These fibers give rise to the extensive anteromedial dopamine terminal system. The branch to the frontal cortex passes along the rostral aspect of the external capsule, and fibers are seen to run into the external capsule, thus contributing to the above-mentioned fiber system within the external capsule. A second branch of the bundle turns more sharply dorsally, to run in a position caudal to the branch to the pregenual cortex. It sweeps caudally above the corpus callosum to ramify into the dense terminal system in the outer layers of the supragenual part of the anteromedial cortex. A third branch runs in a dorsocaudal direction into the septum, contributing to the innervation of this area. Fibers in a ventral position in the bundle first turn dorsally for a short distance and then rostrally to join the medial olfactory tract. Presumably, these fibers give rise to terminals in the olfactory nuclei.

PERIVENTRICULAR SYSTEM

Using the glyoxylic acid method, investigations have revealed a prominent system of catecholamine-containing cell bodies and fibers in the periventricular and periaqueductal gray of the medulla oblongata, pons, mesencephalon, and diencephalon (69,73). It can be regarded as a catecholamine-containing component of the dorsal longitudinal fasciculus of Schütz. Part of the periventricular fibers originate in the neurons of the midline and periventricular catecholamine cell groups, but it is important to remember that other catecholamine neuron systems, such as the locus coeruleus and dorsal medullary cell system (group A2), contribute fibers to the periventricular system as well.

It is well established that the major portion of the midline and periventricular cell system is dopaminergic (20,52; *unpublished data*), but some of the neurons might be noradrenergic (20). On the other hand, the fibers coming from other cell groups such as the locus coeruleus are by all probability noradrenergic. Thus, although the midline and periventricular cell system is regarded as primarily dopaminergic, the periventricular fiber system is mixed noradrenergic and dopaminergic. The relative contributions and projection patterns of the different components are not known in detail, and the description below is therefore by necessity incomplete.

The periventricular fiber system has been distinguished into a dorsal part, the dorsal periventricular system, which can be regarded as a component of the dorsal longitudinal fasciculus of Schütz, and a ventral part, the ventral periventricular system, extending along the periventricular region of the hypothalamus.

Caudally, the dorsal periventricular system (DPS) can be observed in a superficial position at the level of the nucleus of the solitary tract and the dorsal motor nucleus of vagus. The system extends from this area as a rather sparse bundle running rostrally underneath the ependyma of the fourth ventricle. The direction of these fibers is not known; it seems that they either could be axons ascending from the dorsal medullary cell group (A2), or could represent descending fibers, e.g., from the locus coeruleus. At the level of the locus coeruleus, the system increases considerably in width and in number of fibers, in that the locus coeruleus and other pontine and medullary catecholamine cell groups contribute fibers to the system. From the region dorsal and medial to the locus coeruleus, the DPS ascends rostrally underneath the ependyma, occupying the lateral part of the periventricular gray.

The DPS gives off fibers to the raphe nuclei in the pons, and to the inferior and superior colliculi in the mesencephalon (Fig. 4). Fibers run also ventrally from the DPS toward the ventral mesencephalic tegmentum. At the mesodiencephalic junction the DPS splits into several branches (Fig. 4). One component of the DPS runs across the midline in the posterior commissure to reach the pretectal area, and a second component runs immediately in front of the posterior commissure into the habenula. A third component runs rostrally into the paraventricular thalamic nucleus, and a fourth component runs somewhat more ventrally into the parafascicular nucleus. The major portion of the DPS turns, however, ventrally along the periventricular gray of the

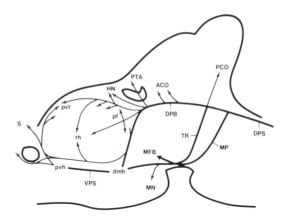

FIG. 4. Schematic representation of the projection routes of the periventricular fiber systems to the tectum, diencephalon, and septum. From Lindvall et al. (73). Abbreviations: ACO, anterior colliculus; dmh, dorso-medial hypothalamic nucleus; DPB, dorsal periventricular catecholamine bundle; DPS, dorsal periventricular catecholamine system; HN, habenular nuclei; MFB, medial forebrain bundle; MN, mammillary nuclei; MP, mammillary peduncle; PCO, posterior colliculus; pf, parafascicular nucleus; PTA, pretectal area; pvh, paraventricular hypothalamic nucleus; pvt, paraventricular thalamic nucleus; rh, rhomboid nucleus; S, septum; TR, tegmental catecholamine radiations; VPS, ventral periventricular catecholamine system.

caudal thalamus through the posterior hypothalamus into the dorsomedial hypothalamic nucleus. At the level of the fasciculus retroflexus fibers from the dorsal tegmental catecholamine bundle join the DPS. These fibers should, at least in part, be responsible for the locus coeruleus innervation of the periventricular hypothalamus (58,60,76). Some of the axons running in the hypothalamic branch of the DPS turn rostrally, dorsal to the dorsomedial hypothalamic nucleus, to form a distinct bundle in the medial zona incerta. At the level of the paraventricular nucleus of the hypothalamus, fibers leave the zona incerta bundle in dorsal direction toward the rhomboid nucleus of the thalamus. Still further rostrally the zona incerta bundle sweeps dorsally and caudally as periventricular thalamic fibers along the paraventricular thalamic nucleus giving off collaterals into this nucleus (Fig. 4).

The ventral periventricular system (VPS) is observed caudally in the region immediately dorsolateral to the interpeduncular nucleus (Fig. 4). In passing above the medial mammillary nucleus, fibers leave the bundle into the nucleus. At the level of the mammillothalamic tract, fibers from the medial part of the MFB leave this bundle, partly as collaterals, in a rostro-medial direction to join the VPS. The VPS thus increases in width and fiber number as it passes in a rostral and somewhat dorsal direction through the posterior hypothalamic area into the dense catecholamine-containing terminal system of the dorsomedial hypothalamic nucleus (Fig. 4). After having received fibers from the hypothalamic branch of the DPS, the VPS continues as a broad ascending hypothalamic catecholamine fiber system dispersed in the lateral aspect of the periventricular nucleus to innervate the paraventricular nucleus and probably the caudal septum and the interstitial nucleus of the stria terminalis. The VPS also contributes fibers to the innervation of the medial thalamus (Fig. 4).

From the above description it is clear that the dorsal and ventral periventricular systems project importantly to several diencephalic nuclei (Fig. 4). The periventricular system gives rise to major innervations in the paraventricular, parafascicular, and rhomboidal nuclei of the thalamus, as well as in the pretectal area and possibly also in the lateral habenular nucleus (73). Evidence for the dopaminergic nature of the innervation in, for example, the lateral habenular nucleus has recently been obtained by immunohistochemical demonstration of tyrosine hydroxylase (53). This is in agreement with our own observations in Vibratome sections incubated in dopamine in the presence of the norepinephrine uptake blocker desipramine. From the recent HRP data of Herkenham and Nauta (47), it seems possible that the dopamine innervation in the lateral habenular nucleus originates in the ventral tegmental area.

TUBEROHYPOPHYSEAL SYSTEM

The cell bodies of the tuberohypophyseal system are located in the arcuate nucleus (primary its rostral half) and the portion of the periventricular nucleus just dorsal to the arcuate nucleus (15,19,40,66). Their axons seem to project in an orderly manner to all parts of the median eminence, the stalk, the neural lobe, and the pars intermedia of the adenohypophysis (Fig. 5; 15,19,59,75,99).

The dopamine innervation of the median eminence and the stem originates in cell bodies situated in the arcuate nucleus and in the part of the periventricular nucleus lying dorsal to the arcuate nucleus (15,19,42,59,66). These tuberoinfundibular dopamine neurons could be distinguished as two groups on the basis of their mode of projection (Fig. 5; 19). One group, situated in the rostral part of the arcuate nuclei, projects more diffusely to all levels of the median eminence and the stem (as well as to the pars intermedia and the neural lobe as mentioned below). The second group, having a more regular dorsoventrally oriented projection, appears to connect each portion of the arcuate nucleus (i.e., the rostral, middle, or caudal portion) with a corresponding part of the ventrally situated median eminence.

The tuberoinfundibular dopamine neurons project to all layers of the median eminence and the stem. The terminals are more abundant in the external layer where they are very densely packed in a palisade-like manner, close to the capillaries of the portal vessels. The fibers have a regular, finely varicose appearance, often ending with a strongly fluorescent droplet-like enlargement. In the internal layer it is likely that part of the fibers are of preterminal nature running parallel to one another in the sagittal and frontal planes. However, part of the fibers appear to ramify together with the

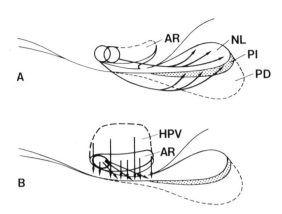

FIG. 5. Organization of the dopamine innervations in the median eminence-pituitary region. A: Arrangement of the dopamine innervation from the arcuate nucleus to the neural lobe and pars intermedia. B: Arrangement of the dopamine innervation from the arcuate and periventricular nuclei to the median eminence. Abbreviations: NL, neural lobe; PI, pars intermedia; PD, pars distalis; AR, arcuate nucleus; HPV, periventricular nucleus.

noradrenergic fibers in this area to form irregular patterns in the deeper layers, partly in association with the capillary loops of the portal vessels. As observed ultrastructurally, the catecholamine fibers in the zona externa do not seem to form any true synaptic connections to other tissue elements, but show sites of close contacts with nonmonoaminergic axons and ependymal cells, as well as with the pericapillary space of the hypophyseal portal vessels (1,48).

Dopamine-containing fibers have been detected by microspectrofluorometric analysis also around the endocrine cells of the pars intermedia, and in the neural lobe and the median eminence (15). In the neurointermediate lobe it seems likely that the norepinephrine detected chemically derives from the peripheral sympathetic vascular supply, and that the central innervation is exclusively dopaminergic. Experiments with small, partial lesions of the arcuate nuclei (19) have provided evidence that the dopamine fibers of the neurointermediate lobe—as well as part of the dopamine fibers in the median eminence—originate in the rostral portion of the arcuate nucleus, the cells innervating the pars intermedia lying immediately rostral to those innervating the neural lobe (Fig. 5A).

The dopamine fibers of the neurointermediate lobe are predominantly of a fine varicose type distributed throughout the parenchyma of the neural lobe and around the endocrine cells of the pars intermedia. These fibers form the densest pattern in the vascular border zone between the two lobes and at the outer margins of the lobules formed by the intermedia cells. From here, the fibers penetrate between the intermedia cells to form a plexus inside the lobules. In a combined fluorescence histochemical and ultrastructural study in the rat, Baumgarten et al. (6) have shown that the dopamine-containing fibers make frequent close contacts (80 to 120Å), without any real membrane thickenings, to neurosecretory axons, pituicyte processes, and pars intermedia cells. This suggests that the direct inhibitory control of the rat pars intermedia is exerted by the tuberohypophyseal dopamine system.

A special feature of the dopamine fibers in the pituitary complex is the occurrence of peculiar, large dopamine-filled droplet-like swellings (14). From the ultrastructural features of these swellings it has been proposed that the tuberohypophyseal dopamine axons—extending out into an environment not protected by a blood-brain barrier—are involved in a continuous degeneration-regeneration process (6; see ref. 30).

INCERTOHYPOTHALAMIC SYSTEM

This fiber system originates in dopamine-containing cell bodies in the dorsal and caudal hypothalamic cell groups (groups A11 and A13) periventricular cells of the A14 cell group (18,73). The neurons probably constitute a second, short intradiencephalic dopamine system of possible importance in the regulation of neuroendocrine functions in the hypothalamus. The fibers are characterized by an unusually low amine concentration and do not show up in specimens processed according to the standard Falck-Hillarp formaldehyde method. The studies related below have been performed with the glyoxylic acid method (18,73). Interestingly, at least part of the incertohypothalamic fiber system has also been demonstrated with immunohistochemistry using tyrosine hydroxylase as a marker for dopaminergic neurons (52).

In the rat the incertohypothalamic system has been topographically distinguished into a caudal and a rostral part (Fig. 6; 18). The caudal part extends from the area of the dopamine cell bodies in the caudal thalamus, the posterior hypothalamic area and the medial zona incerta into the dorsal part of the dorsomedial nucleus and the dorsal and anterior hypothalamic areas. The rostral part, probably originating from the rostral periventricular cell bodies of the A14 cell group, is distributed in the periventricular nucleus of the anterior hypothalamus and in the periventricular, suprachiasmatic, and medial preoptic nuclei, up to the level of the anterior commissure. The system probably extends into the most caudal part of the lateral septal nucleus.

The incertohypothalamic system consists of short, locally projecting neurons whose fibers have an unusual and peculiar fluorescence morphology. The fibers arborize extensively soon after they have left the cell bodies into a network of closely and regularly spaced, very fine varicosities with a remarkably low amine content. Interestingly, the incertohypothalamic system has a prominent projection to the preoptic-anterior hypothalamic region, suggesting an involvement in neuroendocrine mechanisms. In the anterior hypothalamic area the fibers of the incertohypothalamic system constitute

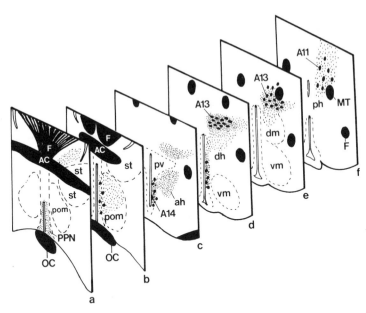

FIG. 6. Distribution of the incertohypothalamic fiber system at 6 representative frontal levels (a–f). The localization of the catecholamine-containing cell groups A11, A13, and A14 is also indicated. From Björklund et al. (18). Abbreviations: AC, anterior commissure; ah, anterior hypothalamic nucleus; dh, dorsal hypothalamic area; dm, dorsomedial hypothalamic nucleus; F, fornix; MT, mammillothalamic tract; OC, optic chiasm; ph, posterior hypothalamic nucleus; pom, medial preoptic nucleus; PPN, periventricular preoptic nuclei; pv, periventricular hypothalamic nucleus; st, interstitial nucleus of the stria terminalis; vm, ventromedial nuclear group.

the predominating type of catecholamine innervation, whereas in the preoptic areas, as well as in the anterior periventricular and the dorsomedial nuclei, they occur intermingled with dense plexuses of norepinephrine-containing fibers. In the anterior hypothalamic and preoptic areas the incertohypothalamic fibers form dense, basket-like patterns around nonfluorescent neuronal perikarya.

PERIGLOMERULAR DOPAMINE NEURONS

In the rat olfactory bulb, periglomerular cells containing a catecholamine were first demonstrated by Dahlström et al. (29). Periglomerular cells have also been shown to accumulate exogenous norepinephrine (65), and Lidbrink et al. (67) obtained pharmacological support for the idea that these cells are dopaminergic. More detailed analyses of the organization of the catecholamine-containing periglomerular cells have recently been performed using immunohistochemistry (44,51). The dopamine-synthesizing enzymes tyrosine hydroxylase and dopa decarboxylase were found in periglomerular cell bodies and dendrites. Dopamine-β-hydroxylase was not present in the cells, indicating that they are dopaminergic. The majority of periglomerular cells were, however, unlabeled after incubation with tyrosine hydroxylase-antiserum, and it has been calculated that the presumed dopamine cells constitute 8% to 22% of all periglomerular neurons (44).

Presumed dopamine-containing fibers have been followed into the glomeruli, and it has been assumed that these processes mainly represent dendrites of the periglomerular cells, which is supported by electron microscopic immunohistochemistry (44). Dendrites containing dopamine have previously been demonstrated in the substantia nigra (16), and evidence for a release of dopamine from the dendrites of nigral neurons has recently been presented (57,61). It has been suggested (44) that dopamine is released from the periglomerular cells at dendrodendritic synapses with mitral cells (see refs. 89,91), where dopamine would then act as an inhibitory transmitter (see refs. 84,92,94,95).

RETINAL DOPAMINE SYSTEM

Dopaminergic interneurons have been described in the retina of many submammalian and mammalian species, including the rat (35,63,78; for review see ref. 36). Most of these neurons have their cell bodies in the inner nuclear layer, among the amacrine cells. In the rat the terminals are located exclusively in a band at the outer border of the inner plexiform layer. In other species, notably New World monkeys and teleost fishes, a second terminal plexus is found in the outer plexiform layer (37,38,63). In these species Dowling and Ehinger (34) have shown that the dopamine neurons make synapses with amacrine cells in the inner plexiform layer and with bipolar and horizontal cells in the outer plexiform layer. In addition, the dopamine-containing processes were found to be postsynaptic to synapses from processes of amacrine cells in the inner plexiform layer. The retinal dopamine neuron thus seems to be an interesting example of a neuron where the dopamine-containing processes are both pre- and postsynaptic. This arrangement can be regarded as analogous to that observed for the dopamine neurons of the substantia nigra (16).

There are observations to indicate that dopamine might be released from the retina upon light stimulation, and that the effect of dopamine in the retina probably is inhibitory. On these grounds it has been suggested that the dopaminergic interneurons might participate in lateral interactions and feedback loops in the retina. In the outer plexiform layer of goldfish, dopamine will reduce the surrounding effects exerted by the horizontal cells on the bipolars. This points to a role for the dopaminergic neurons in the lateral inhibition in the retina (45).

CONCLUSIONS

During recent years much novel information about the organization of central dopamine neurons has been gathered. This includes both more data on well-known systems as well as the findings of previously unknown dopamine neuron systems. Despite this, more work is still required before the organizational features of the central dopamine neurons are clarified in detail. Certain neuron systems such as the periventricular system, and certain brain regions, above all the lower brainstem, are still incompletely mapped. For example, it seems likely that the mesencephalic dopamine neurons have also descending projections. In fact, Domesick et al. (33), using the auto-radiographic tracing method, have described descending projections from these neurons to medial and median zones of the mesencephalic tegmentum and to the mesencephalic raphe nuclei.

An interesting new aspect of the organization of central dopamine neurons is given by the recent finding of an overlap of the neocortical projection fields of the mediodorsal thalamic nucleus and the mesencephalic dopaminergic neurons in the prefrontal cortex of the rat (7,11,31,32). This convergence seems to be a constant feature of the prefrontal cortex and has been demonstrated also in two other species from different orders, the opossum and tree shrew (31,32). The finding of a group of mesencephalic dopamine neurons whose cortical projection fields are correlated with those of a thalamic nucleus points to a much more precise and "specific" organization of the dopamine systems than has previously been known. To what extent such a "specificity" exists also for other dopamine systems in the brain remains to be clarified.

ACKNOWLEDGMENT

This work was supported by a grant from the Swedish Medical Research Council (04X-4493).

REFERENCES

1. Ajika, K., and Hökfelt, T. (1973): Ultrastructural identification of catecholamine neurones in the hypothalamic periventricular-arcuate nucleus-median eminence complex with special reference to quantitative aspects. *Brain Res.,* 57:97–117.
2. Andén, N.-E., Carlsson, A., Dahlström, A., Fuxe, K., Hillarp, N.-Å., and Larsson, K. (1964): Demonstration and mapping out of nigro-neostriatal dopamine neurons. *Life Sci.,* 3:523–530.
3. Andén, N.-E., Dahlström, A., Fuxe, K., Larsson, K., Olson, L., and Ungerstedt, U. (1966): Ascending monoamine neurons to the telencephalon and diencephalon. *Acta Physiol. Scand.,* 67:313–326.
4. Andén, N.-E., Fuxe, K., Hamberger, B., and Hökfelt, T. (1966): A quantitative study on the nigro-neostriatal dopamine neuron system in the rat. *Acta Physiol. Scand.,* 67:306–312.
5. Avendaño, C., Reinoso-Suarez, F., and Llamas, A. (1976): Projections to gyrus

sigmoideus from the substantia nigra in the cat, as revealed by the horseradish peroxidase retrograde transport technique. *Neurosci. Lett.,* 2:61–65.

6. Baumgarten, H. G., Björklund, A., Holstein, A. F., and Nobin, A. (1972): Organization and ultrastructural identification of the catecholamine nerve terminals in the neural lobe and pars intermedia of the rat pituitary. *Z. Zellforsch.,* 126:483–517.

7. Beckstead, R. M. (1976): Convergent thalamic and mesencephalic projections to the anterior medial cortex in the rat. *J. Comp. Neurol.,* 166:403–416.

8. Bédard, P., Larochelle, L., Parent, A., and Poirier, L. J. (1969): The nigrostriatal pathway: A correlative study based on neuroanatomical and neurochemical criteria in the cat and the monkey. *Exp. Neurol.,* 25:365–377.

9. Ben-Ari, Y., Zigmond, R. E., and Moore, K. E. (1975): Regional distribution of tyrosine hydroxylase, norepinephrine and dopamine within the amygdaloid complex of the rat. *Brain Res.,* 87:96–101.

10. Berger, B., Tassin, J. P., Blanc, B., Moyne, M. A., and Thierry, A. M. (1974): Histochemical confirmation for dopaminergic innervation of the rat cerebral cortex after destruction of the noradrenergic ascending pathways. *Brain Res.,* 81:332–337.

11. Berger, B., Thierry, A. M., Tassin, J. P., and Moyne, M. A. (1976): Dopaminergic innervation of the rat prefrontal cortex: A fluorescence histochemical study. *Brain Res.,* 106:133–145.

12. Bertler, Å., Falck, B., Gottfries, C. G., Ljungren, L., and Rosengren, E. (1964): Some observations on adrenergic connections between mesencephalon and cerebral hemispheres. *Acta Pharmacol. Toxicol.,* 21:283–289.

13. Bertler, Å., and Rosengren, E. (1959): Occurrence and distribution of catecholamines in brain. *Acta Physiol. Scand.,* 47:350–361.

14. Björklund, A. (1968): Monoamine-containing fibres in the neurointermediate lobe of the pig and rat. *Z. Zellforsch.,* 89:573–589.

15. Björklund, A., Falck, B., Hromek, F., Owman, Ch., and West, K. A. (1970): Identification and terminal distribution of the tubero-hypophyseal monoamine fibre systems in the rat by means of stereotaxic and microspectrofluorimetric techniques. *Brain Res.,* 17:1–23.

16. Björklund, A., and Lindvall, O. (1975): Dopamine in dendrites of substantia nigra neurons: Suggestions for a role in dendritic terminals. *Brain Res.,* 83:531–537.

17. Björklund, A., Lindvall, O., and Moore, R. Y. (1978): In: *The Central Catecholamine Neuron,* edited by A. Björklund and R. Y. Moore. Raven Press, New York. To be published.

18. Björklund, A., Lindvall, O., and Nobin, A. (1975): Evidence of an incertohypothalamic dopamine neurone system in the rat. *Brain Res.,* 89:29–42.

19. Björklund, Å., Moore, R. Y., Nobin, A., and Stenevi, U. (1973): The organization of tubero-hypophyseal and reticulo-infundibular catecholamine neuron systems in the rat brain. *Brain Res.,* 51:171–191.

20. Björklund, A., and Nobin, A. (1973): Fluorescence histochemical and microspectrofluorometric mapping of dopamine and noradrenaline cell groups in the rat diencephalon. *Brain Res.,* 51:193–205.

21. Brownstein, M., Saavedra, J. M., and Palkovits, M. (1974): Norepinephrine and dopamine in the limbic system of the rat. *Brain Res.,* 79:431–436.

22. Cajal, S. Ramón (1955): *Histologie du Système Nerveux de l'Homme et des Vertébres, Vol. 2,* pp. 275–278. Consejo Superior de Investigaciones Cientificas, Inst. Ramón y Cajal, Madrid.

23. Carlsson, A., Falck, B., and Hillarp, N.-Å. (1962): Cellular localization of brain monoamines. *Acta Physiol. Scand. [Suppl.],* 196:1–27.

24. Carlsson, A., Lindqvist, M., Magnusson, T., and Waldeck, B. (1958): On the presence of 3-hydroxytyramine in brain. *Science,* 127:471.

25. Carpenter, M. B., and Peter, P. (1972): Nigrostriatal and nigrothalamic fibers in the rhesus monkey. *J. Comp. Neurol.,* 144:93–116.

26. Collier, T. J., and Routtenberg, A. (1976): Entorhinal cortex: Catecholamine fluorescence and Nissl staining of identical sections. *Neuroscience Abstracts, Vol. II, Society for Neuroscience Sixth Annual Meeting,* p. 483, Toronto, Canada.

27. Dahlström, A., and Fuxe, K. (1964): Evidence for the existence of monoamine-

containing neurons in the central nervous system. I: Demonstration of monoamines in the cell bodies of brain stem neurones. *Acta Physiol. Scand. [Suppl. 232]*, 62: 1–55.

28. Dahlström, A., and Fuxe, K. (1965): Evidence for the existence of monoamine neurons in the central nervous system. II: Experimentally induced changes in the intraneuronal amine levels of bulbospinal neuron systems. *Acta Physiol. Scand. [Suppl. 247]*, 64:1–36.

29. Dahlström, A., Fuxe, K., Olson, L., and Ungerstedt, U. (1965): On the distribution and possible function of monoamine nerve terminals in the olfactory bulb of the rabbit. *Life Sci.*, 4:2071–2074.

30. Dellman, H. D., and Rodriguez, E. M. (1970): Herring bodies; an electron microscopic study of local degeneration and regeneration of neurosecretory axons. *Z. Zellforsch.*, 111:293–315.

31. Divac, I., Björklund, A., Lindvall, O., and Passingham, R. E. (1978): Converging projections from the mediodorsal thalamic nucleus and mesencephalic dopaminergic neurons to the neocortex in three species. *J. Comp. Neurol.*, (in press).

32. Divac, I., Lindvall, O., Björklund, A., and Passingham, R. E. (1975): Converging projections from the mediodorsal thalamic nucleus and mesencephalic dopaminergic neurons to the neocortex in three species. *Exp. Brain Res.*, 23:58 (abst.).

33. Domesick, V. B., Beckstead, R. M., and Nauta, W. J. H. (1976): Some ascending and descending projections of the substantia nigra and ventral tegmental area in the rat. *Neuroscience Abstracts, Vol. II, Society for Neuroscience Sixth Annual Meeting*, p. 61, Toronto, Canada.

34. Dowling, J. E., and Ehinger, B. (1975): Synaptic organization of the amine-containing interplexiform cells of the goldfish and cebus monkey retinas. *Science*, 188:270–273.

35. Ehinger, B. (1966): Adrenergic nerves to the eye and to related structures in man and in the cynomolgus monkey. *Invest. Ophthalmol.*, 5:42–52.

36. Ehinger, B. (1976): Biogenic monoamines as transmitters in the retina. In: *Symposium on Retinal Neurotransmitters*, edited by Bonting. Barcelona, Madrid.

37. Ehinger, B., and Falck, B. (1969): Adrenergic retinal neurons of some New World monkeys. *Z. Zellforsch.*, 100:364–372.

38. Ehinger, B., Falck, B., and Laties, A. M. (1969): Adrenergic neurons in teleost retina. *Z. Zellforsch.*, 97:285–297.

39. Fallon, J. H., and Moore, R. Y. (1976): Dopamine innervation of some basal forebrain areas in the rat. *Neuroscience Abstracts, Vol. II, Society for Neuroscience Sixth Annual Meeting*, p. 486, Toronto, Canada.

40. Fuxe, K. (1964): Cellular localization of monoamines in the median eminence and infundibular stem of some mammals. *Z. Zellforsch.*, 61:710–724.

41. Fuxe, K. (1965): Evidence for the existence of monoamine neurons in the central nervous system. IV: Distribution of monoamine nerve terminals in the central nervous system. *Acta Physiol. Scand. [Suppl. 247]*, 64:39–85.

42. Fuxe, K., and Hökfelt, T. (1969): Catecholamines in the hypothalamus and the pituitary gland. In: *Frontiers in Neuroendocrinology*, edited by W. F. Ganong and L. Martini, pp. 47–96. Oxford University Press, New York.

43. Fuxe, K., Hökfelt, T., Johansson, O., Jonsson, G., Lidbrink, P., and Ljungdahl, Å. (1974): The origin of the dopamine nerve terminals in limbic and frontal cortex. Evidence for meso-cortico dopamine neurons. *Brain Res.*, 82:349–355.

44. Halász, N., Hökfelt, T., Ljungdahl, Å., Johansson, O., Ebstein, M., Goldstein, M., Park, D., and Biberfeld, P. (1977): Transmitter histochemistry of the rat olfactory bulb. I. Immunohistochemical localization of monoamine synthesizing enzymes. Support for intrabulbar, periglomerular dopamine neurons. *Brain Res.*, 126:455–474.

45. Hedden, W. L. (1976): The interplexiform cell system. Doctorate thesis, Harvard University, Cambridge, Mass.

46. Hedreen, J. C., and Chalmers, J. P. (1972): Neuronal degeneration in rat brain induced by 6-hydroxydopamine; a histological and biochemical study. *Brain Res.*, 47:1–36.

47. Herkenham, M., and Nauta, W. J. H. (1977): Afferent connections of the habenu-

lar nuclei in the rat. A horseradish peroxidase study with a note on the fiber-of-passage problem. *J. Comp. Neurol.,* 173:123–146.

48. Hökfelt, T. (1973): Possible site of action of dopamine in the hypothalamic pituitary control. *Acta Physiol. Scand.,* 89:606–608.

49. Hökfelt, T., Fuxe, K., and Goldstein, M. (1975): Applications of immunohisto-chemistry to studies on monoamine cell systems with special references to nervous tissues. *Ann. N.Y. Acad. Sci.,* 254:407–432.

50. Hökfelt, T., Fuxe, K., Johansson, O., and Ljungdahl, Å. (1974): Pharmaco-histochemical evidence of the existence of dopamine nerve terminals in the limbic cortex. *Eurp. J. Pharmacol.,* 25:108–112.

51. Hökfelt, T., Halász, N., Ljungdahl, Å., Johansson, O., Goldstein, M., and Park, D. (1975): Histochemical support for a dopaminergic mechanism in the dendrites of certain periglomerular cells in the rat olfactory bulb. *Neurosci. Lett.,* 1:85–90.

52. Hökfelt, T., Johansson, O., Fuxe, K., Goldstein, M., and Park, D. (1976): Im-munohistochemical studies on the localization and distribution of monoamine neuron systems in the rat brain. I. Tyrosine hydroxylase in the mes- and diencepha-lon. *Med. Biol.,* 54:427–453.

53. Hökfelt, T., Johansson, O., Fuxe, K., Goldstein, M., and Park, D. (1977): Im-munohistochemical studies on the localization and distribution of monoamine neuron systems in the rat brain. II. Tyrosine hydroxylase in the telencephalon. *Med. Biol.,* 55:21–40.

54. Hökfelt, T., and Ljungdahl, Å. (1972): Modification of the Falck-Hillarp formal-dehyde fluorescence method using the Vibratome: simple, rapid and sensitive localization of catecholamines in sections of unfixed or formalin fixed brain tissue. *Histochemie,* 29:325–339.

55. Hökfelt, T., Ljungdahl, Å., Fuxe, K., and Johansson, O. (1974): Dopamine nerve terminals in the rat limbic cortex: Aspects of the dopamine hypothesis of schizo-phrenia. *Science,* 184:177–179.

56. Hökfelt, T., and Ungerstedt, U. (1969): Electron and fluorescence microscopical studies on the nucleus caudatus putamen of the rat after unilateral lesions of ascending nigro-neostriatal dopamine neurons. *Acta Physiol. Scand.,* 76:415–426.

57. Jessell, T. M., Cuello, A. C., and Iversen, L. L. (1976): Release of dopamine from dendrites in rat substantia nigra. *Nature,* 260:258–260.

58. Jones, B. E., and Moore, R. Y. (1977): Ascending projections of the locus coeruleus in the rat. II. Autoradiographic study. *Brain Res.,* 127:23–53.

59. Jonsson, G., Fuxe, K., and Hökfelt, T. (1972): On the catecholamine innervation of the hypothalamus, with special reference to the median eminence. *Brain Res.,* 40:271–281.

60. Kobayashi, R. M., Palkovits, M., Kopin, I. J., and Jacobowitz, D. M. (1974): Biochemical mapping of noradrenergic nerves arising from the rat locus coeruleus. *Brain Res.,* 77:269–279.

61. Korf, J., Zieleman, M., and Westerink, B. H. C. (1976): Dopamine release in substantia nigra? *Nature,* 260:257–258.

62. Koslow, S. H., Racagni, G., and Costa, E. (1974): Mass fragmentographic meas-urement of norepinephrine, dopamine, serotonin and acetylcholine in seven dis-crete nuclei of the rat tel-diencephalon. *Neuropharmacology,* 13:1123–1130.

63. Laties, A., and Jacobowitz, D. (1966): A comparative study of the autonomic innervation of the eye in monkey, cat and rabbit. *Anat. Rec.,* 156:383.

64. LaVail, J. H., and LaVail, M. M. (1972): Retrograde axonal transport in the central nervous system. *Science,* 176:1416–1417.

65. Lichtensteiger, W. (1966): Uptake of noradrenaline in periglomerular cells of the olfactory bulb of the mouse. *Nature,* 210:955–956.

66. Lichtensteiger, W. (1970): Katecholaminhaltige Neurone in der neuroendokrinen Steuerung. *Prog. Histochem. Cytochem.,* 1:185–276.

67. Lidbrink, P., Jonsson, G., and Fuxe, K. (1974): Selective reserpine-resistant accu-mulation of catecholamines in central dopamine neurones after DOPA administra-tion. *Brain Res.,* 67:439–456.

68. Lindvall, O. (1975): Mesencephalic dopaminergic afferents to the lateral septal nucleus of the rat. *Brain Res.,* 87:89–95.

69. Lindvall, O., and Björklund, A. (1974): The organization of the ascending catecholamine neuron systems in the rat brain as revealed by the glyoxylic acid fluorescence method. *Acta Physiol. Scand.* [*Suppl.*], 412:1–48.
70. Lindvall, O., and Björklund, A. (1974): The glyoxylic acid fluorescence histochemical method: A detailed account of the methodology for the visualization of central catecholamine neurons. *Histochemistry*, 39:97–127.
71. Lindvall, O., Björklund, A., and Divac, I. (1978): Organization of catecholamine neurons projecting to the frontal cortex in the rat. *Brain Res.*, 142:1–24.
72. Lindvall, O., Björklund, A., Moore, R. Y., and Stenevi, U. (1974): Mesencephalic dopamine neurons projecting to neocortex. *Brain Res.*, 81:325–331.
73. Lindvall, O., Björklund, A., Nobin, A., and Stenevi, U. (1974): The adrenergic innervation of the rat thalamus as revealed by the glyoxylic acid fluorescence method. *J. Comp. Neurol.*, 154:317–348.
74. Lindvall, O., and Stenevi, U. (1978): Dopamine and noradrenaline neurons projecting to the septal area in the rat. *Cell Tissue Res.*, (*in press*).
75. Löfström, A., Jonsson, G., and Fuxe, K. (1976): Microfluorometric quantitation of catecholamine fluorescence in rat median eminence. I. Aspects on the distribution of dopamine and noradrenaline nerve terminals. *J. Histochem. Cytochem.*, 24:415–429.
76. Loizou, L. A. (1969): Projections of the nucleus locus coeruleus in the albino rat. *Brain Res.*, 15:563–566.
77. Maler, L., Fibiger, H. C., and McGeer, P. L. (1973): Demonstration of the nigrostriatal projection by silver staining after nigral injections of 6-hydroxydopamine. *Exp. Neurol.*, 40:505–515.
78. Malmfors, T. (1963): Evidence of adrenergic neurons with synaptic terminals in the retina of rats demonstrated with fluorescence and electron microscopy. *Acta Physiol. Scand.*, 58:99–100.
79. Montagu, K. A. (1957): Catechol compounds in rat tissues and in brains of different animals. *Nature*, 180:244–245.
80. Moore, R. Y., Bhatnagar, R. K., and Heller, A. (1971): Anatomical and chemical studies of nigro-neostriatal projection in the cat. *Brain Res.*, 30:119–135.
81. Moore, R. Y., Björklund, A., and Stenevi, U. (1971): Plastic changes in the adrenergic innervation of the rat septal area in response to denervation. *Brain Res.*, 33:13–35.
82. Nauta, W. J. H. (1978): In: *The Continuing Evolution of the Limbic System Concept*, edited by K. Livingston and O. Hornykiewics. Plenum Press, New York (*in press*).
83. Nauta, H. J. W., Pritz, M. B., and Lasek, R. J. (1974): Afferents to the rat caudoputamen studied with horseradish peroxidase. An evaluation of a retrograde neuroanatomical research method. *Brain Res.*, 67:219–238.
84. Nicoll, R. A. (1969): Inhibitory mechanisms in the rabbit olfactory bulb: Dendrodendritic mechanisms. *Brain Res.*, 14:157–172.
85. Nobin, A., and Björklund, A. (1973): Topography of the monoamine neuron systems in the human brain as revealed in fetuses. *Acta Physiol. Scand* [*Suppl.*], 388:1–40.
86. Palkovits, M., Brownstein, M., Saavedra, J. M., and Axelrod, J. (1974): Norepinephrine and dopamine content of hypothalamic nuclei of the rat. *Brain Res.*, 77:137–149.
87. Pickel, V. M., Joh, T. H., Field, P. M., Becker, C. G., and Reis, D. J. (1975): Cellular localization of tyrosine hydroxylase by immunohistochemistry. *J. Histochem. Cytochem.*, 23:1–12.
88. Pickel, V. M., Joh, T. H., and Reis, D. J. (1975): Immunohistochemical localization of tyrosine hydroxylase in brain by light and electron microscopy. *Brain Res.*, 85:295–300.
89. Pinching, A. J., and Powell, T. P. S. (1971): The neuropil of the glomeruli of the olfactory bulb. *J. Cell Sci.*, 9:347–377.
90. Poirier, L. J., and Sourkes, T. L. (1965): Influence of the substantia nigra on the catecholamine content of the striatum. *Brain*, 88:181–192.

91. Price, J. L., and Powell, T. P. S. (1970): The mitral and short axon cells of the olfactory bulb. *J. Cell Sci.,* 7:631–651.
92. Rall, W., Shepherd, G. M., Reese, T. S., and Brightman, M. W. (1966): Dendrodendritic synaptic pathway for inhibition in the olfactory bulb. *Exp. Neurol.,* 14: 44–56.
93. Saavedra, J. M., and Zivin, I. (1976): Tyrosine hydroxylase and dopamine-β-hydroxylase: Distribution in discrete areas of the rat limbic system. *Brain Res.,* 105:517–524.
94. Shepherd, G. M. (1971): Physiological evidence for dendrodendritic synaptic interactions in the rabbit's olfactory glomerulus. *Brain Res.,* 32:212–217.
95. Shepherd, G. M. (1972): Synaptic organization of the mammalian olfactory bulb. *Physiol. Rev.,* 52:864–917.
96. Shimizu, N., and Ohnishi, S. (1973): Demonstration of nigro-neostriatal tract by degeneration silver method. *Exp. Brain Res.,* 17:133–138.
97. Simon, H., LeMoal, M., Galey, D., and Cardo, B. (1974): Selective degeneration of central dopaminergic systems after injection of 6-hydroxydopamine in the ventral mesencephalic tegmentum of the rat. Demonstration by the Fink-Heimer stain. *Exp. Brain Res.,* 20:375–384.
98. Simon, H., LeMoal, M., Galey, D., and Cardo, B. (1976): Silver impregnation of dopaminergic systems after radiofrequency and 6-OHDA lesions of the rat ventral tegmentum. *Brain Res.,* 115:215–231.
99. Smith, G. C., and Fink, G. (1972): Experimental studies on the origin of monoamine-containing fibres in the hypothalamo-hypophyseal complex of the rat. *Brain Res.,* 43:37–51.
100. Thierry, A. M., Blanc, G., Sobel, A., Stinus, L., and Glowinski, J. (1973): Dopamine terminals in the rat cortex. *Science,* 182:499–501.
101. Thierry, A. M., Stinus, L., Blanc, G., and Glowinski, J. (1973): Some evidence for the existence of dopaminergic neurons in the rat cortex. *Brain Res.,* 50:230–234.
102. Ungerstedt, U. (1971): Stereotaxic mapping of the monoamine pathways in the rat brain. *Acta Physiol. Scand. [Suppl.],* 367:1–48.

Advances in Biochemical Psychopharmacology, Vol. 19,
edited by P. J. Roberts et al.
Raven Press, New York © 1978.

Characteristics of Neuronal Dopamine Uptake

Alan S. Horn

Department of Pharmacy, University of Groningen, Groningen, The Netherlands

Recently it has been shown that certain dopamine (DA) rich brain areas possess an uptake system for exogenous [³H]DA that is different from that responsible for the neuronal uptake of [³H]norepinephrine (NE) (38). In the context of this chapter the term *uptake* is taken to mean the passage or transport of a molecule across a cell membrane rather than a simple binding of the molecule to the external membrane surface.

ANATOMICAL ASPECTS OF NEURONAL DA UPTAKE

The dopaminergic areas of the nervous system in which this process has been studied *in vitro* include:

1. The corpus striatum (5,16,21,38)
2. The substantia nigra (13)
3. The median eminence (6)
4. The olfactory tubercle (24)
5. The nucleus accumbens (24)
6. The septal nuclei (11,12)
7. The retina (7,33).

The uptake of [³H]DA has also been studied *in vitro* in:

8. The limbic cortex (40)
9. The cerebral cortex, hypothalamus, midbrain, medulla oblongata-pons, and cerebellum (38).

BIOCHEMICAL AND PHARMACOLOGICAL PROPERTIES OF THE NEURONAL DA UPTAKE SYSTEM

Early work on the DA uptake system used tissue slices or crude synaptosomal preparations, but more recently Holz and Coyle (21) have studied the properties of this system in purified striatal synaptosomes with [³H]DA.

The DA uptake system has the following properties:

1. It is temperature sensitive. Using the purified synaptosomal preparation investigators showed that there is a break in the Arrhenius plot at

30°C; above this temperature the Q_{10} was 1.7 whereas below it the value was 4.5 (21).

2. In synaptosomes the uptake is linear for up to 2 min (21) and for 5 to 10 min in synaptosome-enriched homogenates (16,38). It is also proportional to the amount of synaptosomal protein.

3. The tissue to medium ratio (T/M) reaches 170 after 2 min (21).

4. The system displays Michaelis-Menten kinetics and has a $K_m = 1.3 \times 10^{-7}$ M for DA and a $V_{max} = 25.3$ pmoles/100 μg protein/2 min at normal physiological concentrations of Na^+ and K^+ (21). The affinity for $(-)$ NA is lower, $K_m = 2.0 \times 10^{-6}$ M (28). In general it is assumed that K_m is a measure of the dissociation constant for the binding of substrate to the uptake sites, and thus K_m may be taken as a reciprocal measure of the affinity of the substrate for the uptake sites. The V_{max} will depend on the type and amount of tissue present and is a measure of the number of amine uptake sites present. The K_m is independent of the total number of uptake sites present (27).

5. The uptake of [^{3}H]DA is dependent on the concentration of Na^+ and to a certain extent on that of K^+ (21).

6. It is possible to replace K^+ by Rb^+, but Cs^+ is less effective; the system does not appear to require Ca^{2+} (16).

7. Veratridine (50 μM) and batrachotoxin (0.5 μM) both effectively inhibited [^{3}H]DA uptake. This inhibition was partly blocked by tetrodotoxin (1.0 μM). The effects with veratridine and batrachotoxin may be due to an increased Na^+ permeability (21).

8. It is known (36) that various other β-phenylethylamine analogues can be taken up by dopaminergic neurons; their structures are shown in Table 1.

TABLE 1. *β-Phenylethylamine analogues taken up by dopaminergic neurons*

Drug	Structure			
	R_1	R_2	R_3	R_4
Dopamine	OH	OH	H	H
Norepinephrine	OH	OH	OH	H
Tyramine	OH	H	H	H
m-Tyramine	H	OH	H	H
α-Methyl-m-tyramine	H	OH	H	CH_3
Octopamine	OH	H	OH	H
m-Octopamine	H	OH	OH	H
Metaraminol	H	OH	OH	CH_3

Data from ref. 36.

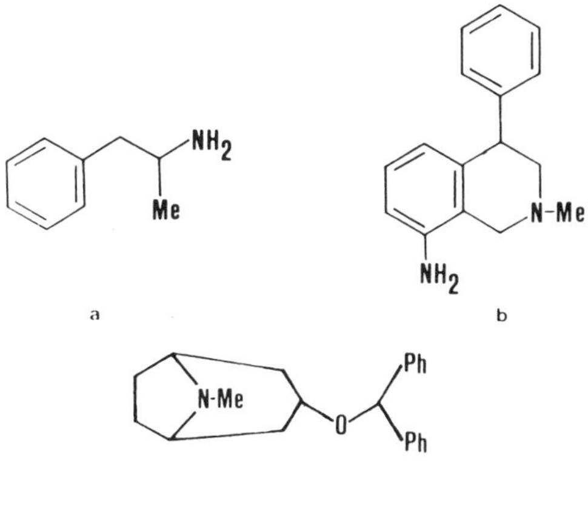

FIG. 1. Chemical structures of (a) amphetamine, (b) nomifensine, and (c) benztropine.

9. The uptake of [³H]DA is potently inhibited *in vitro* by (+)amphetamine, $IC_{50} = 0.5 \times 10^{-7}$ M (24), benztropine, $IC_{50} = 1.2 \times 10^{-7}$ M (23), and nomifensine, $IC_{50} = 1.45 \times 10^{-7}$ M (26) (Fig. 1). This uptake system is much less sensitive than the NA uptake system to inhibition by the tricyclic antidepressants (23). In general the structure-activity relationships for β-phenylethylamine derivatives as inhibitors of [³H]DA uptake are similar to those described for NA uptake (22), i.e.:

(a) phenolic hydroxyl groups in the p and/or m positions enhance uptake site affinity; (b) α-methylation increases affinity; (c) β-hydroxylation decreases affinity; (d) mono- or di-N-methylation decreases affinity; and (e) O-methylation of phenolic hydroxyls produces a marked decrease in affinity.

10. Homogenates of newborn rat corpus striatum show only 10% of the activity of the adult system in transporting [³H]DA. By 4 weeks after birth, however, the activity reaches 75% of the adult level. Kinetic studies show that this increase in uptake is related to an increase in the V_{max} (4).

11. In an attempt to investigate the possible involvement of certain glycoproteins and peptides in the DA transport system, investigators have treated synaptosomes with concanavalin A and trypsin. Neither agent had an effect on [³H]DA uptake (43).

DA UPTAKE AND ITS INHIBITION: NEW DEVELOPMENTS

Recently there has been much discussion in the literature regarding certain aspects of DA uptake and its inhibition by drugs, and it is perhaps useful to try to attempt to clarify some of these points.

In Vivo-in Vitro Inhibition of [³H]DA Uptake

It has been claimed (1) that although one can demonstrate an inhibition of [³H]DA uptake *in vitro* by a drug, this either cannot be done or it is only

TABLE 2. In vivo–in vitro *inhibition* of ³H-DA *into the corpus striatum*

Drug	ED$_{50}$ (μmoles/kg)	Reference
(+) Amphetamine (sl.)	60	37
(−) Amphetamine (sl.)	240	37
(+) Amphetamine (syn.)	< 17	3
Amphetamine (syn.)	< 14	30
Benztropine (sl.)	60	37
Benztropine (syn.)	~78	30
Prolintane (sl.)	55	37

Rats or mice received i.p. injections of the drugs before isolation of striatal tissue and incubation with [³H]DA; sl., slices; syn., synaptosomes. Data taken from (3,30,37). In converting the results from (30) to μmoles/kg, it has been assumed that the quoted values are for the base rather than for the salt.

a weak effect after *in vivo* drug administration which is followed by *in vitro* incubation of striatal preparations with [³H]DA. A careful review of the literature clearly demonstrates that this is, in fact, not the case. This is shown by the results in Table 2 taken from Ross and Renyi (37), who used striatal slices, and Kannengiesser et al. (30) and Carruba et al. (3), who used striatal synaptosomes. The (+) isomer of amphetamine was found to be quite potent, and it is of interest that one can also demonstrate the differential effect of the amphetamine stereoisomers in this *in vivo–in vitro* system (37). It is also noteworthy that two of these groups (30,37) were able to demonstrate an effect with benztropine although others using even higher doses were

Ph-CH$_2$-CH-Pr

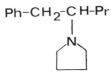

FIG. 2. Chemical structure of prolintane.

not able to do this (1). Prolintane (Fig. 2) was found to be slightly more active than benztropine and d-amphetamine. Other drugs which have been studied by this *in vivo–in vitro* technique include amphetamine analogues (37), fluorinated amphetamines (32), fenfluramine (30), mazindol (3), lithium (39), and certain steroids (44).

Amphetamine Enantiomers and [³H]DA Uptake

Initial *in vitro* studies with the separate enantiomers of amphetamine showed that they were equally potent in inhibiting [³H]DA uptake into homogenates of rat corpus striatum (5). More recent *in vitro* studies by several groups of workers have shown, however, that the (+) isomer is, in fact, four to six times more potent than the (−) isomer in this brain area (8,17,20,24,41). These results also agree with the *in vivo–in vitro* findings (37).

Inhibition of [³H]DA Uptake by Tricyclic Antidepressants

In our studies (23) on the comparative inhibition of [³H]DA and NE-5-hydroxytryptamine (5-HT) uptake into synaptosomal-enriched homogenates of the rat corpus striatum and hypothalamus, respectively, we found that in general the tricyclic antidepressants were weaker inhibitors of DA than of NE and 5-HT uptake (23,25). These studies confirmed earlier reports of other workers who used both *in vivo* and *in vitro* techniques (2,10,29). Our findings were also verified by several other groups using *in vitro* (8,31) and *in vivo–in vitro* techniques (37).

Recently two publications have attempted to place greater emphasis on the possible importance of the inhibition of [³H]DA uptake by the tricyclic antidepressants (9,15). It is somewhat difficult to evaluate the possible clinical significance of the reported effects on [³H]DA uptake of the tricyclics (15) because the single concentration used (1×10^{-5} M) is much in excess of that required to inhibit [³H]NE or 5-HT uptake to the same extent.

INHIBITION OF UPTAKE OR RELEASE?

Several authors (8,19), and in particular Heikkila et al. (18), have pointed out the difficulties in clearly distinguishing between a drug's ability to inhibit the uptake and/or cause the release of ³H-biogenic amines. Heikkila et al. (18) have clearly stated the problem as follows:

Consider first the measurement of [³H] amine uptake. During the time that the [³H] amine is taken up, a releasing agent could cause egress of a portion of the accumulated [³H] amine. The resultant diminution in accumulated [³H] amine could be interpreted as decreased "uptake." Therefore, a releasing agent could be misclassified as an uptake blocker. A second difficulty exists in the experimental verification of a presumed releasing action. If tissue containing [³H] amine is incubated in fresh medium at 37°, there is spontaneous efflux of a portion of the [³H] amine. An agent that blocks the reuptake of [³H] amines could, in theory, augment the net loss from the tissue. Since increased net loss is generally construed as constituting a "releasing" action, it is apparent that an uptake blocker could be misclassified as a releasing agent. Thus, there is reason to suspect that uptake blockade and release can become confounded.

These authors determined dose-response curves for *in vitro* release and inhibition of the uptake of [³H]DA by various drugs. They concluded that cocaine does not produce a significant release of [³H]DA from the striatum even at a concentration as high as 10^{-4}M, i.e., it is an inhibitor of DA uptake. In the case of (+)-amphetamine they are of the opinion that it is mainly a releaser of [³H]DA in the striatum. Using somewhat similar techniques other workers have concluded that amphetamine has a stronger effect on [³H]DA uptake than on release (8,20). Benztropine was found by Orlansky and Heikkila (34) to be predominantly an inhibitor of [³H]DA uptake; this result is also in agreement with the *in vivo* findings of Goodale and Moore (14).

In an attempt to eliminate the ever-present problem of reuptake of released [³H]DA in *in vitro* studies on release, Raiteri et al. (35) have developed a superfusion technique for synaptosomes. They have shown that (+)amphetamine has a dual action, i.e., it inhibits the uptake and also induces the release of [³H]DA from synaptosomes of the corpus striatum.

In conclusion, it can be said that apparently benztropine has its predominant effect on [³H]DA uptake, whereas amphetamine appears to have a mixed action.

CONFORMATION OF DOPAMINE AT ITS UPTAKE SITE

As dopamine is a flexible molecule capable of existing in several conformations (Fig. 3), it is of interest to attempt to obtain information about the preferred conformation at its uptake site. Using several rigid and semirigid analogues of amphetamine, a competitive inhibitor of catecholamine uptake, it has been shown that the preferred conformation for a noncatecholamine as an inhibitor of ³H-DA uptake is probably the fully extended *trans* form (Fig. 3) (22). Similar conclusions were also reached from studies using two rigid analogues of dopamine, 2-amino-6,7-dihydroxy-1,2,3,4-tetrahydronaphthalene (ADTN) and 6,7-dihydroxytetrahydroisoquinoline (Fig. 4). It

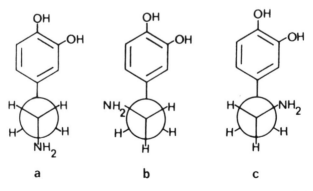

a   b   c

FIG. 3. Newman projections of 3 conformations of dopamine: (a) *trans* or *anti* form, (b) and (c) *gauche* forms.

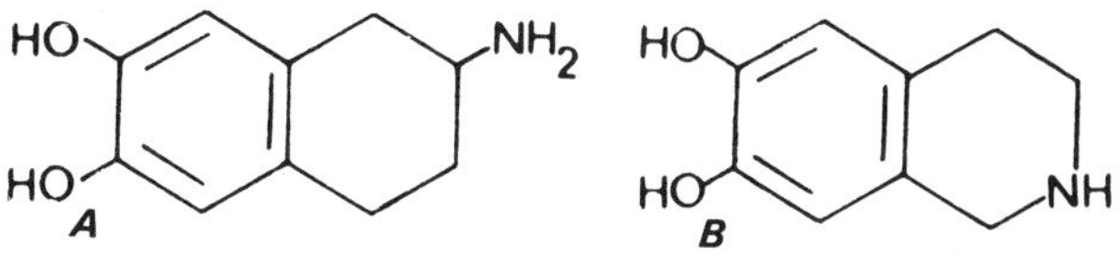

FIG. 4. Chemical structures of (a) 2-amino-6,7-dihydroxy-1,2,3,4-tetrahydronaphthalene (ADTN) and (b) 6,7-dihydroxytetrahydroisoquinoline.

is of interest that the fully extended *trans* form of dopamine is the preferred form in the solid state and in solution (22).

Other authors using catecholamine derivatives of *trans* decalin (Fig. 5) have suggested that the preferred conformation for DA at the uptake site is *gauche* (Fig. 3) (42). A major difficulty in the use of these *trans* decalin derivatives is that a large hydrophobic moiety has been added to the catecholamine molecule in order to reduce flexibility. This may produce interactions at the uptake site that are quite different from the natural ligand. An additional complication due to the presence of the bulky decalin group is that the molecule can approach the uptake site from only one side, rather than having, as dopamine does, a more or less unrestricted access. In general, in order to obtain reliable information from the "rigid-analogue" approach, one must add as little to the molecule as possible in order to produce a more rigid structure. From the evidence available it would appear that it is more likely that the preferred conformation of DA at its uptake site is *trans* rather than *gauche,* but clearly more work needs to be done with other carefully designed rigid analogues of DA.

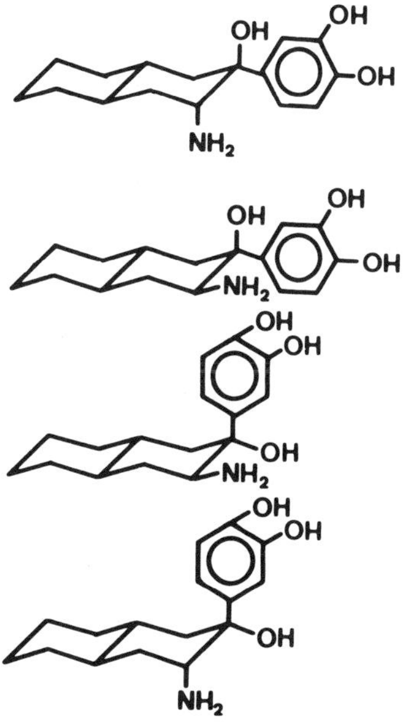

FIG. 5. *Trans* decalin analogues containing the norepinephrine system.

REFERENCES

1. Baumann, P. A., and Maitre, L. (1976): Is drug inhibition of dopamine uptake a misinterpretation of *in vitro* experiments. *Nature*, 264:789–790.
2. Carlsson, A., Fuxe, K., Hamberger, B., and Lindqvist, M. (1966): Biochemical and histochemical studies on the effects of imipramine-like drugs and (+) amphetamine on central and peripheral catecholamine neurons. *Acta Physiol. Scand.*, 67: 481–497.
3. Carruba, M. O., Picotti, G. B., Zambotti, F., and Mantegazza, P. (1977): Mazindol and amphetamine as inhibitors of the uptake and release of ³H-dopamine by rat striatal synaptosomes. *Arch. Pharmacol.*, 298:1–5.
4. Coyle, J. T., and Campochiaro, P. (1976): Ontogenesis of dopaminergic-cholinergic interactions in the rat striatum: A neurochemical study. *J. Neurochem.*, 27:673–678.
5. Coyle, J. T., and Snyder, S. H. (1969): Catecholamine uptake by synaptosomes in homogenates of rat brain: Stereospecificity in different areas. *J. Pharmacol. Exp. Ther.*, 170:221–231.
6. Cuello, A. C., Horn, A. S., Mackay, A. V. P., and Iversen, L. L. (1973): Catecholamines in the median eminence: New evidence for a major noradrenergic input. *Nature*, 243:465–467.
7. Ehringer, B., and Falck, B. (1971): Autoradiography of some suspected neurotransmitter substances: GABA, glycine, glutamic acid, histamine, dopamine and L-dopa. *Brain Res.*, 33:157–172.
8. Ferris, R. M., Tang, F. L. M., and Maxwell, R. A. (1972): A comparison of the capacities of isomers of amphetamine, deoxypipradrol and methylphenidate to inhibit the uptake of tritiated catecholamines into rat cerebral cortex slices, synaptosomal preparations of rat cerebral cortex, hypothalamus and striatum and into adrenergic nerves of rabbit aorta. *J. Pharmacol. Exp. Ther.*, 181:407–416.
9. Friedman, E., Fung, F., and Gershon, S. (1977): Antidepressant drugs and dopamine uptake in different brain regions. *Eur. J. Pharmacol.*, 42:47–51.
10. Fuxe, K., and Ungerstedt, U. (1968): Histochemical studies on the effect of (+)-amphetamine, drugs of the imipramine group and tryptamine on central catecholamine and 5-hydroxytryptamine neurons after intraventricular injection of catecholamines and 5-hydroxtryptamine. *Eur. J. Pharmacol.*, 4:135–144.
11. Garey, R. E. (1976): Regional differences in the high affinity uptake of ³H-dopamine and ³H-norepinephrine in synaptosome rich homogenates of cat brain. *Life Sci.*, 18:411–418.
12. Garey, R. E., and Heath, R. G. (1974): Uptake of catecholamines by human synaptosomes. *Brain Res.*, 79:520–523.
13. Geffen, L. B., Jessell, T. M., Cuello, A. C., and Iversen, L. L. (1976): Release of dopamine from dendrites of rat substantin nigra. *Nature*, 260:258–260.
14. Goodale, D. B., and Moore, K. E. (1975): Benztropine induced release of dopamine from brain *in vivo*. *Neuropharmacology*, 14:585–589.
15. Halaris, A. E., Belendiuk, K. T., and Freedman, D. X. (1975): Antidepressant drugs affect dopamine uptake. *Biochem. Pharmacol.*, 24:1896–1898.
16. Harris, J. E., and Baldessarini, R. J. (1973): The uptake of [³H]-dopamine by homogenates of rat corpus striatum: Effects of cations. *Life Sci.*, 13:303–312.
17. Harris, J. E., and Baldessarini, R. J. (1973): Uptake of [³H]-catecholamines by homogenates of rat corpus striatum and cerebral cortex: Effects of amphetamine analogues. *Neuropharmacology*, 12:669–679.
18. Heikkila, R. E., Orlansky, H., and Cohen, G. (1975): Studies on the distinction between uptake inhibition and release of [³H] dopamine in rat brain tissues slices. *Biochem. Pharmacol.*, 24:847–852.
19. Hendley, E. D., Snyder, S. H., Fawley, J. J., and Lapidus, J. B. (1972): Stereoselectivity of catecholamine uptake by brain synaptosomes: Studies with ephedrine, methylphenidate and phenyl-2-piperidyl carbinol. *J. Pharmacol. Exp. Ther.*, 183: 103–116.
20. Holmes, J. C., and Rutledge, C. O. (1974): A comparison of the effects of d and l amphetamine on the uptake and release of [³H]-norepinephrine, [³H]-dopamine and

[³H]-5-hydroxytryptamine from several regions of rat brain. *Fed. Proc.*, 33:523, 1761.

21. Holz, K. W., and Coyle, J. T. (1974): The effects of various salts, temperature and the alkaloids veratridine and batrachotoxin on the uptake of [³H]-dopamine into synaptosomes from rat striatum. *Mol. Pharmacol.*, 10:746–758.

22. Horn, A. S. (1976): Characteristics of transport in dopaminergic neurons. In: *The Mechanism of Neuronal and Extraneuronal Transport of Catecholamines*, edited by D. M. Paton, pp. 195–214. Raven Press, New York.

23. Horn, A. S., Coyle, J. T., and Snyder, S. H. (1971): Catecholamine uptake by synaptosomes from rat brain: Structure-activity relationships of drugs with differential effects on dopamine and norepinephrine neurons. *Mol. Pharmacol.*, 7:66–80.

24. Horn, A. S., Cuello, A. C., and Miller, R. J. (1974): Dopamine in the mesolimbic system of the rat brain: Endogenous levels and the effects of drugs on the uptake mechanism and stimulation of adenylate cyclase activity. *J. Neurochem.*, 22:265–270.

25. Horn, A. S., and Trace, R. C. A. M. (1974): Structure-activity relations for the inhibition of 5-hydroxytryptamine uptake by tricyclic antidepressants into synaptosomes from serotonergic neurones in rat brain homogenates. *Br. J. Pharmacol.*, 51:399–403.

26. Hunt, P., Kannengiesser, M. H., and Raynaud, J. P. (1974): Nomifensine: A new potent inhibitor of dopamine uptake into synaptosomes from rat brain corpus striatum. *J. Pharm. Pharmacol.*, 26:370–371.

27. Iversen, L. L. (1972): Methods involved in studies of the uptake of biogenic amines. In: *The Thyroid and Biogenic Amines*, edited by T. Rall and I. Kopin, pp. 569–603. North-Holland Publishing Co., Amsterdam.

28. Iversen, L. L., Jarrot, B., and Simmonds, M. A. (1971): Differences in the uptake, storage and metabolism of (+) and (−)-noradrenaline. *Br. J. Pharmacol.*, 43:845–855.

29. Jonason, J., and Rutledge, C. O. (1968): Metabolism of dopamine and noradrenaline in rabbit caudale nucleus *in vitro*. *Acta Physiol. Scand.*, 73:411–417.

30. Kannengiesser, M. H., Hunt, P. F., and Raynaud, J. P. (1976): Comparative action of fenfluramine on the uptake and release of serotonin and dopamine. *Eur. J. Pharmacol.*, 35:35–43.

31. Koe, B. K. (1976): Molecular geometry of inhibitors of the uptake of catecholamines and serotonin in synaptosomal preparations of rat brain. *J. Pharmacol. Exp. Ther.*, 199:649–661.

32. Kouyoumdjian, J. C., Belin, M. F., Barakdjian, J., and Gonnard, P. (1976): Action of some fluorinated amphetamine-like compounds on the synaptosomal uptake of neurotransmitters. *J. Neurochem.*, 27:817–819.

33. Kramer, S. G., Potts, A. M., and Mangnall, Y. (1971): Dopamine: A retinal neurotransmitter. II—Autoradiographic localization of [³H]-dopamine in the retina. *Invest. Ophthalmol.*, 10:617–624.

34. Orlansky, H., and Heikkila, R. E. (1974): An evaluation of various antiparkinsonian agents as releasing agents and uptake inhibitors for ³H-dopamine in slices of rat neostriatum. *Eur. J. Pharmacol.*, 29:284–291.

35. Raiteri, M., Bertollini, A., Angelini, F., and Levi, G. (1975): d-Amphetamine as a releaser or reuptake inhibitor of biogenic amines in synaptosomes. *Eur. J. Pharmacol.*, 34:189–195.

36. Ross, S. B. (1976): Structural requirements for uptake into catecholamine neurons. In: *The Mechanism of Neuronal and Extraneuronal Transport of Catecholamines*, edited by D. M. Paton, pp. 67–93. Raven Press, New York.

37. Ross, S. B., and Renyi, A. L. (1975): Inhibition of the uptake of ³H-dopamine and ¹⁴C-5-hydroxytryptamine in mouse striatum slices. *Acta Pharmacol. Toxicol.*, 36:56–66.

38. Snyder, S. H., and Coyle, J. T. (1969): Regional differences in [³H]-norepinephrine and [³H]-dopamine uptake into rat brain homogenates. *J. Pharmacol. Exp. Ther.*, 165:78–86.

39. Stefanini, E., Argiolas, A., Gessa, G. L., and Fadda, F. (1976): Effect of lithium on dopamine uptake by brain synaptosomes. *J. Neurochem.*, 27:1237–1239.

40. Tassin, J. P., Thierry, A. M., Blanc, G., and Glowinski, J. (1974): Evidence for a specific uptake of dopamine by dopaminergic terminals of the rat cerebral cortex. *Naunyn Schmiedebergs Arch. Pharmacol.,* 282:239–244.
41. Thornburg, J. E., and Moore, K. E. (1973): Dopamine and norepinephrine uptake by rat brain synaptosomes: Relative inhibitory potencies of 1 and d-amphetamine and amantadine. *Res. Commun. Chem. Pathol. Pharmacol.,* 5:81–89.
42. Tuomisto, L., Tuomisto, J., and Smissman, E. E. (1974): Dopamine uptake in striatal and hypothalamic synaptosomes: Conformational selectivity of the inhibition. *Eur. J. Pharmacol.,* 25:351–361.
43. Wang, Y. J., Gurd, J. W., and Mahler, H. R. (1975): Topography of high affinity uptake systems. *Life Sci.,* 17:725–734.
44. Wirz-Justice, A., Hackmann, E., and Lichsteiner, M. (1974): The effect of oestradiol dipropionate and progesterone on monoamine uptake in rat brain. *J. Neurochem.,* 22:187–189.

Advances in Biochemical Psychopharmacology, Vol. 19,
edited by P. J. Roberts et al.
Raven Press, New York © 1978.

Studies on Dopamine Uptake and Release in Synaptosomes

M. Raiteri, F. Cerrito, A. M. Cervoni, R. del Carmine, M. T. Ribera, and *G. Levi

*Institute of Pharmacology, Catholic University, and *Cellular Biology Laboratory, Rome, Italy*

Isolated nerve endings are particularly suitable for characterizing the mechanisms of neurotransmitter transport, not only because they are a relatively pure, metabolically functioning, presynaptic preparation, but also because of the possibility of accurately controlling the many experimental variables which may influence the transport parameters.

In many cases, the studies performed with synaptosomes have searched the confirmation of the existence of processes evidenced or hypothesized in experiments on living animals. In other instances, however, experiments with isolated nerve endings have led to the characterization of processes, for example, the homoexchange of GABA (53,67), or the carrier-mediated release of catecholamines (66), that could hardly be identified in *in vivo* experiments.

In the present chapter we shall discuss some recent data on dopamine (DA) transport in synaptosomes isolated from the corpus striatum. Since DA uptake has been treated in detail in other reports (23,37,41,42) and also in this volume, our attention will be mainly focused on DA release, and we shall be concerned with only a few aspects of DA uptake, directly connected with our release studies.

UPTAKE INHIBITORS VERSUS RELEASERS OF DOPAMINE

The problem of classifying a compound as an uptake inhibitor or as a releaser of a given neurotransmitter is still a matter of controversy. The discrimination is particularly difficult in *in vivo* experiments or when complex preparations of cerebral tissue, such as brain slices, are utilized. The difficulty is largely due to the intimate connection existing between the processes of release and reuptake, which take place almost concomitantly. As a consequence, it may occur that a drug which inhibits the reuptake of the neurotransmitter released, indirectly increases the neurotransmitter overflow and may erroneously be considered as a releaser. The importance of the problem is indicated by the fact that, even using relatively simple brain preparations, such as homogenates or synaptosomes, the same drug has been proposed to act through uptake inhibition by some authors and as a direct releaser by others (9,26,64,69,90).

An exact discrimination between the two mechanisms of action is important. Although uptake inhibitors and releasers both increase the concentration of the transmitter in the synaptic cleft, they may affect differently some presynaptic events: for example, uptake inhibitors may favor the activation of presynaptic receptors and thus cause inhibition of synthesis and/or of release of the neurotransmitter, whereas releasers may enhance neurotransmitter synthesis (18,21,50,52,72,80).

Drugs affecting DA transport at nerve endings provide a good example of this controversy. It has been recently proposed by de Belleroche and Bradford (26,27) that amphetamine is not a releaser of DA, as it is generally believed, but a pure DA uptake inhibitor, causing indirect release through inhibition of DA reuptake. However, Fig. 1 shows that in striatal synaptosomes, superfused in conditions preventing drug effects on reuptake (63), amphetamine was a strong releaser of the ^{3}H-DA previously taken up by the particles. Figure 2 also shows that the release of the DA synthesized from radioactive tyrosine was strongly stimulated.

Besides being a direct releaser, amphetamine is probably also an uptake inhibitor of DA, as reported by several authors (37,39,64,65,69,78). It is interesting to recall that when synaptosomes from hypothalamus, cerebellum, or pons-medulla prelabeled with ^{3}H-norepinephrine (^{3}H-NE) were superfused in conditions preventing drug effects on reuptake, amphetamine was devoid of releasing activity, suggesting that the drug, generally considered to be both an uptake inhibitor and a direct releaser of NE, affects NE transport essentially through an inhibition of its reuptake (64).

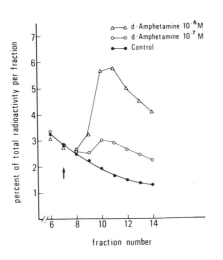

FIG. 1. Effect of D-amphetamine on the release of ^{3}H-DA from striatal synaptosomes. Crude synaptosomal fractions were washed once with 0.32 M sucrose, resuspended in 0.32 M glucose at a protein concentration of about 6–8 mg/ml, diluted 1:10 in Krebs-Ringer medium, and prelabeled with 0.1 μM ^{3}H-DA for 10 min at 37°C. Then 1-ml aliquots of the suspension were placed on Millipore filters laying at the bottom of parallel superfusion chambers, washed with 10 ml of medium, and superfused with glucose-containing oxygenated medium at 37°C, at a rate of about 0.5 ml/min. Fractions were collected every minute. When indicated by the arrow, the superfusion medium was replaced either with identical medium (controls) or with medium containing D-amphetamine. The incubation and superfusion media contained 12.5 μM nialamide and 1 mM ascorbic acid. The radioactivity of each fraction is expressed as percentage of the total radioactivity recovered (total fractions plus filter). Each curve is the average of 3 experiments.

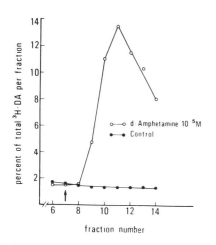

FIG. 2. Effect of D-amphetamine on the release of DA synthesized from ³H-tyrosine. Crude synaptosomal fractions from rat corpus striatum were superfused on Millipore filters with a Krebs-Ringer medium containing 0.5 µM L-[2,3-³H]tyrosine (5.5 µCi/ml) for 10 min at 37°C. After they were washed with 10 ml of standard, tyrosine-free medium, they were superfused and treated with D-amphetamine as described in the legend for Fig. 1 except that no MAO inhibitors were present. Fractions were collected every minute and the radioactivity present as DA was determined in each fraction and in the superfused filter by the method of Smith et al. (77). Average of 2 experiments run in triplicate are presented.

Recently Baumann and Maitre (9) challenged the existence of DA uptake inhibitors and proposed that drugs such as benztropine and nomifensine, which are thought to inhibit DA uptake (43,44), are in fact pure DA releasers. According to the authors, the inhibition of DA uptake, observed with benztropine or nomifensine *in vitro,* results from stimulation of the release of the radioactive DA just taken up. Baumann and Maitre based their conclusion on the observation that the inhibitory activity of these drugs on ³H-DA uptake by striatal homogenates was accompanied by a proportional depletion of the total DA content. However, they did not determine with direct experiments whether or not the drugs tested could release the ³H-DA taken up by the nerve endings. Figure 3 shows that in superfusion conditions, nomifensine (up to 10^{-5} M) was unable to stimulate the release of the ³H-DA previously taken up by striatal synaptosomes. Similar results were obtained when the release of DA was studied in striatal synaptosomes preincubated with radioactive tyrosine: nomifensine (10^{-5} M) did not alter the spontaneous

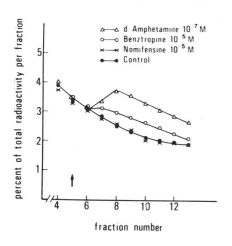

FIG. 3. Effects of amphetamine, benztropine, and nomifensine on ³H-DA release from striatal synaptosomes. Experimental details as in the legend for Fig. 1. Each curve is the average of 2–4 duplicate experiments.

release of the radioactive amine (*unpublished observations*). Benztropine had a modest stimulatory activity on the release of the ^{3}H-DA taken up only at high concentration (10^{-5} M). Our results indicate that the releasing activity can not account for uptake inhibition. It should also be noted that amphetamine, which was a good releaser of ^{3}H-DA even at 10^{-7} M (Fig. 3), is a weaker uptake inhibitor than either nomifensine or benztropine (44,46).

The depletion of DA observed by Baumann and Maitre with nomifensine and benztropine could be due to some factors not considered by the authors. In the preparation used by Baumann and Maitre (crude homogenate), a large amount of DA (exceeding that contained in synaptosomes) is present in the extracellular fluid (60). This free amine is likely to be accumulated by the synaptosomes during incubation, but its uptake will be prevented when uptake inhibitors are present. Similarly, the reuptake of the spontaneously released DA will be prevented by DA uptake inhibitors. It is difficult to establish which of these factors is quantitatively more important; however, both of them may contribute to the depletion observed by Baumann and Maitre in drug-treated synaptosomes, as compared to incubated controls.

In conclusion, the problem of discriminating between true releasers and reuptake inhibitors of a given transmitter is better approached utilizing synaptosomes superfused in conditions in which the process of release can be "separated" from that of reuptake, and any effect of the drug under study on neurotransmitter reuptake can be minimized. A drug which does not exhibit any releasing activity in these conditions can be considered as a pure uptake inhibitor, if active in uptake inhibition tests. However, if a drug exhibits a strong releasing activity, its potency as an uptake inhibitor may be overestimated in uptake inhibition tests, since uptake inhibition could be partly accounted for by the concomitant release of the neurotransmitter just taken up.

EFFECTS OF PHENYLETHYLAMINES ON DOPAMINE UPTAKE AND RELEASE

Besides the well-known "major" biogenic amines (NE, DA, and 5-HT), the brain contains as normal constituents several phenylethylamine derivatives (octopamine, β-phenylethylamine, phenylethanolamine, p-tyramine, etc.) which have gained increasing interest in recent years (2,3,16,17,31,65, 73,88). These amines, normally present at concentrations much lower than those of NE, DA, or 5-HT, are metabolically related to the major biogenic amines; their concentration has been reported to increase in some pathological conditions and under the effect of some drugs. As far as the function of the "trace" amines is concerned, they have been hypothesized to be either true neurotransmitters or co-transmitters (together with a major amine) or modulators of the neurotransmission mediated by catecholamines and serotonin (2,3,16,31,73).

Since the trace amines are structurally related to the major biogenic amines, the possibility exists that they modulate (in physiological conditions) or unbalance (in pathological conditions) the aminergic transmission by interfering with the transport systems of catecholamines and serotonin. Phenylethylamines are generally inhibitors of the uptake and stimulators of the release of catecholamines and serotonin in central nerve endings (4–6, 33,37,42,45,55,64,65,89). The potencies of the different compounds as uptake inhibitors or release stimulators of a given biogenic amine vary considerably depending on the substituents present in the phenylethylamine structure.

Table 1 summarizes the effects of various phenylethylamines (including some synthetic compounds) on the uptake and release of ^{3}H-DA in rat striatal synaptosomes. The good correlation between the rank of potency of the compounds examined as uptake inhibitors and as release stimulators may suggest that part of the uptake inhibition originates from the concomitant release of the radioactive amine just taken up. Such a possibility was considered by Heikkila et al. (39) in the case of ^{3}H-DA uptake inhibition by amphetamine in striatal slices.

The data reported in Table 1 indicate that the potency toward uptake inhibition and release stimulation was increased by the presence of phenolic hydroxyl groups in the phenylethylamine molecule, in keeping with the results obtained by Horn (42) in uptake inhibition studies.

The presence of a β-hydroxyl group dramatically decreased the ability to stimulate the release or to inhibit the uptake of ^{3}H-DA (compare phenyl-

TABLE 1. *Relative potencies of phenylethylamines as releasers and as uptake inhibitors of catecholamines and serotonin in rat striatal synaptosomes*

Compound tested	p	m	β	α	Release stimulation Release rate[a]	Uptake inhibition $IC_{50}(10^{-7}$ M)	Relative potency
Dopamine	OH	OH	H	H	12.8	6.1	7.4
m-Tyramine	H	OH	H	H	8.0	18	2.6
L-Norepinephrine	OH	OH	OH	H	6.8	19	2.3
p-Tyramine	OH	H	H	H	6.5	25	1.8
D-Amphetamine	H	H	H	CH_3	6.0	23	2.0
p-OH-D-Amphetamine	OH	H	H	CH_3	5.7	32	1.4
β-Phenylethylamine	H	H	H	H	2.2	45	1.0
D,L-Octopamine	OH	H	OH	H	2.1	157	0.3
p-Cl-Phenylethylamine	Cl	H	H	H	0.5	165	0.3
D,L-Phenylethanolamine	H	H	OH	H	0.2	729	0.06

[a] The release rates (percent radioactivity released per min) were calculated from the data of Fig. 2 of ref. 65. The concentration of the releasing agents was 5×10^{-7} M. IC_{50} = concentration giving 50% inhibition of 0.1 μM ^{3}H-dopamine uptake (the drugs were added simultaneously with the radioactive amine for 5 min). Relative potencies were calculated as reciprocals of the IC_{50} values, giving the value of 1 to β-phenylethylamine. Data from refs. 65 and 68.

ethanolamine with β-phenylethylamine, octopamine with p-tyramine, and NE with DA).

The introduction of a chloro-group in the *para* position of the phenyl ring led to a decrease in potency toward both uptake inhibition and release.

On the contrary, phenylethylamines with an α-methyl group were generally stronger uptake inhibitors and release stimulators of ³H-DA than the corresponding nonmethylated compounds. It was previously found that in the case of noradrenergic nerve endings, α-methylation strikingly reduced the releasing activity toward ³H-NE in hypothalamic synaptosomes, D-amphetamine being inactive and p-OH-D-amphetamine showing only a very modest activity (64,65,69).

The release of DA elicited by phenylethylamines is the final result of a complex series of events which may differ among the various compounds, depending on their physicochemical properties (for a more extensive discussion see ref. 68). That the phenylethylamines must enter into nerve endings in order to cause DA release is demonstrated by the fact that when the entry is blocked, the releasing activity is inhibited. Figure 4 shows that the stimulation of ³H-DA release induced by several phenylethylamines in striatal synaptosomes was abolished or strongly inhibited when the DA carrier blocker nomifensine (44,74) was present together with the releasing amine in the superfusion fluid.

It would thus appear that nomifensine prevents the releasing effect of phenylethylamines because it precludes their entry into nerve endings through

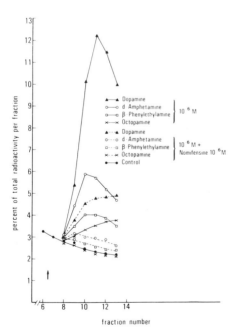

FIG. 4. Effect of nomifensine on the release of ³H-DA induced by different phenylethylamines. The effect of nomifensine was tested by adding the drug together with DA, D-amphetamine, β-phenylethylamine, or octopamine to the superfusion fluid (*arrow*). Other experimental details as in the legend for Fig. 1. Each curve is the average of 1–4 experiments run in triplicate.

the membrane carrier. However, it was reported that nonphenolic phenyl-ethylamines are poor substrates for the NE carrier and can enter noradrenergic nerve terminals by passive diffusion (71). It is likely that phenylethyl-amines lacking phenolic hydroxyl groups, such as β-phenylethylamine and D-amphetamine, enter more easily by diffusion than by the carrier also into dopaminergic nerve endings. In this case, the data of Figure 4 could be interpreted as inhibition by nomifensine of a carrier-mediated efflux of the ^{3}H-DA displaced from its storage sites by the nonphenolic phenylethylamines. Another consequence of this reasoning is that, in normal conditions, the DA released by phenylethylamines exits from nerve endings by a carrier-mediated process. A similar conclusion had been previously reached in the case of NE release (66).

As mentioned above, the trace amines are normal brain constituents and their concentration can increase under various conditions affecting their metabolic pathways. The fact that catecholamine carrier blockers were able to inhibit the phenylethylamine-induced release of DA and NE raises the possibility that the carrier-mediated release of the major biogenic amines, which may be stimulated by the endogenous trace amines (both in physiological and in pathological conditions), represents an as yet unexplored target of the action of those neuroactive drugs whose effects are generally attributed only to their ability to inhibit amine reuptake.

RELEASE INDUCED BY ALTERATIONS OF THE SODIUM GRADIENT

Release Induced by a Decrease of Extracellular Sodium

Figures 5 and 6 show that when striatal synaptosomes prelabeled with ^{3}H-DA were superfused with media containing decreasing [Na^+], ^{3}H-DA release increased proportionally with the decrease of the [Na^+]. The fact that the stimulation of DA release by Na^+ deprivation was obtained in superfusion conditions, preventing the reuptake of the spontaneously released amine (63), excludes that the inhibition of the Na^+-dependent reuptake plays a major role in determining the effect observed. Since the carrier-mediated uptake of biogenic amines depends on the inward Na^+ gradient across the nerve ending membrane (15,41,45), the stimulation of ^{3}H-DA release observed with decreasing extracellular [Na^+] may be due to the inversion of the Na^+ gradient, which would favor a carrier-mediated outward transport of DA. If this were the case, a blocker of the DA carrier should inhibit the release induced by low Na^+. In keeping with this expectation, nomifensine almost abolished the release of ^{3}H-DA elicited by the absence of Na^+ (Figure 6). It had been previously reported that desipramine strongly inhibited the release of radioactive NE evoked by an Na^+-free medium in heart preparations (12,57) and in hypothalamic synaptosomes (66), both from normal animals

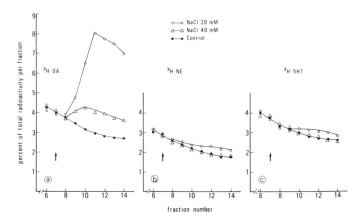

FIG. 5. Effect of decreasing the concentration of external Na$^+$ on biogenic amine release. The experiments on ^{3}H-DA and ^{3}H-5-HT were performed on striatal crude synaptosomal preparations, those on ^{3}H-NE on hypothalamic crude synaptosomes. When indicated by the arrows, the superfusion medium containing 128 mM NaCl was substituted with a medium containing 20 or 40 mM NaCl (sucrose replaced the NaCl omitted). Other experimental details as in the legend for Fig. 1. Each curve is the average of 2–4 triplicate experiments.

and from animals reserpinized in the presence of a MAO inhibitor. All these results support the concept that cytoplasmic catecholamines can exit from nerve endings through a carrier having characteristics similar to that operating during uptake.

The DA release system was much more sensitive than those of NE and 5-HT to Na$^+$ deprivation. Figure 5 shows that the release of ^{3}H-NE from hypothalamic synaptosomes or of ^{3}H-5-HT from striatal synaptosomes was

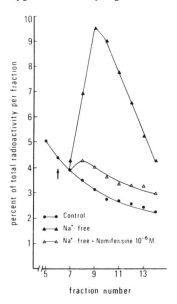

FIG. 6. Effect of nomifensine on the release of ^{3}H-DA from striatal synaptosomes induced by lack of Na$^+$. The effect of nomifensine was tested by adding the drug to a Na$^+$-free medium. Experimental details as in the legend for Fig. 1. Each curve is the average of 2–3 experiments in duplicate.

almost unaffected by a decrease in concentration of NaCl down to 20 mM, whereas ³H-DA release was already substantially increased with a medium containing 40 mM NaCl.

Assuming that the intrasynaptosomal ionic concentrations are the same in the three populations of nerve endings and that the radioactive amines taken up mix homogeneously with the endogenous pools, the fact that the DA outward transport apparently takes place with a $[Na^+]_i/[Na^+]_o$ lower than that required by the noradrenergic and serotoninergic systems may have several explanations. For example: (a) the DA carriers per nerve terminal might be more numerous and/or have higher mobility than either the NE or the 5-HT carriers; (b) DA might be or become relatively more available in the cytoplasm than NE or 5-HT. Whatever the explanation, our results seem to indicate that the three aminergic systems examined have a different sensitivity to the Na⁺ gradient across the nerve ending membrane and that dopaminergic nerve terminals are capable of performing outward transport in the presence of a relatively low Na⁺ gradient.

Release Induced by Ouabain

The Na⁺ gradient across the synaptosomal membrane can be lowered not only by reducing the extracellular [Na⁺], but also by increasing the intracellular concentration of this ion. Ouabain or lack of K⁺ was reported to increase intrasynaptosomal [Na⁺] through an inhibition of the Na⁺-K⁺-ATPase (1,15,84).

Figure 7 shows that ouabain stimulated ³H-DA release from superfused striatal synaptosomes. The stimulatory effect of ouabain was almost entirely blocked by nomifensine, suggesting the involvement of the DA carrier. Interestingly, the release of ³H-NE from superfused hypothalamic synaptosomes was almost unaffected by the same concentration (10⁻⁴ M) of ouabain (54), in keeping with the idea that noradrenergic nerve terminals require relatively large changes in the Na⁺ gradient to allow carrier-mediated release.

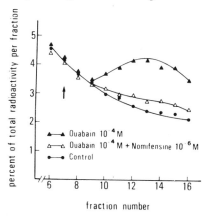

FIG. 7. Effect of nomifensine on the release of ³H-DA induced by ouabain from striatal synaptosomes. The effect of nomifensine was tested by adding the drug together with ouabain to the superfusion fluid (*arrow*). Experimental details as in the legend for Fig. 1. Each curve is the average of 4 duplicate experiments.

As shown in the section on calcium-dependent release, the stimulation of DA release induced by veratridine was only modestly affected by nomifensine. Evidently, an increase of intracellular [Na$^+$] is not sufficient to trigger a carrier-mediated release. The rate of increase of intrasynaptosomal [Na$^+$] and the availability of the amine in the cytoplasm are probably important factors in determining the mechanism by which the amine exits through the plasma membrane. The sudden increase of intracellular [Na$^+$] caused by veratridine (85) may not stimulate a carrier-mediated release because, in normal conditions, the amine free in the cytoplasm is very little and because the influx of Ca^{2+} accompanying the veratridine-induced depolarization (13) triggers the release of DA directly from vesicles into the extracellular space, possibly by exocytosis. In keeping with this hypothesis is the finding that veratridine could elicit a Ca^{2+}-*independent* carrier-mediated release of ^{3}H-NE from reserpinized atria, prelabeled in the presence of an MAO inhibitor, i.e., in conditions in which the cytoplasmic concentration of the amine was increased (58). On the other hand, the increase of internal [Na$^+$] indirectly caused by ouabain is probably less rapid than that caused by veratridine. Moreover, vesicular DA may be shifted toward the cytoplasm during ouabain treatment because the binding of DA to striatal synaptic vesicles seems to be inhibited by high [Na$^+$] (61). Thus, the parallel increase of intracellular [Na$^+$] and of cytoplasmic DA could explain the nomifensine-sensitive release of ^{3}H-DA evoked by ouabain (Fig. 7).

CALCIUM-DEPENDENT RELEASE

It is known that the depolarization-induced release of neurotransmitters from central nerve endings is Ca^{2+} dependent (7,8,13,22,51). The critical event triggering transmitter release seems to be an increased availability of intraterminal [Ca^{2+}] (13,20,22,25,40).

Comparative data on the Ca^{2+} dependence of the release of aminergic transmitters in synaptosomes are lacking. Figure 8 summarizes the results obtained when hypothalamic synaptosomes, prelabeled with ^{3}H-NE, and striatal synaptosomes, prelabeled either with ^{3}H-DA or with ^{3}H-5-HT, were simultaneously stimulated with 56 mM KCl, in the presence or in the absence of Ca^{2+}. All three amines showed a Ca^{2+}-dependent release. However, although the Ca^{2+} dependence of NE and 5-HT release was complete for the entire duration of the stimulus, in the case of DA a relatively slow Ca^{2+}-independent component was detectable. The nature of this component, which was present also when the Ca^{2+}-free medium contained EDTA, will be discussed elsewhere (Raiteri et al., *in preparation*).

A comparison of the effects of the Ca^{2+} ionophore A23187 on biogenic amine release showed that a low concentration of A23187 (5.10^{-7} M) elicited a substantial release of ^{3}H-DA, but did not affect significantly the release of the other two amines (Raiteri et al., *in preparation*). These results

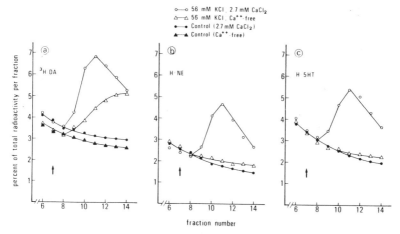

FIG. 8. Calcium dependence of ^{3}H-biogenic amines release from synaptosomes depolarized with 56 mM KCl. Striatal synaptosomes (prelabeled with 0.1 μM ^{3}H-DA or ^{3}H-5-HT) or hypothalamic synaptosomes (prelabeled with 0.1 μM ^{3}H-NE) were treated (*arrow*) during superfusion with a medium containing 56 mM KCl (substituting an equimolar concentration of NaCl). The whole superfusion was carried out with media lacking CaCl$_2$ in the experiments marked as Ca^{2+}-free. Other experimental details as in the legend for Fig. 1. Each curve is the average of 2 triplicate experiments (b and c) or of 5 triplicate experiments (a).

suggest that the concentration of Ca^{2+} necessary to trigger DA release may be much lower than that required for NE or 5-HT.

So that more quantitative information on the Ca^{2+} dependence of DA release could be obtained, striatal synaptosomes prelabeled with ^{3}H-DA were stimulated with 56 mM KCl in the presence of decreasing [Ca^{2+}] (Fig. 9). The stimulation of release was only modestly decreased when the extracellular [Ca^{2+}] was lowered from 2.7 mM down to 0.2 mM. In contrast, the K$^+$-induced

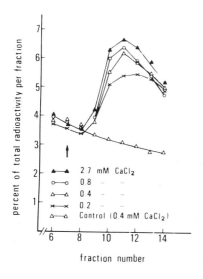

FIG. 9. Influence of external Ca^{2+} concentration on ^{3}H-DA release from striatal synaptosomes depolarized with 56 mM KCl. Synaptosomes prelabeled with 0.1 μM ^{3}H-DA were treated (*arrow*) during superfusion with media containing 56 mM KCl and various concentrations of Ca^{2+}. Other experimental details as in the legend for Fig. 1. Each curve is the average of 2–4 triplicate experiments.

release of ^{3}H-NE was 90% decreased under comparable conditions of Ca^{2+} deprivation (22).

The data presented above, showing that the stimulus-coupled release of DA can take place even in the presence of very low $[Ca^{2+}]$, raise the possibility that dopaminergic nerve terminals may be less responsive to drugs such as barbiturates or diphenylhydantoin, which were reported to depress Ca^{2+} influx into depolarized nerve endings and to inhibit the high K^+-induced release of GABA and NE (14,24,38,62,79).

As far as the mechanism involved in the Ca^{2+}-dependent release of biogenic amines in the CNS, some evidence supporting the existence of an exocytotic-like release has been recently obtained. For example, synaptosomes depolarized in the presence of Ca^{2+} were found to release biogenic amines largely unmetabolized (51,56,70).

In order to ascertain whether the released amines could exit from the plasma membrane independently of the carrier, we analyzed the Ca^{2+}-dependent release of NE and DA after blocking the amine carriers with specific drugs. In these conditions, the release of ^{3}H-DA elicited by high K^+, veratridine, or the ionophore A23187 remained largely unchanged in nomifensine-treated synaptosomes (Fig. 10). Analogous results had been obtained with NE (66).

Evidence in favor of an exocytotic release in central nerve endings has been provided also by morphological studies (32).

One important aspect of the depolarization-induced release of biogenic amines concerns the identification of the intrasynaptosomal pool(s) susceptible to the releasing stimuli. In the case of NE and DA, evidence has been

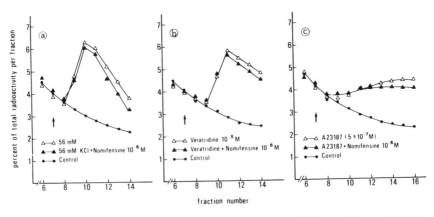

FIG. 10. Effect of nomifensine on the release of ^{3}H-DA induced by high K^+, veratridine, or A23187 from striatal synaptosomes. Synaptosomes prelabeled with 0.1 μM ^{3}H-DA were treated (*arrow*), after superfusion with standard medium, with media containing 56 mM KCl (a), 10^{-5} M veratridine (b), or 5.10^{-7} M A23187 (c), both in the presence and in the absence of nomifensine. Other experimental details as in the legend for Fig. 1. The curves presented are the average of 8 duplicate experiments (a and b) or of 4 triplicate experiments (c).

provided that the most recently synthesized amine is preferentially released by depolarizing agents, both *in vivo* and *in vitro* (10,11,49,75).

In apparent contrast with these data, de Belleroche et al. (27) reported recently that electrical stimulation or high K^+ was incapable of eliciting the release of ^{14}C-DA from striatal synaptosomes previously incubated with radioactive tyrosine or DOPA. The depolarizing stimuli could only evoke the release of unlabeled DA. In order to explain the unexpected result, the authors hypothesized that the depolarizing stimuli affect a small DA pool at rapid turnover which can be replaced only by newly formed unlabeled DA, but not by the radioactive DA stored in the synaptosomes. In contrast with the findings of de Belleroche et al., we found that high K^+ could release radioactive DA from superfused synaptosomes previously incubated with tritiated DOPA or tyrosine (not shown). In order to rule out the possibility that the release observed was due to recently synthesized ^3H-DA spontaneously released and taken up again during incubation (in this case it would behave as exogenous DA), we treated the synaptosomes with the radiolabeled precursors in superfusion conditions preventing the reuptake of the spontaneously released "newly" formed ^3H-DA. Also in these conditions 56 mM KCl stimulated the release of the radioactive amine (Fig. 11).

The DA present in nerve terminals in physiological conditions originates

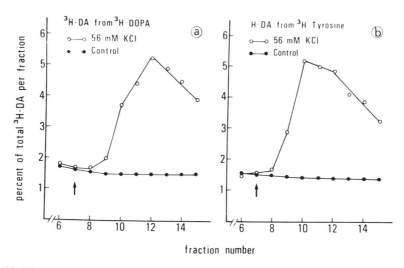

FIG. 11. Effect of high K^+ on the release of DA synthesized from radioactive DOPA or tyrosine. Crude synaptosomal fractions from rat corpus striatum were superfused on Millipore filters with a Krebs-Ringer medium containing 0.5 μM L-3,4-dihydroxy(ring 2,5,6 ^3H)phenylalanine (5.5 μCi/ml) (a) or 0.5 μM L-[2,3-^3H] tyrosine (5.5 μCi/ml) (b) for 10 min at 37°C. After being washed with 10 ml of standard medium they were superfused with the same medium and then treated (*arrows*) with a medium containing 56 mM KCl. The 1-min fractions were collected into a protective solution containing 1% ascorbic acid, 1.5% EDTA, and 0.001% DA (10), and the radioactivity present as DA was determined in each fraction and in the superfused filters by the method of Smith et al. (77). Other experimental details as in the legend for Fig. 1 except that no MAO inhibitors were present throughout the experiment. Each curve is the average of 4 experiments run in triplicate.

not only from synthesis, but also from reuptake of the amine released. The problem of the compartmentation and of the functional significance of the amine taken up is therefore of interest. Since depolarizing stimuli are effective toward the DA taken up by nerve endings, it can be reasonably assumed that newly synthesized and newly taken up amine can occupy the same intra-synaptosomal pool.

PRESYNAPTIC CONTROL OF DOPAMINE RELEASE

It is now well accepted that the release of NE from peripheral noradrenergic nerve endings is modulated by a negative feedback mechanism localized presynaptically and involving α-receptors (36,52,80,82). Some studies performed with brain slices seem to suggest the existence of a similar mechanism also in the CNS (28,30,81).

According to several authors, presynaptic autoregulatory systems would operate also toward the release of acetylcholine (35) and of other biogenic amines, including DA (18,21,30,47,72,87). Moreover, evidence has been provided for the involvement of presynaptic receptors of cholinergic nature in the control of NE or DA release from central nerve endings (34,86). In conclusion, there seems to be a tendency to consider presynaptic feedback inhibition as a general mechanism for the control of the release of aminergic neurotransmitters. However, substantial differences seem to exist among the various systems, so that the evidence in favor of a unitary mechanism for the modulation of amine release is far from conclusive.

First of all, it should be noted that the studies on the DA system support the existence of a presynaptic control of the *synthesis* of the amine (19,47, 48,72,87). As far as DA release, if an autoregulatory mechanism similar to that of NE existed, one would expect dopaminergic agonists, like apomorphine, to decrease the stimulus-evoked release; on the contrary, neuroleptics should antagonize apomorphine and, by themselves, increase DA release. We have summarized in Table 2 the data of the literature on the effects of apomorphine and of some neuroleptics on the stimulus-evoked release of ^{3}H-DA from striatal preparations. The inhibitory effect of apomorphine found by Farnebo and Hamberger (30) was fairly weak; moreover, it could not be confirmed by other authors, under identical or different experimental conditions (7,29). The data concerning neuroleptics are very contradictory. Also in this case, the results obtained by Farnebo and Hamberger (30) with chlorpromazine could not be reproduced by Dismukes and Mulder (29). Under somewhat different experimental conditions, Seeman and Lee (76) found neuroleptics to inhibit rather than increase DA release, and this result was confirmed by other authors, both in striatal slices (29) and in synaptosomes (47). The existence of a diphasic effect (inhibition at low and activation at high concentrations, or vice versa) can hardly be accepted on the basis of the data of Table 2. Paradoxically, apomorphine, which should in-

TABLE 2. *Effect of apomorphine and neuroleptics on the stimulus-coupled release of dopamine in the rat corpus striatum*

Drug	Concentration (μM)	Tissue preparation	Type of stimulus	^{3}H-DA release % change	Reference
Apomorphine	1	Slices	Electrical	−20	30
	10	"	"	−10	30
	1	"	Same as Seeman & Lee (76)	0	29
	10	"	Same as Farnebo & Hamberger (30)	0	29
	0.01–1	"	Electrical	0	7
Chlorpromazine	1	Slices	Electrical	+35	30
	0.7	"	"	−50	76
	0.1–2	"	Same as Farnebo & Hamberger (30) and Seeman & Lee (76)	0	29
	0.1	"	Electrical	−32	59
	0.	"	Not specified	+60	7
	10	"	" "	strong inhib.	7
	0.9	Synaptosomes	Protoveratrine	−50	47
Haloperidol	0.1	Slices	Electrical	−50	76
	0.1	"	"	−22	59
	10	"	"	+53	59
	1	"	Same as Seeman & Lee (76)	−35	29
	10	"	Electrical	−67	29
Fluphenazine	0.05	Slices	Electrical	−50	76
	0.1	"	Same as Seeman & Lee (76)	0	29
	1	"	Electrical	−24	29

hibit DA release, had little or no effect, whereas neuroleptics, which should stimulate DA release, were in most cases inhibitory. The expected antagonism between apomorphine and neuroleptics toward the stimulus-coupled DA release was either not found or not investigated (29,30,47).

We have attempted to gain information on the presynaptic control of DA release with superfused synaptosomes. This experimental procedure should be particularly suitable for the following reasons: (a) synaptosomes are a relatively pure presynaptic preparation; (b) in superfusion, the transmitter released is rapidly removed and any autoinhibition of release is minimized. Therefore, presynaptic receptors are completely available to agonists (which should decrease the stimulus-evoked release) or antagonists (which should *not* stimulate the release because the system is already disinhibited).

The validity of the procedure seems supported by experiments on the presynaptic control of NE release in hypothalamic synaptosomes. In these experiments, exogenous NE (in the presence of desipramine to prevent its uptake) inhibited ^{3}H-NE release elicited by 24 mм KCl. Phentolamine had no effect by itself and antagonized the inhibitory effect of exogenous NE (*unpublished results*).

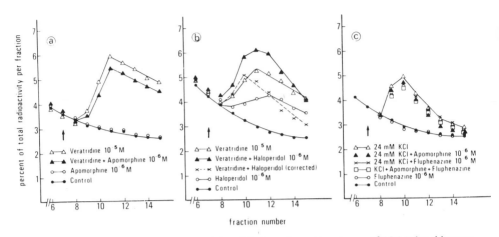

FIG. 12. Effect of apomorphine, haloperidol, and fluphenazine on the release of ³H-DA induced by veratridine or high K⁺ in striatal synaptosomes. Synaptosomes prelabeled with 0.1 μM ³H-DA were superfused with standard medium and then treated (arrows) either with standard medium (controls) or with new media as indicated in the figure. a: The curves presented are the average of 3 experiments run in triplicate. b; The dashed curve was obtained by subtracting the release induced by haloperidol in standard medium from that elicited by haloperidol in veratridine-containing medium. Each curve is the average of 2 triplicate experiments. c: Each curve is the average of 3 experiments run in triplicate. Other experimental details as in the legend for Fig. 1.

In the case of DA, in most of the experiments carried out, apomorphine showed an inhibitory activity on the stimulus-coupled release but, in the several experimental conditions tested (stimulation with veratridine, 56 mM or 24 mM KCl, in the presence of various Ca²⁺ concentrations, with or without pretreatment with the drug), the inhibitory effect, present in 7 out of 10 experiments, never exceeded the value of 10% to 20% (see, for example, Fig. 12a). Not even the removal from the superfusion media of ascorbic acid, recently reported to inhibit the interaction between DA and its receptors (83), increased the apomorphine effect. When DA was utilized as an antagonist (in the presence of nomifensine to prevent its uptake), no effect could be detected.

The behavior of neuroleptics was similar to that observed by Dismukes and Mulder (29) with electrically stimulated superfused striatal slices. Haloperidol increased the ³H-DA spontaneous release and decreased the release elicited by veratridine (after correction for the effect on spontaneous release) (Fig. 12b). Fluphenazine (10⁻⁶ M) was devoid of effect on the spontaneous release and had hardly any inhibitory activity on the stimulus-evoked release. In any case, no clear antagonism could be observed between apomorphine and the neuroleptics tested (Fig. 12c). It should be noted that the conditions are far from optimal for detecting an antagonism between the two types of drugs.

In conclusion, although the existence of a direct control of DA release through presynaptic receptors can not be entirely excluded, the data obtained with exogenous DA and, in particular, those concerning neuroleptics militate against a similarity between the noradrenergic and dopaminergic systems. It is possible that DA release is modulated indirectly through the presynaptic control of the synthesis of the neurotransmitter.

SUMMARY

The following conclusions can be drawn from the results presented:

1. The superfusion method used allows one to determine whether or not a drug is a direct releaser of DA or a reuptake inhibitor. We could demonstrate that amphetamine and high K^+ release "newly taken up" and "newly synthesized" DA from striatal synaptosomes. Moreover, the existence of pure DA uptake inhibitors, recently challenged by some authors (9), has been confirmed.

2. The potency of several phenylethylamine derivatives as uptake inhibitors or as release stimulators of DA was found to vary profoundly, depending on the structural modifications. A good parallelism was found between changes in releasing activity and uptake inhibition potency. For example, the introduction of phenolic hydroxyl or α-methyl groups enhanced, whereas β-hydroxylation and p-chloro-substitution decreased both activities. The release of DA induced by phenylethylamines was prevented by the DA carrier blocker nomifensine, suggesting that the released DA exited from synaptosomes through the membrane carrier.

3. Alterations of the Na^+ gradient across the synaptosomal membrane, induced by omission of extracellular Na^+ or by ouabain, enhanced the carrier-mediated nomifensine-sensitive release of DA. The other aminergic systems (NE and 5-HT) were much less sensitive to changes in the Na^+ gradient.

4. Depolarization of synaptosomes by high K^+ triggered the release of both "newly taken up" and "newly synthesized" DA. This release was largely Ca^{2+} dependent, but a relatively slow Ca^{2+}-independent component was clearly apparent. The depolarization-induced release of NE and 5-HT was totally dependent on the presence of Ca^{2+} in the extracellular fluid. A substantial release of DA was elicited by concentrations of the ionophore A23187 or of Ca^{2+} (in depolarized synaptosomes) at which the release of NE and 5-HT was unaffected. The Ca^{2+}-dependent release of DA (induced by high K^+, veratridine, or A23187) was not affected by a carrier blockade and may occur by an exocytotic-like process.

5. The effects of apomorphine and neuroleptics on the stimulus-coupled release of DA do not support the existence of a presynaptic receptor-mediated inhibitory control of DA release similar to that described for NE.

ACKNOWLEDGMENTS

The authors wish to thank Miss Gianna Casazza for collaboration. The investigation was partly supported by Research Grant No. CT76.01555.04

from the Italian National Research Council and by Grant No. 922 from the North Atlantic Treaty Organization.

REFERENCES

1. Archibald, J. T., and White, T. D. (1974): Rapid reversal of internal Na$^+$ and K$^+$ contents of synaptosomes by ouabain. *Nature,* 252:595–596.
2. Axelrod, J., and Saavedra, J. M. (1974): Octopamine, phenylethanolamine, phenylethylamine and tryptamine in the brain. *Ciba Found. Symp.,* 22:51–59.
3. Axelrod, J., and Saavedra, J. M. (1977): Octopamine. *Nature,* 265:501–504.
4. Azzaro, A. J., and Rutledge, C. O. (1973): Selectivity of release of norepinephrine, dopamine and 5-hydroxytryptamine by amphetamine in various regions of rat brain. *Biochem. Pharmacol.,* 22:2801–2813.
5. Baker, G. B., Raiteri, M., Bertollini, A., del Carmine, R., Keane, P. E., and Martin, I. L. (1976): Interaction of 2-phenylethylamine with dopamine and noradrenaline in the central nervous system of the rat. *J. Pharm. Pharmacol.,* 28:456–458.
6. Baldessarini, R. J. (1971): Compounds antagonistic to norepinephrine retention by rat brain homogenates. *Biochem. Pharmacol.,* 20:1769–1780.
7. Baldessarini, R. J. (1975): Release of catecholamines. In: *Biochemistry of Biogenic Amines, Vol. 3, Handbook of Psychopharmacology,* edited by L. L. Iversen, S. D. Iversen, and S. H. Snyder, pp. 37–137. Plenum Press, New York.
8. Baldessarini, R. J., and Kopin, I. J. (1967): Tritiated norepinephrine: Release from brain slices by electrical stimulation. *Science,* 152:1630–1631.
9. Baumann, P. A., and Maitre, L. (1976): Is drug inhibition of dopamine uptake a misinterpretation of *in vitro* experiments? *Nature,* 264:789–790.
10. Besson, M. J., Cheramy, A., Feltz, P., and Glowinski, J. (1969): Release of newly synthesized dopamine from dopamine-containing terminals in the striatum of the rat. *Proc. Natl. Acad. Sci. U.S.A.,* 62:741–748.
11. Besson, M. J., Cheramy, A., Feltz, P., and Glowinski, J. (1971): Dopamine: Spontaneous and drug-induced release from the caudate nucleus in the cat. *Brain Res.,* 32:407–424.
12. Blaszkowski, T. P., and Bogdanski, D. F. (1972): Evidence for sodium-dependent outward transport of the ^{3}H-norepinephrine mobilized by calcium at the adrenergic synapse. Inhibition of transport by desipramine. *Life Sci.,* 11:867–876.
13. Blaustein, M. P. (1975): Effects of potassium, veratridine and scorpion venom on calcium accumulation and transmitter release by nerve terminals *in vitro. J. Physiol.,* 247:617–655.
14. Blaustein, M. P., and Hector, C. A. (1975): Barbiturate inhibition of calcium uptake by depolarized nerve terminals *in vitro. Mol. Pharmacol.,* 11:369–378.
15. Bogdanski, D. F., Blaszkowski, T. P., and Tissari, A. H. (1970): Mechanisms of biogenic amine transport and storage. IV. Relationship between K$^+$ and the Na$^+$ requirement for transport and storage of 5-hydroxytryptamine and norepinephrine in synaptosomes. *Biochim. Biophys. Acta,* 211:521–532.
16. Boulton, A. A. (1974): Amines and theories in psychiatry. *Lancet,* II:52–53.
17. Boulton, A. A., and Baker, G. B. (1975): The subcellular distribution of β-phenylethylamine, p-tyramine and tryptamine in rat brain. *J. Neurochem.,* 25:477–481.
18. Carlsson, A., Kehr, W., Lindqvist, M., Magnusson, T., and Atack, C. V. (1972): Regulation of monoamine metabolism in the central nervous system. *Pharmacol. Rev.,* 24:371–384.
19. Christiansen, J., and Squires, R. F. (1974): Antagonistic effects of apomorphine and haloperidol on rat striatal synaptosomal tyrosine hydroxylase. *J. Pharm. Pharmacol.,* 26:367–369.
20. Colburn, R. W., Thoa, N. B., and Kopin, I. J. (1976): Influence of ionophores which bind calcium on the release of norepinephrine from synaptosomes. *Life Sci.,* 17:1395–1400.
21. Costa, E., and Trabucchi, M. (1975): Regulation of brain dopamine turnover rate:

pharmacological implications. In: *Catecholamines and Behavior*, edited by A. J. Friedhoff, pp. 201–227. Plenum Press, New York.

22. Cotman, C. W., Haycock, J. W., and White, W. F. (1976): Stimulus-secretion coupling processes in brain: Analysis of noradrenaline and gamma-aminobutyric acid release. *J. Physiol.*, 254:475–505.

23. Coyle, J. T., and Snyder, S. H. (1969): Catecholamine uptake by synaptosomes in homogenates of rat brain: Stereospecificity in different areas. *J. Pharmacol. Exp. Ther.*, 170:221–231.

24. Cutler, R. W. P., and Dudzinski, D. S. (1974): Effect of pentobarbital on uptake and release of ^{3}H-GABA and ^{14}C-glutamate by brain slices. *Brain Res.*, 67:546–548.

25. De Belleroche, J. S., and Bradford, H. F. (1973): The synaptosome: An isolated, working, neuronal compartment. *Prog. Neurobiol.*, 1:275–298.

26. De Belleroche, J. S., and Bradford, H. F. (1976): Transport of amino acids and catecholamines in relation to metabolism and transmission. *Transport phenomena in the nervous system. Physiological and pathological aspects. Adv. Exp. Med. Biol.*, 69:395–404.

27. De Belleroche, J. S., Bradford, H. F., and Jones, D. G. (1976): A study of the metabolism and release of dopamine and amino acids from nerve endings isolated from sheep corpus striatum. *J. Neurochem.*, 26:561–571.

28. Dismukes, R. K., and Mulder, A. H. (1976): Cyclic AMP and α-receptor-mediated modulation of noradrenaline release from rat brain slices. *Eur. J. Pharmacol.*, 39: 383–388.

29. Dismukes, R. K., and Mulder, A. H. (1977): Effects of neuroleptics on release of ^{3}H-dopamine from slices of rat corpus striatum. *Naunyn-Schmiedeberg's Arch. Pharmacol.*, 297:23–29.

30. Farnebo, L. O., and Hamberger, B. (1971): Drug-induced changes in the release of ^{3}H-amines from field-stimulated rat brain slices. *Acta Physiol. Scand. [Suppl.]*, 371: 35–44.

31. Fisher, J. E., and Baldessarini, R. J. (1971): False neurotransmitters and hepatic failure. *Lancet*, II:75.

32. Fried, R. C., and Blaustein, M. P. (1976): Synaptic vesicles recycling in synaptosomes *in vitro. Nature*, 261:255–256.

33. Fuller, R. W., and Molloy, B. B. (1974): Recent studies with 4-chloroamphetamine and some analogues. *Adv. Biochem. Psychopharmacol.*, 10:195–203.

34. Giorguieff, M. F., Le Floc'h, M. L., Glowinski, J., and Besson, M. J. (1977): Involvement of cholinergic presynaptic receptors of nicotinic and muscarinic types in the control of the spontaneous release of dopamine from striatal dopaminergic terminals in the rat. *J. Pharmacol. Exp. Ther.*, 200:535–544.

35. Hadhazy, P., and Szerb, J. C. (1977): The effect of cholinergic drugs on ^{3}H-acetylcholine release from slices of rat hippocampus, striatum and cortex. *Brain Res.*, 123:311–322.

36. Häggendal, J. (1970): Some further aspects on the release of the adrenergic transmitter. In: *New Aspects of Storage and Release Mechanisms of Catecholamines, Bayer-Symposium II*, edited by H. J. Schumann and G. Kroneberg, pp. 100–109. Springer-Verlag, Berlin.

37. Harris, J. E., and Baldessarini, R. J. (1973): Uptake of ^{3}H-catecholamines by homogenates of rat corpus striatum and cerebral cortex: Effects of amphetamine analogues. *Neuropharmacology*, 12:669–679.

38. Haycock, J. W., Levy, W. B., and Cotman, C. W. (1977): Pentobarbital depression of stimulus-secretion coupling in brain. Selective inhibition of depolarization-induced calcium-dependent release. *Biochem. Pharmacol.*, 26:159–161.

39. Heikkila, R. E., Orlanski, H., and Cohen, G. (1975): Studies on the distinction between uptake inhibition and release of ^{3}H-dopamine in rat brain tissue slices. *Biochem. Pharmacol.*, 24:847–852.

40. Holz, R. W. (1975): The release of dopamine from synaptosomes from rat striatum by the ionophores X537A and A23187. *Biochim. Biophys. Acta*, 375:138–152.

41. Holz, R. W., and Coyle, J. T. (1974): The effects of various salts, temperature and the alkaloids veratridine and batrachotoxin on the uptake of ^{3}H-dopamine into synaptosomes from rat striatum. *Mol. Pharmacol.*, 10:746–758.

42. Horn, A. S. (1973): Structure-activity relations for the inhibition of catecholamine uptake into synaptosomes from noradrenaline and dopaminergic neurones in rat brain homogenates. *Br. J. Pharmacol.,* 47:332–338.
43. Horn, A. S., Coyle, J. T., and Snyder, S. H. (1971): Catecholamine uptake by synaptosomes from rat brain. Structure-activity relationships of drugs with differential effects on dopamine and norepinephrine neurons. *Mol. Pharmacol.,* 7:66–80.
44. Hunt, P., Kennengiesser, M. H., and Raynaud, J. P. (1974): Nomifensine: A new potent inhibitor of dopamine uptake into synaptosomes from rat brain corpus striatum. *J. Pharm. Pharmacol.,* 26:370–371.
45. Iversen, L. L. (1971): The uptake of biogenic amines. In: *Biogenic Amines and Physiological Membranes in Drug Therapy,* edited by J. Biel and L. G. Abood, pp. 259–327. Marcel Dekker, New York.
46. Iversen, L. L. (1973): Catecholamine uptake processes. *Br. Med. Bull.,* 29:130–135.
47. Iversen, L. L., Rogawski, M. A., and Miller, R. J. (1976): Comparison of the effects of neuroleptic drugs on pre- and post-synaptic dopaminergic mechanisms in the rat striatum. *Mol. Pharmacol.,* 12:251–262.
48. Kerh, W., Carlsson, A., Lindqvist, M., Magnusson, T., and Atack, C. (1972): Evidence for a receptor mediated feedback control of striatal tyrosine hydroxylase activity. *J. Pharm. Pharmacol.,* 24:744–747.
49. Kopin, I. J., Breeze, G. R., Krauss, R., and Weise, V. K. (1968): Selective release of newly synthesized norepinephrine from the cat spleen during sympathetic nerve stimulation. *J. Pharmacol. Exp. Ther.,* 161:271–278.
50. Kuczenski, R. (1975): Effects of catecholamine releasing agents on synaptosomal dopamine biosynthesis: Multiple pools of dopamine or multiple forms of tyrosine hydroxylase? *Neuropharmacology,* 14:1–10.
51. Lane, J. D., and Aprison, M. H. (1977): Calcium-dependent release of endogenous serotonin, dopamine and norepinephrine from nerve endings. *Life Sci.,* 20:665–672.
52. Langer, S. Z. (1974): Presynaptic regulation of catecholamine release. *Biochem. Pharmacol.,* 23:1793–1800.
53. Levi, G., and Raiteri, M. (1974): Exchange of neurotransmitter amino acids at nerve endings can simulate high affinity uptake. *Nature,* 250:735–737.
54. Levi, G., Roberts, P. J., and Raiteri, M. (1976): Release and exchange of neurotransmitters in synaptosomes: Effects of the ionophore A23187 and of ouabain. *Neurochem. Res.,* 1:409–416.
55. Maxwell, R. A., Ferris, R. M., and Burcsu, J. E. (1976): Structural requirements for inhibition of noradrenaline uptake by phenylethylamine derivatives, desipramine, cocaine and other compounds. In: *The Mechanism of Neuronal and Extraneuronal Transport of Catecholamines,* edited by D. M. Paton, pp. 95–153. Raven Press, New York.
56. Mulder, A. H., Van den Berg, W. B., and Stoof, J. C. (1975): Calcium-dependent release of radiolabeled catecholamines and serotonin from rat brain synaptosomes in a superfusion system. *Brain Res.,* 99:419–424.
57. Paton, D. M. (1973): Mechanism of efflux of noradrenaline from adrenergic nerves in rabbit atria. *Br. J. Pharmacol.,* 49:614–627.
58. Paton, D. M. (1976): Effect of veratridine alkaloids on the efflux of extragranular noradrenaline from rabbit atria. *J. Neurochem.,* 27:1271–1272.
59. Perkins, N. A., and Westfall, T. C. (1976): Drug-induced alterations in the field-stimulated release of ^{3}H-dopamine from slices of rat striatum and median eminence. Society for Neuroscience Sixth Annual Meeting, Toronto, Canada. *Neurosci. Abstr.,* 2:717.
60. Philippu, A., and Heyd, W. (1970): Release of dopamine from subcellular particles of the striatum. *Life Sci.,* 9:361–373.
61. Philippu, A., Matthaei, H., and Lentzen, H. (1975): Uptake of dopamine into fractions of pig caudate nucleus homogenates. *Naunyn-Schmiedeberg's Arch. Pharmacol.,* 287:181–190.
62. Pincus, J. H., and Lee, S. H. (1972): Diphenylhydantoin and norepinephrine release. *Neurology (Minneap.),* 22:410.
63. Raiteri, M., Angelini, F., and Levi, G. (1974): A simple apparatus for studying

the release of neurotransmitters from synaptosomes. *Eur. J. Pharmacol.,* 25:411–414.

64. Raiteri, M., Bertollini, A., Angelini, F., and Levi, G. (1975): d-Amphetamine as a releaser or reuptake inhibitor of biogenic amines in synaptosomes. *Eur. J. Pharmacol.,* 34:189–195.

65. Raiteri, M., del Carmine, R., Bertollini, A., and Levi, G. (1977): Effect of sympathomimetic amines on the synaptosomal transport of noradrenaline, dopamine and 5-hydroxytryptamine. *Eur. J. Pharmacol.,* 41:133–143.

66. Raiteri, M., del Carmine, R., Bertollini, A., and Levi, G. (1977): Effect of desmethylimipramine on the release of ³H-norepinephrine induced by various agents in hypothalamic synaptosomes. *Mol. Pharmacol.,* 13:746–758.

67. Raiteri, M., Federico, R., Coletti, A., and Levi, G. (1975): Release and exchange studies relating to the synaptosomal uptake of GABA. *J. Neurochem.,* 24:1243–1250.

68. Raiteri, M., and Levi, G. (1978): Release mechanisms for catecholamines and serotonin in synaptosomes. In: *Reviews in Neuroscience, Vol. 3,* edited by S. Ehrenpreis and I. J. Kopin, pp. 77–130. Raven Press, New York.

69. Raiteri, M., Levi, G., and Federico, R. (1975): d-Amphetamine and the release of ³H-norepinephrine from synaptosomes. *Eur. J. Pharmacol.,* 28:237–240.

70. Raiteri, M., Levi, G., and Federico, R. (1975): Stimulus-coupled release of unmetabolized ³H-norepinephrine from rat brain synaptosomes. *Pharmacol. Res. Commun.,* 7:181–187.

71. Ross, S. B. (1976): Structural requirements for uptake into catecholamine neurons. In: *The Mechanism of Neuronal and Extraneuronal Transport of Catecholamines,* edited by D. M. Paton, pp. 67–93. Raven Press, New York.

72. Roth, R. H., Walters, J. R., and Morgenroth, V. H. (1974): Effects of alteration in impulse flow on transmitter metabolism in central dopaminergic neurons. In: *Neuropsychopharmacology of Monoamines and Their Regulatory Enzymes,* edited by E. Usdin, pp. 369–384. Raven Press, New York.

73. Sabelli, H. C., Mosnaim, A. D., and Vazquez, A. J. (1974): Phenylethylamine: Possible role in depression and antidepressive drug action. In: *Neurohumoral Coding of Brain Function,* edited by R. D. Myers and R. R. Drucker-Colin, pp. 331–357. Plenum Press, New York.

74. Schacht, U., and Heptner, W. (1974): Effect of nomifensine (Hoe 984), a new antidepressant, on uptake of noradrenaline and serotonin and on release of noradrenaline in rat brain synaptosomes. *Biochem. Pharmacol.,* 23:3413–3422.

75. Sedvall, G. C., Weise, V. K., and Kopin, I. J. (1968): The rate of norepinephrine synthesis measured *in vivo* during short intervals: Influence of adrenergic nerve impulse activity. *J. Pharmacol. Exp. Ther.,* 159:274–282.

76. Seeman, P., and Lee, T. (1975): Antipsychotic drugs: Direct correlation between clinical potency and presynaptic action on dopamine neurons. *Science,* 188:1217–1219.

77. Smith, J. E., Lane, J. D., Shea, P. A., McBride, W. J., and Aprison, M. H. (1975): A method for concurrent measurement of picomole quantities of acetylcholine, choline, dopamine, norepinephrine, serotonin, 5-hydroxytryptophan, 5-hydroxyindoleacetic acid, tryptophan, tyrosine, glycine, aspartate, glutamate, alanine, and gamma-aminobutyric acid in single tissue samples from different areas of rat central nervous system. *Anal. Biochem.,* 64:149–169.

78. Snyder, S. H., Kuhar, M. J., Green, A. I., Coyle, J. T., and Shaskan, E. G. (1970): Uptake and subcellular localization of neurotransmitters in the brain. *Int. Rev. Neurobiol.,* 13:127–157.

79. Sohn, R. S., and Ferrendelli, J. A. (1973): Inhibition of Ca⁺⁺ transport into rat brain synaptosomes by diphenylhydantoin (DPH). *J. Pharmacol. Exp. Ther.,* 185:272–275.

80. Starke, K. (1977): Regulation of noradrenaline release by presynaptic receptor systems. *Rev. Physiol. Biochem. Pharmacol.,* 77:1–124.

81. Starke, K., and Montel, H. (1973): Involvement of α-receptors in clonidine-induced inhibition of transmitter release from central monoamine neurons. *Neuropharmacology,* 12:1073–1080.

82. Stjärne, L. (1973): Alpha-adrenoceptor mediated feed-back control of sympathetic neurotransmitter secretion in guinea-pig vas deferens. *Nature [New Biol.]*, 241:190–191.

83. Thomas, T. N., and Zemp, J. W. (1977): Inhibition of dopamine sensitive adenylate cyclase from rat brain striatal homogenates by ascorbic acid. *J. Neurochem.*, 28: 663–665.

84. Tissari, A., and Bogdanski, D. F. (1971): Biogenic amine transport. VI. Comparison of the effects of ouabain and K^+ deficiency on the transport of 5-hydroxytryptamine and norepinephrine by synaptosomes. *Pharmacology*, 5:225–234.

85. Ulbricht, W. (1969): The effect of veratridine on excitable membranes of nerve and muscle. *Ergebn. Physiol.*, 61:18–71.

86. Westfall, T. C. (1974): Effect of muscarinic agonists on the release of ^{3}H-norepinephrine and ^{3}H-dopamine by potassium and electrical stimulation from rat brain slices. *Life Sci.*, 14:1641–1652.

87. Westfall, T. C., Besson, M. J., Giorguieff, M. F., and Glowinski, J. (1976): The role of presynaptic receptors in the release and synthesis of ^{3}H-dopamine by slices of rat striatum. *Naunyn-Schmiedeberg's Arch. Pharmacol.*, 292:279–287.

88. Willner, J., LeFevre, H. F., and Costa, E. (1974): Assay by multiple ion detection of phenylethylamine and phenylethanolamine in rat brain. *J. Neurochem.*, 23:857–859.

89. Wong, D. T., Horng, J. S., and Fuller, R. W. (1973 : Kinetics of serotonin accumulation into synaptosomes of rat brain: Effects of amphetamine and chloroamphetamines. *Biochem. Pharmacol.*, 22:311–322.

90. Ziance, R. J., Azzaro, A. J., and Rutledge, C. O. (1972): Characteristics of amphetamine-induced release of norepinephrine from rat cerebral cortex *in vitro*. *J. Pharmacol. Exp. Ther.*, 182:284–294.

Advances in Biochemical Psychopharmacology, Vol. 19,
edited by P. J. Roberts et al.
Raven Press, New York © 1978.

Compartmentation of Synaptosomal Dopamine

J. S. de Belleroche and H. F. Bradford

*Department of Biochemistry, Imperial College of Science and Technology,
London SW7 2AZ England*

STRIATAL SYNAPTOSOMES

Synaptosomes obtained from the corpus striatum of sheep or rat by differential and discontinuous sucrose gradient centrifugation (10,26) have
the characteristic properties and appearance (Fig. 1) common to synaptosomes obtained from other brain regions (31), and like the striatal nerve
endings from which they are derived, are rich in dopamine. When incubated
in Krebs-bicarbonate medium containing glucose (10 mM), for instance,
these synaptosomes show high and linear respiration during at least 90 min
of incubation (21). Depolarizing agents such as electrical pulses, veratrine,
and raised K^+ stimulate respiration and the release of transmitters, dopamine,
glutamate, and GABA (21).

SYNAPTOSOMAL DOPAMINE AND ITS MEASUREMENT

The release of endogenous dopamine from incubated striatal synaptosomes
by depolarizing agents is accompanied by an increased synthesis of dopamine. The latter has been measured as the increase in levels of endogenous
dopamine and [^{14}C]dopamine formed from [^{14}C]tyrosine (21,22) and the increased activity of tyrosine hydroxylase that occur in response to stimulation
(37,44,45).

In order to follow both the changes in turnover of synaptosomal dopamine
and the release in response to drugs or depolarizing stimuli, we measured
both endogenous dopamine and dopamine labeled from the radioactively
labeled precursors L-tyrosine and L-DOPA. These precursors differentially
labeled pools of synaptosomal dopamine, whose progress could be followed
during stimulation. The minimal rates of dopamine synthesis from tyrosine
were similar to those obtained for caudate nucleus *in vivo* (18,30) and
those measured in striatal slices (5). Separation of dopamine from its
precursors and metabolites and its subsequent analysis were carried out by
automated ion-exchange chromatography with "on line" scintillation counting (22).

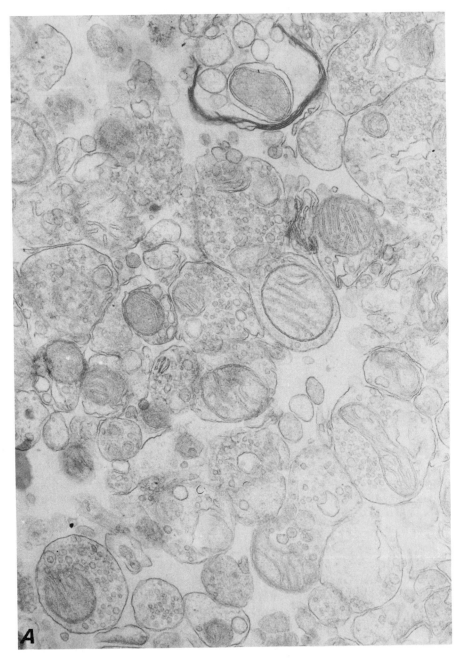

FIG. 1. Synaptosomes of sheep corpus striatum. Synaptosomes were incubated at 37°C for 30–60 min in Krebs-bicarbonate medium. Suspensions of synaptosomes were fixed at 4°C with veronal acetate-buffered 1% OsO₄ for 1 hr, sedimented, dehydrated, embedded in Araldite, and stained with uranyl acetate and lead citrate. a: × 37,500; b: × 46,000; c: × 94,500. b and c are reproduced from ref. 21.

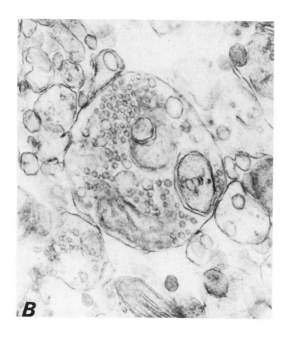

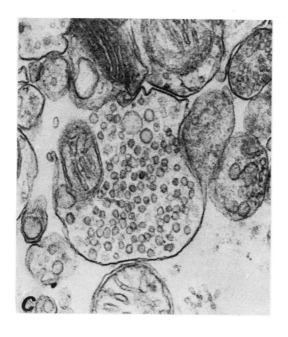

COMPARTMENTATION OF SYNAPTOSOMAL DOPAMINE AND ITS PRECURSORS

Compartmentation of Tyrosine

Although both L-DOPA and L-tyrosine are precursors of synaptosomal dopamine, only L-tyrosine added as a continuous label significantly labeled the synaptosomal pool released by depolarization (Fig. 2). This occurred even though dopamine was labeled from L-[U-^{14}C]DOPA at a rate six to seven times more rapid than from tyrosine (21). Even when L-[U-^{14}]DOPA was provided as a precursor, the increased synthesis of dopamine in response to stimulation largely utilized endogenous precursor and therefore resulted in a decrease in the specific activity of synaptosomal dopamine (Fig. 3). Endogenous tyrosine was found to be present at a concentration of 20 nmoles/100 mg protein which would be adequate to provide the dopamine

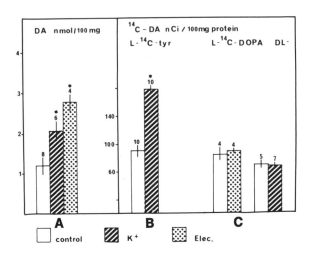

FIG. 2. Dopamine release from striatal synaptosomes. a: Endogenous dopamine. Synaptosome beds were incubated at 37°C for 40 min in Krebs-bicarbonate medium containing 10 mM glucose and 0.5 mM L-ascorbate. Potassium stimulation (K$^+$) was carried out by adding KCl made up in the above saline to give a final concentration of 56 mM (from 6 mM) at 30 min. Electrical stimulation (Elec.) was by application of square-wave electrical pulses of 10 V, 0.4 msec duration, and alterating in polarity at 100/sec for the final 10 min of incubation. Dopamine release to the medium was measured fluorimetrically (39), following extraction with alumina (2). Data are taken from ref. 21. b: Dopamine labeled from [^{14}C]tyrosine. Synaptosomes were incubated at 37°C in Krebs-bicarbonate medium containing 10 mM glucose, 0.5 mM L-ascorbate, 0.1 mM nialamide, and 2.5 µCi L-[U-^{14}C]tyrosine (495 mCi/mmole) for 30 min. Potassium stimulation as in (a). Samples were acidified, and nonisotopic carrier dopamine and norepinephrine and an internal radioactive standard (valine) were added. Analysis was carried out by ion-exchange chromatography linked to "on line" scintillation counting (22). Data are taken from ref. 20. c: Dopamine labeled from [^{14}C]DOPA. Synaptosome beds were incubated at 37°C for 40 min in Krebs-bicarbonate medium (5 ml) containing 10 mM glucose, 0.5 mM L-ascorbate, and the radioactively labeled precursor, 1 µCi L-DOPA (10 mCi/mmole) or 1 µCi DL-DOPA (51 mCi/mmole) as indicated. The beds were then transferred to fresh medium with no isotope and were incubated for a further 20 min at 37°C. K$^+$ and electrical stimulation as in (a) for the final 10 min of incubation. Extraction and analysis were carried out as in (b). Data are from ref. 21. Values are means ± SEM with the number of experiments indicated.

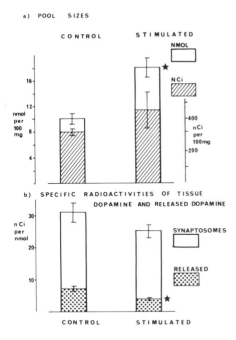

FIG. 3. Specific radioactivity of synaptosomal dopamine. Synaptosome beds were incubated at 37°C in Krebs-bicarbonate medium containing 10 mM glucose, 0.5 mM L-ascrobate, and 3.9 μM DL-3,4-dihydroxyphenyl-[2-^{14}C]alanine (51 mCi/mmole) for 40 min. The beds were then drained and transferred to fresh Krebs bicarbonate medium containing 10 mM glucose, 0.5 mM-L-ascorbate, and no isotope with no further additions (control) or in 56 mM K$^+$ (stimulated). Incubation was carried out for 10 min. The synaptosomes were then analyzed fluorometrically for dopamine (plain histograms) and for radioactively labeled dopamine (hatched histograms) (Fig. Ia) in the same extract by means of the automated analytical procedure and an "on line" scintillation counter. Specific radioactivities (nCi/nmole) of these synaptosome extracts are shown (plain histogram) in Fig. 1b for control and stimulated samples, specific radioactivities of dopamine released during incubation are shown (spotted histograms) for control and stimulated samples. Dopamine was measured fluorometrically by the hydroxyindole method following purification on alumina and in separate samples for radioactivity. The values are means ± SEM for 4–7 samples. The asterisk indicates that the stimulated value is significantly different from the control with p < 0.01. Data from ref. 20.

which was formed. The specific radioactivity of dopamine released by K$^+$ stimulation under these conditions also showed a significant decrease (40%) compared to that released by controls. Both endogenous and externally applied tyrosine were found to label dopamine synthesized in response to depolarization.

The exogenous tyrosine used to synthesize dopamine released by stimulation appears to be "recently taken up," as loading with L-[^{14}C]tyrosine prior to a 20-min incubation, including 10 min stimulation, did not result in significant labeling of released dopamine, whereas continuous labeling with tyrosine did. The synaptosome is therefore able to compartment "recently taken up" tyrosine and use it for dopamine synthesis and release in preference to other pools of tyrosine. This compartmentation of synaptosomal tyrosine has also been suggested by Katz et al. (33) and Kapatos and Zigmond (32) who, from measurement of tyrosine hydroxylation, have shown that tyrosine can be taken up by synaptosomes and used to synthesize dopamine without equilibrating with the whole pool of synaptosome tyrosine.

The depolarizing alkaloid veratrine, which increases the sodium permeability of synaptosomes (7) and stimulates their release of catecholamine (8,45) and amino acid transmitters (20), also accelerates dopamine synthesis from externally supplied tyrosine (45), which again appears not to mix rapidly with the internal tyrosine pool.

Compartmentation of DOPA

A further implication which follows from the above observations is the existence of two separate compartments of tyrosine hydroxylase, DOPA decarboxylase, and DOPA. A possible explanation of the data could come from the fact that L-DOPA may be decarboxylated in both dopaminergic and in nondopaminergic terminals which contain aromatic amino acid decarboxylase, e.g., noradrenergic and serotonergic nerve endings which are likely to be present in the preparation. However, since there was negligible formation, for instance, of norepinephrine from [^{14}C]DOPA or tyrosine in the striatal synaptosomes (21), dopamine formed by the preparation was likely to be mainly the product of dopaminergic nerve endings.

Turnover of Dopamine Pools

The observation that pulse labeling of synaptosomes with tyrosine was not sufficient exposure to label the "functional" pool of tyrosine producing the dopamine released in response to stimulation during the subsequent 20-min period indicates that this pool is turning over rapidly. This is supported by estimations of rate of turnover of the "functional" pool as opposed to the "total" pool *in vivo*. Thus, rates of turnover of the "total" pool (approximately 30 nmoles/100 mg protein/hr) are similar to those found for its equivalent in synaptosomes. In contrast, the rate of turnover of the "functional" pool *in vivo* (which accounts for 23% of the tissue content) is about 70 nmoles/g/hr (30). The equivalent "functional" pool in synaptosomes would turnover in less than 4 min. Sympathetic ganglia (17) and rat hemidiaphragm (47) have been shown to use externally supplied choline to synthesize acetylcholine in response to stimulation, in preference to choline loaded immediately prior to stimulation. Consequently, in these and other systems, such as cerebral cortex (14) and *Torpedo* electric organ (23,54), the most recently synthesized acetylcholine is released in response to stimulation.

COMPARTMENTATION OF DOPAMINE REVEALED BY AMPHETAMINE ACTION

Amphetamine has the marked effect of "releasing" dopamine from synaptosomes (3,21); the ED$_{50}$ of the process has been estimated as 0.5×10^{-4} M by Azzaro and Rutledge (3). In our experiments, D-amphetamine (1.2×10^{-4} M) caused a decrease of 25% in the total synaptosomal dopamine during 40 min incubation, and this may be attributable to the inhibition of tyrosine hydroxylase which occurs in synaptosomes at and above this concentration (27,36) and *in vivo* after 5 mg/kg injections of D-amphetamine sulfate (6).

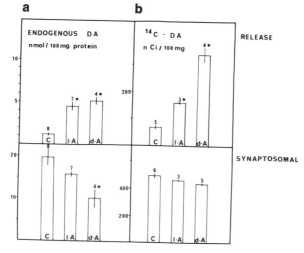

FIG. 4. The effect of amphetamine on synaptosomal dopamine. a: Experimental details as for Fig. 2a. D- or L-Amphetamine (1.2 × 10⁻⁴ M) were present throughout incubation as indicated by d-A and l-A, respectively, control incubations are indicated by C. b: Experimental details as for Fig. 2b, using 3.9 μM-3,4-dihydroxyphenyl-[2-¹⁴C]alanine (51 mCi/mmole) for pulse labeling. The final 20-min incubation was carried out in the presence of D- or L-amphetamine (1.2 × 10⁻⁴ M). Values are means ± SEM for the number of experiments indicated. Data from ref. 21.

Amphetamine is able to facilitate the outflow of [¹⁴C]dopamine which is formed from [¹⁴C]DOPA (Fig. 4), whereas, as emphasized above, depolarizing agents cause the release of unlabeled dopamine. Further evidence for compartmentation of dopamine metabolism was indicated by the action of amphetamine in releasing 60% of the [¹⁴C]dopamine formed from [¹⁴C]DOPA during the 40 min incubation. In contrast, only 30% of the unlabeled endogenous dopamine was measured in the same time (21). The dopamine pool formed from exogenous DOPA was therefore highly susceptible to the action of amphetamine in synaptosome preparations.

Dopamine Pool Affected by Amphetamine

The compartment of dopamine which is released by the action of amphetamine appears to be distinct from that affected by depolarizing agents. In fact, the releasing action of amphetamine could be due to blocking of dopamine uptake. The D-amphetamine-induced release of [¹⁴C]dopamine from synaptosomes labeled from [¹⁴C]DOPA was measured over short periods of incubation (1 to 3 min). Influx of externally applied [³H]dopamine could also be followed, thus allowing simultaneous monitoring of both influx and efflux (19). Under these conditions, amphetamine did not affect the efflux of [¹⁴C]dopamine but did competitively inhibit the uptake of [³H]dopamine. Therefore, the continuous cycling of a large synaptosomal pool of dopamine apparently occurs, which leads to an accumulation of dopamine in the medium when the uptake process is blocked. This exchange of dopamine has been studied by Azzaro and Rutledge (3) by following the exchange of unlabeled external dopamine with intracellular [^{3}H]dopamine. Extrapolating from ED_{50} values for the exchange reactions, which are affected by amphetamine, Kuczenski (36) has also suggested that the synaptosomal pool of dopamine which is susceptible to amphetamine action is large, compared to the pool involved in depolarizing action.

RELEASE OF TYROSINE-LABELED DOPAMINE MEDIATED THROUGH PRESYNAPTIC RECEPTORS

The concept that presynaptic receptors exist on catecholamine nerve terminals originated from experiments with noradrenergic synapses in the sympathetic nervous system. It was found that alpha blockers such as phenoxybenzamine and phentolamine increase the release of norepinephrine elicited by nerve stimulation at both α- and β-receptor mediated synapses [reviewed by Langer (38) and Burnstock and Costa (12)]. In this case the agents were not acting as inhibitors of uptake since other compounds which block uptake did not increase outflow in this way. The most acceptable explanation for this effect has been that the α-receptor blocker prevented the negative feedback effect of norepinephrine on its own release. In addition to these α-receptors, dopamine and muscarinic and nicotinic receptors modulating the release of norepinephrine have been proposed for adrenergic nerve endings.

Parallel conclusions have been reached concerning presynaptic α receptors for norepinephrine release in the cerebral cortex, and for presynaptic dopamine receptors in the caudate nucleus which affect the release of dopamine. The latter proposal offers an explanation for the increased striatal turnover of dopamine which occurs *in vivo* in response to dopamine antagonists (e.g., neuroleptics) and the decreased turnover which is caused by agonists such as apomorphine. The proposal that the receptors occupy a presynaptic site is borne out by the increased turnover of striatal dopamine that follows lesions of the nigrostriatal tract, which is antagonized by apomorphine (34). In further support, dopamine and apomorphine inhibition of dopamine synthesis can be shown in striatal slices and synaptosomes (37,44), which are antagonized by neuroleptics (16,53), and also neuroleptics on their own affect dopamine release in striatal slices (15,24,48). The assumption in these experiments was that when the dopaminergic tract is functional, or when apomorphine is applied, dopaminergic activity is high and dopamine synthesis is inhibited. On the other hand, it was assumed that lesions resulting in cessation of impulse flow or the application of dopamine antagonist prevents the feedback inhibition by dopamine of synthesis, thus showing the persistence of receptors in the striatum.

Cholinergic receptors located on dopaminergic terminals of the striatum have also been suggested by studies on striatal slices where acetylcholine blocks potassium-stimulated release of isotopically labeled dopamine; this effect in turn is blocked by muscarinic receptor antagonists (50,53). The mediation of this effect through a presynaptic site is a likely explanation, although an indirect action through a cholinergic or other nondopaminergic intrinsic neuron cannot be ruled out. However, this explanation would still require a receptor on the dopaminergic terminal. Recently a stimulatory effect of acetylcholine on dopaminergic systems mediated through a nicotinic receptor has also been reported in both striatal slices and superfused cat caudate (25). The *in vitro* effects are consistent with *in vivo* observations where both muscarinic and nicotinic receptors have been implicated. These concern the action of acetylcholine on dopaminergic cells in the striatum (9,42), either activating or inhibiting discharge activity, respectively. Drugs such as physostigmine which favor cholinergic systems increase firing of dopamine-sensitive cells (28) and increase striatal dopamine turnover. Systemically administered physostigmine, oxotremorine, and choline increase striatal and limbic dopamine turnover (46). In contrast, drugs which block muscarinic receptors, e.g., atropine, decrease the rate of dopamine utilization (1).

More direct evidence for the existence of presynaptic receptors comes from the effects of acetylcholine and dopaminergic agents on metabolism and release of dopamine in synaptosome preparations, i.e., supposedly properties of the presynaptic terminal only. In the case of the acetylcholine receptors, direct estimation of the size of the populations of the two types of receptors can be obtained through binding studies, using, for instance, α-bungarotoxin and atropine for nicotinic and muscarinic receptors, respectively.

EFFECT OF ACETYLCHOLINE ON SYNAPTOSOMAL DOPAMINE

Receptor-Mediated Dopamine Release

Acetylcholine (3×10^{-4} M) in the presence of neostigmine (0.15 mg/ml) stimulated the release of [^{14}C]dopamine by 70% when L-[U-^{14}C]tyrosine was used as precursor (Table 1). At the same time, it stimulated the formation of isotopically labeled dopamine by 25%. These effects were similar to those produced by K$^+$ stimulation. Acetylcholine also increased the turnover of dopamine labeled from [^{14}C]DOPA, as measured by the increased formation of [^{14}C]dopamine and DOPAC. However, there was no change in the size of the endogenous pool of dopamine (Table 2).

The effect of acetylcholine antagonists on the release of labeled dopamine formed from [^{14}C]tyrosine was further investigated. The muscarinic receptor antagonist atropine (1.3×10^{-4} M) potentiated the action of acetylcholine on [^{14}C]dopamine release by 72% and enhanced the control release of [^{14}C]dopamine (Fig. 5). The effects due to K$^+$ stimulation were unaffected

TABLE 1. *Radioactive labeling of synaptosomal dopamine with* L-[U-14C]tyrosine

	nCi [14C]dopamine/100 mg protein	
	Released dopamine	Total dopamine
Control	90.9 ± 9.5 (10)	603.1 ± 53.0 (6)
K+ (56 mM)	178.7 ± 7.7 (10)[a]	794.4 ± 69.3 (6)[b]
Acetylcholine (0.3 mM) with neostigmine (0.15 mg/ml)	147.8 ± 12.7 (7)[a]	736.5 ± 65.2 (6)[b]

Rat corpus striatum synaptosomes were incubated at 37°C in Krebs-bicarbonate medium containing 10 mM glucose, 0.5 mM L-ascorbate, 0.1 mM nialamide, and 2.5 μCi L-[U-14C]tyrosine (495 mCi/mmole) for 30 min. Potassium or acetylcholine with neostigmine was added after 20 min. The values are means ± SEMs with the number of experiments in brackets. Data from ref. 20.
[a] Denotes that the value is significantly greater than the control $p < 0.01$.
[b] Denotes that the value is significantly greater than the control $p < 0.05$.

by atropine. One interpretation of these findings is that atropine was preventing an acetylcholine-induced inhibition of dopamine release. The enhanced control release could be due to atropine's preventing the action of external acetylcholine, whose endogenous levels are high in the striatum, and any released acetylcholine would not be destroyed in the presence of neostigmine. The nicotinic receptor antagonists hexamethonium (3×10^{-4} M) and α-bungarotoxin (1.9×10^{-7} M) blocked rather than stimulated the acetylcholine stimulation of dopamine release. The release due to K+ was unaffected by hexamethonium but was reduced by α-bungarotoxin. It seems fairly clear from these experiments that the action of acetylcholine in releasing dopamine from synaptosome preparations is mediated through a nicotinic receptor.

TABLE 2. *Synaptosomal dopamine, [14C]dopamine, and [14C]DOPAC formation from [14C]DOPA*

	DA nmoles/100 mg protein	DA nCi/100 mg protein	DOPAC nCi/100 mg protein	No. of experiments
Control	10.12 ± 0.84	315.4 ± 19.8	128.0 ± 18.0	7
K+ 0.56 mM	17.89 ± 1.47 [a]	450.6 ± 112.5	88.0 ± 15.6	4
ACh. 0.1 mM, neostigmine	10.02 ± 0.24	459.1 ± 43.6 [a]	197.1 ± 26.9 [a]	5

Sheep striatal synaptosome beds were incubated at 37°C in Krebs-bicarbonate medium containing 10 mM glucose, 0.5 mM L-ascorbate, and 3.9 μM DL-3,4-dihydroxyphenyl-[2-14C]alanine (51 mCi/mmole) for 40 min. The beds were then drained and placed in fresh medium as used above, except that DOPA was omitted, and incubation was continued for a further 10 min. The fresh medium contained either no additions (control) or K+ at 56 mM or acetylcholine (0.1 mM) in the presence of neostigmine (0.1 mg/ml). Dopamine was analyzed fluorometrically and dopamine and DOPAC were analyzed for radioactivity by means of combined automated analysis. Values are means ± SEM for the number of experiments indicated at the side. Data from ref. 20.
[a] $p < 0.01$.

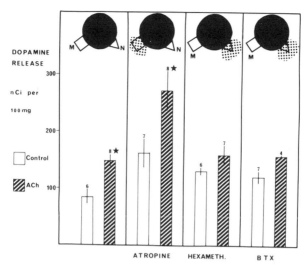

FIG. 5. The effect of acetylcholine and muscarinic and nicotinic agonists on dopamine release. Rat corpus striatum synaptosomes were incubated at 37°C in Krebs-bicarbonate medium containing 10mM glucose, 0.5 mM L-ascorbate, 0.1 mM nialamide, neostigmine bromide (0.1 mg/ml), and 2.5 μCi L-[U-^{14}C]tyrosine (495 mCi/mmole) for 30 min. Additions were made after the first 20 min. The final concentrations of added compounds were acetylcholine (0.3 mM), atropine (0.129 mM), hexamethonium (0.298 mM), and α-bungaro-toxin (0.188 μM), indicated as BTX. The values are means ± SEMs with the number of experiments indi-cated by the bars. The asterisk indicates that the values were significantly greater than the appropriate controls, with $p < 0.02$. Data from ref. 20.

Potassium-Acetylcholine Interactions

Acetylcholine also had the effect of reducing the dopamine released in response to K$^+$. A reduction of 65% was found in the presence of atropine and 95% in the presence of hexamethonium (Figs. 6 and 7). The reduction

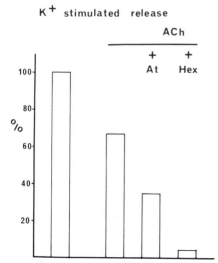

FIG. 6. The effect of acetylcholine on K$^+$-stimulated release of [^{14}C]dopamine. Experimental details as for Fig. 5. K$^+$ was added after 20 min to give a final concentration of 56 mM. The response to K$^+$ stimulation in the presence of acetylcholine and its antagonists is shown as a percentage of response (100%) shown in the absence of acetylcholine. The SEMs are 8%–15% for 3–7 experiments. Data from ref. 20. Acetylcholine in the presence of hexa-methonium significantly inhibited K$^+$-stimulated re-lease, $p < 0.05$.

SYNAPTOSOMAL DOPAMINE nCi per 100 mg protein

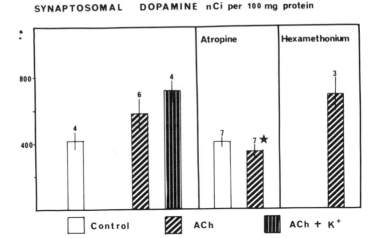

FIG. 7. The effect of acetylcholine and its antagonists on synaptosomal dopamine. Experimental details as for Fig. 5. The asterisk denotes that the value is significantly reduced ($p < 0.01$) compared to the effect of acetylcholine with no antagonist present. The control histogram shows the level of [^{14}C]dopamine when no neostigmine is present in the incubation medium. Data from ref. 20.

in K^+-stimulated release caused by added acetylcholine was greatest when only the muscarinic receptors were exposed, i.e., when hexamethonium was present and therefore occupying the nicotinic sites. The acetylcholine inhibition of both acetylcholine and K^+-stimulated release appeared to be blocked by a muscarinic receptor. Acetylcholine has also been shown to block the K^+-stimulated release of preloaded [^{3}H]dopamine from striatal slices (50).

Effect of Acetylcholine on Dopamine Synthesis

An index of the effect of acetylcholine and its antagonists on dopamine synthesis came from the measurement of synaptosomal total dopamine formed in the presence of nialamide (10^{-4} M). Metabolism of dopamine formed from L-[U-^{14}]tyrosine by synaptosomes is principally to DOPAC via monamine oxidase. A stimulatory effect of acetylcholine on dopamine synthesis is indicated by the observation that neostigmine alone enhanced dopamine synthesis, acetylcholine increased synthesis further, but the combined effect of acetylcholine and neostigmine was totally abolished by prior addition of atropine. The enhanced synthesis due to neostigmine could be due to a response to release of endogenous acetylcholine which would be more potent in the presence of neostigmine. Any muscarinic effect would be inhibited by atropine. Hexamethonium did not reduce the effect of added neostigmine plus acetylcholine. Part of the muscarinically mediated response to acetylcholine *in vivo* could therefore be attributed to this presynaptic action.

Receptor Binding Studies

Binding studies were carried out on striatal synaptosomes to obtain independent evidence for the presence of specific nicotinic and muscarinic receptors. Estimation of nicotinic receptors was made by measuring the binding of [^{3}H-diacetyl]-α-bungarotoxin that was inhibited by pretreatment with D-tubocurarine (1.3×10^{-3} M) or hexamethonium (10 mM). Specific nicotinic binding sites were found to be present at a concentration of 11 fmoles/mg protein (Table 3) using either antagonist. This value is compa-

TABLE 3. *Cholinergic receptors in striatal synaptosomes*

Nicotinic receptors	
Specific binding of [^{3}H]-α-bungarotoxin	11.2 ± 1.0 fmoles/mg protein
	N = 13
Muscarinic receptors	
Specific binding of [^{3}H]-N-methyl-atropine	1.65 ± 0.5 pmoles/mg protein
	N = 6

Binding of [^{3}H]-α-bungarotoxin: Rat striatal synaptosomes were incubated at 37°C in Krebs-bicarbonate medium containing 10 mM glucose and 16 mM [^{3}H]-α-bungarotoxin (5 Ci/mmole) for 30 min. Similar incubations were carried out in the presence of 1.3 mM D-tubocurarine or 10 /mM hexamethonium. Free toxin was removed by 3 washes in a large excess of saline. The specific binding was taken as the binding that was displaceable by hexamethonium or D-tubocurarine. Values are means ± SEMs for N experiments. Binding of [^{3}H]-N-methyl-atropine: Suspensions of rat striatal synaptosomes in Krebs-Henseleit medium were incubated at 32°C for 15 min in 2.5 nM [^{3}H]-N-methyl-atropine (2.2 Ci/mmole). This incubation was also carried out in the presence of an excess of N-methyl-atropine (10 μM). Free reagent was removed by 3 washes in a large excess of saline. Specific binding was taken as that which was displaceable by excess atropine. Data are taken from ref. 20 and Luqmani and Bradford, *unpublished results*.

rable to that found for whole rat brain homogenate, which was estimated to be 0.75 fmoles/mg tissue (40), i.e., 7.5 fmoles/mg protein approximately.

Muscarinic receptors were estimated by a similar method using [^{3}H]-N-methyl-atropine as the labeled ligand to obtain total binding sites (Y. Luqmani and H. F. Bradford, *unpublished results*), and from this value was subtracted the binding of the labeled ligand in the presence of N-methyl-atropine (0.01 mM) to obtain a measure of the specific binding. The number of muscarinic receptors in this preparation appears to outnumber the nicotinic sites by two orders of magnitude, as has been shown in a number of regions of the CNS (11,29).

Conclusions from the Acetylcholine-Dopamine Interactions

Our own evidence from studies with striatal synaptosomes strongly supports the proposal that presynaptic cholinergic receptors controlling dopamine release exist on striatal nerve terminals. This strengthens the case previously made from the experiments employing *in vivo* caudate and striatal slice preparations (25,50,53). It appears that both muscarinic and nicotinic acetylcholine receptors are present. This follows from their high-affinity binding of specific agents as well as from their effects on dopamine release and turnover. The nicotinic receptor appears to mediate a stimulatory effect on dopamine release, whereas a muscarinic receptor appears to inhibit the release of dopamine. This may well be the mechanism by which acetylcholine inhibited the nicotine-induced release of [³H]dopamine *in vitro* (51) which is blocked by atropine (52).

A model to account for the effects of acetylcholine on dopamine release and its inhibitory effect on K⁺-stimulated release would have three sites at which acetylcholine interacts on the nerve terminals: a muscarinic site, a nicotinic site, and a site influencing the effects of K⁺ depolarization. The first two are self-explanatory and interactions at these sites would lead to changes which induce inhibition or stimulation of release. These two sites are likely to be separate from the third, since K⁺ stimulation is unaffected by the presence of the acetylcholine antagonists. The action of K⁺ stimulation is reduced only when extracellular acetylcholine is added at the same time, and this reduction is greatest when nicotinic sites are blocked. Therefore, added acetylcholine appears to affect processes also influenced by K⁺ and presumably linked to the membrane depolarization that occurs. It is unlikely that atropine or hexamethonium acts through the same mechanism since atropine did not reduce the K⁺ effect on either dopamine or GABA release.

Origin of the Cholinergic Effect *In Vivo*

Should these cholinergic influences on dopamine release be occurring *in vivo* as we would predict to be the case, then the origin of the acetylcholine producing these effects could be the intrinsic cholinergic neurons of the striatum, since most striatal acetylcholine is thought to be in these cells as deduced from histochemical and lesion studies (13,41). The electrophysiology of the intrinsic neurons of the striatum, which have been estimated as comprising 95% of the terminals of this region (49), has not been easy to establish since the cells are less easily penetrated by electrodes. Therefore, the majority of cells which are encountered will be of extrinsic origin, and these have been shown to respond in most cases to acetylcholine with muscarinic responses. Evidence of nicotinic receptors on the intrinsic neurons has been shown by Misgeld and Okada (43) who measured evoked potentials in the caudate, which were blocked by D-tubocurarine and unaffected by atropine. Although these receptors are mediating postsynaptic responses, it is possible that their characteristics are common to the presynaptic receptors as well. The acetylcholine presynaptic receptors could either form part of the postsynaptic region of an axoaxonic synapse, a serial synapse (35), or a symmetrical synapse (4), or simply be the sites of action of acetylcholine diffusing from local cholinergic nerve endings.

ACKNOWLEDGMENTS

We thank the M.R.C. for financing this work (M.R.C. Programme Grant), Dr. D. G. Jones for the electron microscopy, Elsevier Publishing Co., for allowing Tables 1 and 2 and Fig. 3 to be used, and Pergamon Press for allowing Figs. 1b and 1c to be used.

REFERENCES

1. Anden, N.-E., and Bedard, P. (1971): Influences of cholinergic mechanisms on the function and turnover of brain dopamine. *J. Pharm. Pharmacol.,* 23:460–462.
2. Anton, A. H., and Sayre, D. F. (1962): A study of the factors affecting the aluminium oxide trihydroxyindole procedure for the analysis of catecholamines. *J. Pharmacol. Exp. Ther.,* 138:360–375.
3. Azzaro, A. J., and Rutledge, C. O. (1973): Selectivity of release of norepinephrine, dopamine and 5-hydroxytryptamine by amphetamine in various regions of rat brain. *Biochem. Pharmacol.,* 22:2801–2813.
4. Bak, I. J., Choi, W. B., Hassler, K. G., Usunoff, K. G., and Wagner, A. (1975): Fine structural synaptic organization of the corpus striatum and substantia nigra in rat and cat. *Adv. Neurol.,* 9:25–41.
5. Besson, M. J., Cheramy, A., Feltz, P., and Glowinski, J. (1969): Release of newly synthesized dopamine from dopamine-containing terminals in the striatum of the rat. *Proc. Natl. Acad. Sci. U.S.A.,* 62:741–748.
6. Besson, M. J., Cheramy, A., and Glowinski, J. (1971): Effects of some psychotropic drugs on dopamine synthesis in the rat striatum. *J. Pharmacol. Exp. Ther.,* 177:196–205.
7. Blaustein, M. P., and Goldring, J. M. (1975): Membrane potentials in pinched-off presynaptic nerve terminals monitored with a fluorescent probe: Evidence that synaptosomes have potassium diffusion potentials. *J. Physiol. (Lond.),* 247:589–615.
8. Blaustein, M. P., Johnson, E. M., Jr., and Needleman, P. (1972): Calcium dependent norepinephrine release from presynaptic nerve endings *in vitro. Proc. Natl. Acad. Sci. U.S.A.,* 69:2237–2240.
9. Bloom, F. E., Costa, E., and Salmoiraghi, G. C. (1965): Anaesthesia and the responsiveness of individual neurons of the caudate nucleus of the cat to acetylcholine, norepinephrine and dopamine administered by microelectrophoresis. *J. Pharmacol. Exp. Ther.,* 150:244–252.
10. Bradford, H. F. (1969): Respiration *in vitro* of synaptosomes from mammalian cerebral cortex. *J. Neurochem.,* 16:675–684.
11. Burgen, A. S. W., Hiley, C. R., and Young, J. M. (1974): The properties of muscarinic receptors in mammalian cerebral cortex. *Br. J. Pharmacol.,* 51:279–285.
12. Burnstock, G., and Costa, M. (1975): Adrenergic neuroeffector transmission. In: *Adrenergic Neurones,* pp. 58–61. Chapman & Hall, Ltd., London.
13. Butcher, S. G., and Butcher, L. L. (1974): Origin and modulation of acetylcholine activity in the neostriatum. *Brain Res.,* 71:167–171.
14. Chakrin, L. M., Marchbanks, R. M., Mitchell, J. F., and Whittaker, V. P. (1972): The origin of the acetylcholine released from the surface of the cortex. *J. Neurochem.,* 19:2727–2736.
15. Chéramy, A., Beeson, M. J., and Glowinski, J. (1970): Increased release of dopamine from striatal dopaminergic terminals in the rat after treatment with a neuroleptic: Thioproperazine. *Eur. J. Pharmacol.,* 10:206–214.
16. Christiansen, J., and Squires, R. F. (1974): Antagonistic effects of apomorphine and haloperidol on rat striatal synaptosomal tyrosine hydroxylase. *J. Pharm. Pharmacol.,* 26:367–369.
17. Collier, B., and Katz, H. S. (1971): The synthesis, turnover and release of surplus acetylcholine in sympathetic ganglion. *J. Physiol. (Lond.),* 214:537–552.

18. Costa, E., and Neff, N. H. (1966): Isotopic and non-isotopic measurements of the rate of catecholamine biosynthesis. In: *Biochemistry and Pharmacology of the Basal Ganglia*, edited by E. Costa, L. J. Cote, and M. D. Yahr, pp. 141–155. Raven Press, New York.
19. de Belleroche, J. S., and Bradford, H. F. (1976): Transport of amino acids and catecholamines in relation to metabolism and transmission. In: *Transport Phenomena in the Nervous System*, edited by G. Levi, L. Battistin, and A. Lajtha, pp. 395–404. Plenum Press, New York.
20. de Belleroche, J. S., and Bradford, H. F. (1978): Biochemical evidence for the presence of presynaptic receptors on dopaminergic nerve terminals. *Brain Res.* 8, 142:53–68.
21. de Belleroche, J. S., Bradford, H. F., and Jones, D. A. (1976): A study of the metabolism and release of dopamine and amino acids from nerve endings isolated from sheep corpus striatum. *J. Neurochem.*, 26:561–571.
22. de Belleroche, J. S., Dykes, C. R., and Thomas, A. J. (1976): The automated separation and analysis of dopamine, its amino acid precursors and metabolites and the application of the method to the measurement of specific radioactivities of dopamine in striatal synaptosomes. *Anal. Biochem.*, 71:193–203.
23. Dunnant, Y., Gautron, J., Israel, M., Lesbats, B., and Manaranche, R. (1972): Les compartiments d'acetylcholine de l'organe electrique de la torpille et leurs modifications par la stimulation. *J. Neurochem.*, 19:1987–2002.
24. Farnebo, L.-O., and Hamberger, B. (1971): Drug-induced changes in the release of ^{3}H-monoamines from field stimulated rat brain slices. *Acta Physiol. Scand.* [*Suppl.*], 371:35–44.
25. Giorguieff, M. F., Le Floc'h, M. L., Westfall, T. C., Glowinski, J., and Beeson, M. J. (1976): Nicotinic effect of acetylcholine on the release of newly synthesised [^{3}H]-dopamine on rat striatal slices and cat caudate nucleus. *Brain Res.*, 106:117–131.
26. Gray, E. G., and Whittaker, V. P. (1962): The isolation of nerve endings from brain: An electron microscopic study of cell fragments derived by homogenisation and centrifugation. *J. Anat.*, 96:79–88.
27. Harris, J. E., and Baldessarini, R. J. (1973): Amphetamine induced inhibition of tyrosine hydroxylase in homogenates of rat striatum. *J. Pharm. Pharmacol.*, 25:755–757.
28. Hertz, A., and Zieglgänsberger, W. (1968): The influence of microiontophoretically applied biogenic amines, cholinomimetics and procaine on synaptic excitation in the corpus striatum. *Int. J. Neuropharmacol.*, 7:221–230.
29. Hiley, C. R., and Burgen, A. S. V. (1974): The distribution of muscarinic receptor sites in the nervous system of dogs. *J. Neurochem.*, 22:159–162.
30. Javoy, F., and Glowinski, J. (1971): Dynamic characteristics of the "functional compartment" of dopamine in dopaminergic terminals of the rat striatum. *J. Neurochem.*, 18:1305–1311.
31. Jones, D. G. (1975): Synaptosomes as structural units. In: *Synapses and Synaptosomes*, pp. 98–134. Chapman and Hall, London.
32. Kapatos, G., and Zigmond, M. (1977): Dopamine biosynthesis from L-tyrosine and L-phenylalanine in rat brain synaptosomes: Preferential use of newly accumulated precursors. *J. Neurochem.*, 28:1109–1119.
33. Katz, I., Lloyd, T., and Kaufman, S. (1976): Studies on phenylalanine and tyrosine hydroxylation by rat brain tyrosine hydroxylase. *Biochem. Biophys. Acta*, 445:567–578.
34. Kehr, W., Carlsson, A., Lindqvist, M., Magnusson, T., and Atack, C. (1972): Evidence for a receptor-mediated feedback control of tyrosine hydroxylase activity. *J. Pharm. Pharmacol.*, 24:744–746.
35. Kemp, J. M., and Powell, T. P. S. (1971): The synaptic organization of the caudate nucleus. *Philos. Trans. R. Soc. Lond.* [*Biol.*], 262:403–412.
36. Kuczenski, R. (1975): Effects of catecholamine releasing agents on synaptosomal dopamine biosynthesis: Multiple pools of dopamine or multiple forms of tyrosine hydroxylase? *Neuropharmacology*, 14:1–10.
37. Kuczenski, R., and Segal, D. S. (1974): Intrasynaptosomal conversion of tyrosine

to dopamine as an index of catecholamine biosynthetic capacity. *J. Neurochem.,* 22:1039–1044.

38. Langer, S. Z. (1974): Presynaptic regulation of catecholamine release. *Biochem. Pharmacol.,* 23:1793–1800.
39. Laverty, R., and Taylor, K. M. (1968): A fluorometric assay of catecholamines and related compounds. *Anal. Biochem.,* 22:269–279.
40. Lowy, J., McGregor, J., Rosenstone, J., and Schmidt, J. (1976): Solubilization of an α-bungarotoxin-binding component of rat brain. *Biochemistry,* 15:1522–1527.
41. Lynch, G. S., Lucas, P. A., and Deadwyler, S. A. (1972): The demonstration of acetylcholinesterase containing neurones within the caudate nucleus of the rat. *Brain Res.,* 45:617–621.
42. McLennan, H., and York, D. H. (1966): Cholinergic mechanisms in the caudate nucleus. *J. Physiol. (Lond.),* 187:163–175.
43. Misgeld, U., and Okada, Y. (1976): Evoked potentials in striatal slices of the rat: A tool for the investigation of intrinsic connections. First meeting of the European Society of Neurochemistry, Bath.
44. Patrick, R. L., and Barchas, J. D. (1974): Regulation of catecholamine synthesis in rat brain synaptosomes. *J. Neurochem.,* 23:7–15.
45. Patrick, R. L., Snyder, T. E., and Barchas, J. D. (1975): Regulation of dopamine synthesis in rat brain striatal synaptosomes. *Mol. Pharmacol.,* 11:621–631.
46. Perez-Cruet, J., Gessa, G. L., Tagliamonte, A., and Tagliamonte, P. (1971): Evidence for a balance in the basal ganglia between cholinergic and dopaminergic activity. *Fed. Proc. Am. Soc. Exp. Biol.,* 30: No. 127.
47. Potter, L. T. (1970): Synthesis, storage and release of [14C]-acetylcholine in isolated rat diaphragm muscles. *J. Physiol. (Lond.),* 206:145–166.
48. Seeman, P., and Lee, T. (1975): Antipsychotic drugs: Direct correlation between clinical potency and presynaptic action on dopamine neurons. *Science,* 188:1217–1219.
49. Tennyson, V. M. (1975): Fluorescence and electron microscope studies on the caudate nucleus following chronic isolation. *Neurosci. Res. Program Bull.,* 13:381–385.
50. Westfall, T. C. (1974): Effect of muscarinic agonists on the release of 3H-norepinephrine and 3H-dopamine by potassium and electrical stimulation from rat brain slices. *Life Sci.,* 14:1641–1652.
51. Westfall, T. C. (1974): Effect of nicotine and other drugs on the release of [3H]-norepinephrine and [3H]-dopamine from rat brain slices. *Neuropharmacology,* 13:693–700.
52. Westfall, T. C. (1974): The effect of cholinergic agents on the release of [3H] dopamine rat striatal slices by nicotine, potassium and electrical stimulation. *Fed. Proc.,* 33:524.
53. Westfall, T. C., Besson, M. J., Giorguieff, M. F., and Glowinski, J. (1976): The role of presynaptic receptors in the release and synthesis of [3H]-dopamine by slices of rat striatum. *Naunyn-Schmiedeberg's Arch. Pathol. Pharmacol.,* 292:279–287.
54. Zimmerman, H. (1976): Separation of cholinergic synaptic vesicles of different functional states by density gradient centrifugation. First meeting of the European Society of Neurochemistry, Bath.

Advances in Biochemical Psychopharmacology, Vol. 19,
edited by P. J. Roberts et al.
Raven Press, New York © 1978.

Regulations of the Activity of the Nigrostriatal Dopaminergic Pathways by Cortical, Cerebellar, and Sensory Neuronal Afferences

J. Glowinski, A. Niecoullon, and *A. Chéramy

Groupe NB (INSERM U. 114), College of France, Paris, Cedex 5 France

During the past few years, we have developed a new approach for studying the *in vivo* release of dopamine (DA) from nerve terminals of the nigrostriatal dopaminergic neurons in the cat (24). It consists of the use of a push-pull cannula and continuous labelling of the dopaminergic terminals with L-^{3}H-tyrosine. Indeed, when introduced at a constant rate into the push-pull cannula, the labeled precursor is selectively converted into ^{3}H-DA in these nerve terminals, and the newly formed ^{3}H-amine, which is preferentially released, can be estimated in successive superfusate fractions. Due to the high specific activity of L-^{3}H-tyrosine (40 to 50 Ci/mmole) and to an elaborate technique of separation of ^{3}H-DA from L-^{3}H-tyrosine and all radioactive metabolites, quantities as low as 0.5 pg of ^{3}H-DA can be easily detected. In our hands, this isotopic approach was much more rapid and sensitive than the radioenzymatic estimation of DA released in superfusates (6). Both in *encéphale isolé* and in halothane-anesthetized cats, the spontaneous release of ^{3}H-DA rapidly reaches a steady-state level after the onset of labeling. The ^{3}H-amine release is reduced by local application of tetrodotoxin (5.10^{-7} M) and completely abolished by acute electrocoagulation of the substantia nigra, a procedure which interrupts nerve firing in dopaminergic fibers. Conversely, the depolarization of the dopaminergic nerve terminals by local application of potassium chloride (30 mM) or by mechanical or electrical stimulation of the dopaminergic fibers stimulates the release of the ^{3}H-transmitter (24).

Recent findings suggest that DA is released not only from nerve terminals, but also from dendrites. In fact, Geffen et al. (14) first demonstrated that ^{3}H-DA previously taken up in slices of the rat substantia nigra was released by potassium through a calcium-dependent process. The stimulating effect of potassium was more pronounced in slices prepared from the pars reticulata which is rich in dendrites than in those prepared from the pars compacta

---

* A. Chéramy is a research fellow from Rhône Poulenc Company

which contains the dopaminergic cell bodies. Similar results were obtained when DA was directly estimated in the superfusing medium (9). The dendritic release of DA was confirmed *in vivo* in the cat (25). Indeed, we detected a spontaneous release of ^{3}H-DA when L-^{3}H-tyrosine was continuously delivered to a push-pull cannula precisely introduced into the substantia nigra. The amount of ^{3}H-DA released, which closely depends on the location of the cannula within the substantia nigra, is almost identical to that observed in the caudate nucleus. It is stimulated under potassium depolarization and by drugs such as amphetamine and benztropine which also favor the release of ^{3}H-DA from nerve terminals. However, the mechanisms involved in the release process of DA from nerve terminals and dendrites may be different, since tetrodotoxin does not reduce the release of ^{3}H-DA in the substantia nigra in contrast to that observed in the caudate nucleus (25).

One way to further explore the regulatory processes controlling the release of DA from dopaminergic terminals and dendrites is to estimate simultaneously the changes in ^{3}H-DA release in the caudate nucleus and in the substantia nigra induced by various stimuli which may directly or indirectly influence the activity of the dopaminergic neurons. We will summarize some of the results obtained in experiments in which we stimulated various cortical areas or cerebellar nuclei. This is of particular interest since the cerebral cortex and the cerebellum are the two main structures involved with the basal ganglia in the control of sensory motor behavior. Furthermore, the effects of various sensory stimuli will be described and compared with those induced by electrical stimulation of the cortical areas or cerebellar nuclei.

CHANGES IN DA RELEASE FROM DOPAMINERGIC NERVE TERMINALS AND DENDRITES INDUCED BY ELECTRICAL STIMULATION OF CORTICAL AREAS

Messages originating from the cerebral cortex may influence the nigrostriatal dopaminergic neurons in several ways. Indeed, neurons from various cortical areas converge to the striatum. Whereas those located in motor areas (4 and 6) project bilaterally, those which originate from other cortical areas exhibit an ipsilateral projection (4,22,42). A corticothalamostriatal neuronal loop could also be involved since the thalamic intralaminar nuclei contain terminals of cortical neurons (10,30) and cell bodies of neurons which innervate the striatum; some of them are cholinergic (37,41). Finally, a direct corticonigral pathway which originates mainly from the motor cortex has been described (1,35).

In a first series of experiments, we investigated the effects of punctuate electrical stimulations applied in one motor cortex on the release of ^{3}H-DA in the ipsilateral and contralateral caudate nuclei and in the ipsilateral substantia nigra (Table 1) (29). For this purpose, three push-pull cannulas were implanted in halothane-anesthetized cats, and ^{3}H-DA released

TABLE 1. *Comparison of the changes in ³H-DA release from terminals and dendrites of the two dopaminergic pathways induced by various stimuli*

	Motor cortex	Dentate nuclei	Somatic stimuli
Ipsilateral caudate	+	−	+
Ipsilateral nigra	+	+	−
Contralateral caudate	+	+	−
Contralateral nigra	No data	−	+

The stimuli consisted of a unilateral electrical stimulation of the motor cortex, the cerebellar dendate nucleus, or the right forelimb (somatic stimuli). Release of ³H-DA was simultaneously estimated as described in Fig. 1 in the ipsilateral and contralateral caudate nuclei and substantia nigra. These stimuli activated (+) or reduced (−) the release of ³H-DA in the various structures examined.

from each site was estimated during the continuous delivery of ³H-tyrosine to each push-pull cannula. The stimulus consisted of a train of shocks (train duration, 100 msec; duration of each shock, 0.5 msec; frequency, 300 Hz) delivered during 10 min at a frequency of 0.2 Hz. Applied in the cortical motor area 4, this stimulus (which induced a flexion of the contralateral forelimb) enhanced the release of ³H-DA in both the ipsilateral and the contralateral caudate nuclei. It also activated the release of ³H-DA from dopaminergic dendrites in the ipsilateral substantia nigra. These effects, which were similar in amplitude, were seen not only during the stimulation but also for a long time (at least 40 min) after the end of the stimulation.

To check if the symmetric changes in ³H-DA release seen in both caudate nuclei were induced by activation of the bilateral corticostriatal projections, we repeated the experiments in animals in which the rostral part of the corpus callosum was transected a few hours before the stimulation (29). This was done because the contralateral projections pass through the corpus callosum. As expected, this transection abolished the enhanced release of ³H-DA evoked in the contralateral caudate nucleus but not that induced in the ipsilateral structure. Since the corticostriatal projections which originate from other cortical areas are mainly ipsilateral, we also examined the effects of a unilateral punctuate electrical stimulation of visual areas (areas 18 and 19) (29). This 10-min stimulation enhanced the release of ³H-DA in the ipsilateral caudate nucleus and in the ipsilateral substantia nigra in a way similar to that observed under stimulation of the motor cortex but had very little effect on the ³H-amine release in the contralateral caudate nucleus.

Changes in DA metabolites were detected in the rat substantia nigra after electrical stimulation of the medial forebrain bundle by Korf et al. (21). According to these authors, these changes reflect an enhanced release of DA from dendrites induced by antidromic activation. The pronounced and persistent stimulation of ³H-DA release seen in the cat substantia nigra under

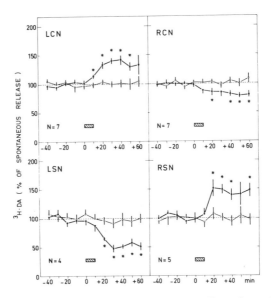

FIG. 1. Effects of unilateral electrical stimulation of the dentate cerebellar nucleus on the release of ³H-DA from the two caudate nuclei and the two substantia nigrae. Four push-pull cannulas were simultaneously implanted in the left (LCN) and the right (RCN) caudate nuclei and in the left (LSN) and right (RSN) substantia nigrae. The four structures were perfused with an artificial CSF containing L-3,5-³H-tyrosine. ³H-DA was estimated in 10-min successive superfusate fractions. The right cerebellar dentate nucleus was stimulated (*hatched bars*) for 10 min (train duration 100 msec; shock duration 0.5 msec; frequency in the train 300 Hz) delivered at a frequency of 0.2 Hz, and the intensity was adjusted in each experiment at the threshold of the apparent movement, from 3 to 6 V. In each animal and for each cannula, ³H-DA in each successive fraction was expressed as a percentage of an average spontaneous release calculated from the 5 fractions collected before the stimulation. Data are the mean ± SEM of results obtained with groups of N animals. *$p < 0.05$ when compared with corresponding control values (*open circles*) obtained in 5 non-stimulated animals. (From ref. 26.)

electrical stimulation of the motor or of the visual cortex directly reveals that the dendritic release of ³H-DA can be modulated by nigral afferent neuronal systems and that it may have a functional significance. This effect is very likely mediated by the corticonigral pathway which projects mainly to the pars compacta. As will be described more extensively latter, the activation of DA release in the substantia nigra generally decreases the activity of the dopaminergic neurons and thus reduces the release of DA from nerve terminals. This has been observed after the nigral application of amphetamine or of benztropine (7), treatments which mimic the effect induced by the direct application of DA into the substantia nigra (8). However, the activation of the dendritic release of ³H-DA induced by the stimulation of cortical areas was associated with an activation of ³H-DA release from nerve terminals. In this case, the two effects may be independent since the first one can be attributed to the activation of the corticonigral projection and the second one to the stimulation of the corticostriatal projection.

The corticostriatal neurons could directly or indirectly interact with the dopaminergic terminals and modulate DA transmission through a presynaptic influence. In fact, converging data suggest that the corticostriatal projection exerts a direct effect on dopaminergic terminals. The pathway originating from the motor cortex is very likely glutamatergic. Indeed, the high-affinity uptake of L-glutamic acid measured in striatal sucrose homogenates is significantly reduced after extensive lesion of the frontal cortex in the rat, suggesting a degeneration of glutamatergic terminals (11). Furthermore, striatal cells sensitive to L-glutamic acid are activated during stimulation of the motor cortex and these effects are blocked by glutamic acid diethyl-ester, a compound used as a blocker of glutamatergic receptors (40). Finally, as shown in our laboratory by Giorguieff et al. (15), L-glutamic acid stimulates the release of ^{3}H-DA synthesized from L-^{3}H-tyrosine in rat striatal slices. This mimicks in some ways the *in vivo* effect induced by the stimulation of the motor cortex. The *in vitro* release of ^{3}H-DA induced by L-glutamic acid was not blocked by cholinergic antagonists. This excluded the intervention of striatal cholinergic interneurons which may be directly influenced by the corticostriatal neurons. Moreover, this effect was still detected in the presence of tetrodotoxin, suggesting that glutamatergic receptors are located on dopaminergic terminals.

The corticostriatal glutamatergic neurons may not be the only ones involved in the presynaptic control of DA release from dopaminergic terminals. Indeed, on the basis of *in vitro* release experiments, we have also established the presence of muscarinic and nicotinic receptors on dopaminergic terminals (16,17), and Pollard et al. (31) have recently demonstrated the existence of enkephalin-binding sites on these terminals.

CHANGES IN ^{3}H-DA RELEASE FROM DOPAMINERGIC TERMINALS AND DENDRITES INDUCED BY STIMULATION OF CEREBELLAR NUCLEI

For many years, it was thought that the basal ganglia and the cerebellum had independent relationships with the cerebral motor cortex. The main neuronal outputs from these structures project onto the ventralateral nucleus of the thalamus (3), from which originate neurons innervating the cerebral motor cortex (36). Thus, it was assumed that no important pathways were connecting the basal ganglia and the cerebellum. Nevertheless, a projection originating from the substantia nigra and innervating the cerebellar cortex (area IV) has been described (5). Furthermore, Snider et al. (38) have recently demonstrated the existence of neuronal pathways originating in cerebellar nuclei and projecting into the substantia nigrae. According to these authors, some neurons originating in the cerebellar dentate and interposate nuclei innervate the contralateral substantia nigra, whereas others located in the fastigial nucleus project mainly in the ipsilateral substantia nigra and to a lesser extent to the contralateral structure. Moreover, Snider and Snider (39) detected slight asymmetric changes in DA levels in the right and left forebrains of rats a few weeks after unilateral electrolytic lesions of some cerebellar nuclei.

These observations led us to examine the effects of a unilateral electrical stimulation of the dentate and fastigial cerebellar nuclei on the release of DA from dopaminergic terminals and dendrites (26). Halothane-anesthetized cats were implanted with four push-pull cannulas to determine the effects of these stimulations on the release of ^{3}H-DA in each caudate nucleus and each substantia nigra. A train of monophasic electric shocks delivered for 10 min at a frequency of 0.2 Hz into the dentate nucleus induced asymmetric effects on ipsilateral and contralateral dopaminergic neurons. An enhanced release of ^{3}H-DA from dopaminergic terminals was associated with a reduction of the dendritic release of the ^{3}H-transmitter in the contralateral dopaminergic pathway. Conversely, a decreased release of ^{3}H-DA from terminals was associated with a stimulation of dendritic release of the ^{3}H-amine in the ipsilateral dopaminergic pathway. These effects were particularly pronounced 10 to 20 min after the end of the stimulus and persisted for at least 60 min. Furthermore, the changes in the dendritic release of ^{3}H-DA were even more striking than those observed in nerve terminals. Different results were obtained when the stimulus was applied in the fastigial nucleus since significant changes in the release of ^{3}H-DA from terminals and dendrites were seen only in the ipsilateral side. However, the responses were similar to that observed in the contralateral side after stimulation of the dentate nucleus: an increased release of ^{3}H-DA from terminals corresponded to a decreased dendritic release of the ^{3}H-transmitter.

These experiments revealed that messages delivered from specific nuclei of the cerebellum influenced in a complex and different way the activity of the two nigrostriatal dopaminergic pathways. They confirmed and extended the original findings of Snider et al. (38) on the relationships between the cerebellar nuclei and the substantia nigra. Indeed, as indicated by the enhanced release of ^{3}H-DA from terminals, the activation of the contralateral dopaminergic pathway induced by the stimulation of the dentate nucleus is likely mediated by the dentate-nigral contralateral projection. On the other hand, the activation of the ipsilateral dopaminergic pathway induced by the stimulation of the fastigial nucleus may involve the ipsilateral projection which connects this nucleus and the ipsilateral substantia nigra. An alternative hypothesis is that these effects are mediated by the thalamostriatal neurons (37,41) or the thalamocorticostriatal neuronal loop (4,20,22,36,42) since fibers originating from both cerebellar nuclei project into the intralaminar nuclei and the nucleus ventralis lateralis of the thalamus (3). This hypothesis may be excluded since in this case similar responses should be observed under stimulation of these two cerebellar nuclei. Moreover, as previously shown, the messages delivered from the motor cortex induced symmetric responses in the two caudate nuclei, and they activate as well the release of ³H-DA from terminals and from dendrites in the ipsilateral dopaminergic neurons. This is in contrast to that observed under stimulation of the cerebellar nuclei.

Reciprocal relationships exist between the two dopaminergic pathways, i.e., the activity of one pathway may be influenced by the activity of the contralateral pathway. Indeed, we have shown that the interruption of the activity of one dopaminergic pathway induced by a nigral electrocoagulation, or a unilateral nigral application of DA, amphetamine, or benztropine stimulates the activity of the contralateral dopaminergic neurons as revealed by the increased release of ³H-DA in the contralateral caudate nucleus (27). Conversely, the activation of one dopaminergic pathway induced by the ipsilateral application of neuroleptics or of serotonin in the substantia nigra reduces the activity of the contralateral dopaminergic neurons. Since no anatomical connection has yet been described between the dentate nucleus and the ipsilateral substantia nigra, the reduced activity of the ipsilateral dopaminergic neurons seen under stimulation of this cerebellar nucleus could result from the direct activation of the contralateral dopaminergic pathway. On this basis, the activation of the ipsilateral dopaminergic pathway evoked by the stimulation of the fastigial nucleus should decrease the activity of the contralateral dopaminergic neurons. However, no significant effects were seen in the contralateral side. This may be related to an antagonistic influence resulting from the activation of the "minor" projection connecting the fastigial nucleus and the contralateral substantia nigra. Further experiments are required to confirm these interpretations. In particular, the mesencephalic connections involved in the relationships between the two dopaminergic pathways must be identified. Polysynaptic neuronal pathways could be implicated, since to our knowledge no direct connection has yet been shown between the two substantia nigrae.

As already mentioned, the increased dendritic release of ³H-DA induced by the unilateral nigral application of amphetamine or benztropine is responsible for the reduced release of ³H-DA from terminals in corresponding dopaminergic neurons as observed after the nigral application of DA. This effect may be mediated through dopaminergic autoreceptors as suggested by electrophysiological microiontophoretic studies (2). In fact, numerous dendrodendritic contacts have been seen in the substantia nigra (9,19); they could be involved in the reciprocal inhibition of the dopaminergic neurons as suggested by Groves et al. (18). Alternatively, the inhibition of the activity of the dopaminergic neurons triggered by the enhanced release of DA from dendrites could be related to an interaction of DA with nigral neuronal afferences. As revealed by the presence of a DA-sensitive adenylate cyclase on terminals of the striatonigral pathways, dopaminergic receptors are located on some of these nigral afferences (13,33). Moreover, DA has been shown to favor the release of GABA in the substantia nigra both *in vitro* in the rat (34) and *in vivo* in the cat (Gauchy and Besson, *unpublished observations*). Therefore, the changes in the dendritic release of ^{3}H-DA induced by the stimulation of the dentate and fastigial cerebellar nuclei may be responsible for the opposite changes in the release of ^{3}H-DA from nerve terminals, i.e., for the changes in the activity of the dopaminergic neurons. In fact, whatever the dopaminergic pathway involved, the increased dendritic release of DA was associated with a reduction of the activity of the dopaminergic neurons (as reflected by the reduced release of ^{3}H-DA from nerve terminals) or vice versa. This hypothesis is further supported by the close similarity of the time courses of the opposite changes in ^{3}H-DA release observed in each substantia nigra and the corresponding caudate nucleus. Moreover, in most cases the effects on the dendritic release of ^{3}H-DA were more pronounced than those observed in nerve terminals. Thus it can be assumed that the changes in the activity of the dopaminergic neurons induced by the stimulation of the dentate or the fastigial nuclei are related to regulatory influences of corresponding cerebellonigral projections on the release of DA from nigral dopaminergic dendrites.

As it will be shown, the effects induced by sensory messages on the dendritic release of DA and on the activity of the two dopaminergic pathways further support these various hypotheses.

CHANGES IN ^{3}H-DA RELEASE FROM DOPAMINERGIC NERVE TERMINALS AND DENDRITES INDUCED BY SENSORY STIMULI

Sensory stimuli were used to further demonstrate the occurrence of simultaneous and opposite changes in the release of DA from dendrites and terminals of corresponding dopaminergic pathways in physiological states (28). Two types of stimuli were selected; the first one consisted of a 10-min electrical stimulation of the paw of the right forelimb in halothane (2%) anesthetized cats. For this purpose, a pair of electrodes was implanted in the paw and the intensity of the stimulus (monophasic square pulses, 4 to 6 V, 0.5 msec, 0.25 Hz) was adjusted just below the threshold of the apparent muscle contraction. The second stimulus consisted of exposing the right eye to a series of light flashes delivered during 10 min with a frequency of 0.2 Hz, the left eye being obturated. In both cases, a significant activation (170% and 130%, respectively) of ^{3}H-DA release was observed in the contralateral substantia nigra when compared to the release of ^{3}H-DA measured in corresponding 10-min superfusate fractions of control animals. This effect was associated with a simultaneous reduction of ^{3}H-DA release from the dopaminergic terminals in the corresponding caudate nucleus. Reverse responses were seen in the ipsilateral side: the reduction of the dendritic release of ^{3}H-DA was associated with an activation of the ^{3}H-amine release from nerve terminals. These effects detected as early as the end of the stimuli persisted from 20 to 40 min at least later on. As observed under stimulation of the cerebellar nuclei, the time courses of the opposite changes in ^{3}H-DA release from dendrites and nerve terminals were similar.

These results confirm that the activity of the dopaminergic neurons (or more precisely the extent of DA release in the caudate nucleus) is inversely correlated to the extent of the dendritic release of the transmitter in several physiological states. They also support our initial observations concerning the reciprocal control of the activity of the dopaminergic pathways (27). As after the unilateral stimulation of the cerebellar dentate nuclei, the unilateral sensory stimuli induced opposite effects on the two dopaminergic pathways. However, in this case, the ipsilateral pathway was activated whereas the activity of the contralateral pathway was reduced. As already discussed, the opposite fluctuations in the activity of the two dopaminergic pathways very likely result from the respective opposite changes in the dendritic release of DA.

Since a balance between the activity of the two dopaminergic pathways is triggered by physical or pharmacological manipulation of the activity of one pathway, the effects induced by unilateral sensory stimuli may be initiated by inputs preferentially delivered to one substantia nigra. However, nearly identical evoked potentials have been recorded in the two substantia nigrae during unilateral somatic or visual stimuli (12). Further electrophysiological studies in which the firing rate of dopaminergic cells is specifically recorded should be made to correlate more precisely electrophysiological and biochemical data. In any case, the asymmetric responses in the activity of the two dopaminergic pathways evoked by the somatic and visual stimuli raised several questions concerning the nature of the polysynaptic pathways involved. Indeed, such results could not have been predicted from the present knowledge of the neuronal circuits thought to be responsible for the delivery of somatic or visual stimuli to the basal ganglia.

There was already some indication that the dopaminergic neurons were affected by sensory stimuli since Portig and Vogt (32) observed an increase in the levels of homovanillic acid in the perfusates of the cat lateral ventricle during electrical stimulation of the paws. Furthermore, the role of the dopaminergic neurons in sensory motor coordination has already been emphasized by recent experiments. Ljungberg and Ungerstedt (23) observed that the unilateral degeneration of the nigrostriatal dopaminergic pathway, which induced a pronounced deviation in movements and posture on the side ipsilateral to the lesion, was associated with a marked deficiency in the ability to orient toward sensory stimuli presented to the contralateral side. The asymmetric responses in the activity of the two dopaminergic pathways induced by unilateral sensory stimuli provide further evidence for a contribution of the dopaminergic neurons in the regulation of sensory motor integration.

CONCLUSION

Several conclusions may be drawn from this series of studies on the reactivity of the two dopaminergic pathways to cortical, cerebellar, or sensory influences:

1. There is little doubt that DA is released from dendrites in the substantia nigra and not from recurrent collaterals of the dopaminergic neurons. The nigral release of DA is not reduced when sodium channels are blocked by tetrodotoxin; moreover, in several circumstances (cerebellar and sensory influences), it is affected in a way which is just the opposite to that observed in corresponding dopaminergic nerve terminals.

2. The changes in the dendritic release of DA seem to govern the activity of the dopaminergic neurons. As indicated by the result obtained under stimulation of various cerebellar nuclei or under somatic or visual stimuli, the extent of DA release from nerve terminals appears to be inversely correlated to the extent of the dendritic release of the transmitter. Neuronal afferences projecting into the substantia nigra may initially control the dendritic release of DA, which is then involved in the control of the activity of the dopaminergic neurons. Several mechanisms may contribute to this local regulatory process. They include the interaction of DA either with autoreceptors or with dopaminergic receptors on some nigral afferences or dendrodendritic contacts between several dopaminergic neurons. Such a model, which may not be the only one involved, will explain the long-term post-effects seen in the changes in ^{3}H-DA release from nerve terminals in the various situations examined. It is also supported by the similarity of the effects induced on the release of DA from nerve terminals by the nigral application of DA or of amphetamine and benztropine and those initiated by cerebellar or sensory influences which directly or indirectly increase the dendritic release of DA.

3. As already reported, interneuronal regulatory processes are involved in a reciprocal control of the activity of the two dopaminergic pathways. They can be triggered by affecting the dendritic release of DA in one substantia nigra. Such a balance between the activity of the two dopaminergic pathways is observed under unilateral sensory stimuli or unilateral stimulation of the cerebellar dentate nuclei, but not under stimulation of motor or visual areas of the cerebral cortex.

4. Besides the nigral local circuits involved in the control of the activity of the two dopaminergic pathways, neuronal circuits may independently contribute to the regulation of DA release from nerve terminals by affecting directly these terminals. This may be the case for the bilateral corticostriatal glutamatergic projection which may synapse on dopaminergic terminals.

5. The two dopaminergic pathways react to unilateral sensory stimuli, to unilateral stimulation of the dentate cerebellar nuclei, or to unilateral stimulation of the motor cortex. This confirms that these neurons are influenced by structures involved in the control of sensory motor functions. However, since

the responses observed in these different situations are different, there is little doubt that in all cases distinct neuronal pathways are involved. The identification of these various pathways and better elucidation of their role in the control of the activity of each dopaminergic pathway in physiological states should contribute to progress in this field.

ACKNOWLEDGMENTS

This research was supported by grants from INSERM (No. 75.5.153.6) and DRME (76,329) and Rhône-Poulenc Company.

REFERENCES

1. Afifi, A. K., Bahuth, N. B., Kaelber, W. W., Mikhael, E., and Nassar, S. (1974): The cortico-nigral fibre tract. An experimental Fink-Heimer study in cats. *J. Anat.*, 118:469–476.
2. Aghajanian, G. K., and Bunney, B. S. (1977): Dopamine "autoreceptors." Pharmacological characterization by microiontophoretic single cell recording studies. *Naunyn-Schmiedeberg's Arch. Pharmacol.*, 297:1–7.
3. Angaut, P., and Bowsher, D. (1970): Ascending projections of medial cerebellar (fastigial) nucleus: An experimental study in the cat. *Brain Res.*, 24:49–68.
4. Carman, J. B., Cowan, W. M., Powell, T. P. S., and Webster, K. E. (1965): A bilateral cortico-striate projection. *J. Neurol. Neurosurg. Psychiatry*, 28:71–77.
5. Chan-Palay, V. (1977): *Cerebellar Dentate Nucleus: Organization, Cytology and Transmitters*, p. 202. Springer-Verlag, Berlin.
6. Chéramy, A., Bioulac, B., Besson, M. J., Vincent, J. D., Glowinski, J., and Gauchy, C. (1975): Radioenzymatic estimation of catecholamines released from the caudate nucleus in the cat and in the monkey. In: *Neuropsychopharmacology*, edited by J. R. Boissier, H. Hippius, and P. Pichot, pp. 493–498. Excerpta Medica, Amsterdam.
7. Chéramy, A., Nieoullon, A., and Glowinski, J. (1978): In vivo changes in dopamine release in the caudate nucleus and the substantia nigra of the cat induced by nigral application of various drugs including GABAergic agonists and antagonists. In: *Interactions Between Putative Neurotransmitters in the Brain*, edited by S. Garattini, J. F. Pujol, and R. Samanin, pp. 175–190. Raven Press, New York.
8. Chéramy, A., Nieoullon, A., Michelot, R., and Glowinski, J. (1977): Effect of intranigral application of dopamine and substance P on the in vivo release of newly synthesized ^{3}H-dopamine in the ipsilateral caudate nucleus of the cat. *Neurosci. Lett.*, 4:105–109.
9. Cuello, A. C., and Iversen, L. L. (1978): Interactions of dopamine with other neurotransmitters in the rat substantia nigra: A possible functional role of dendritic dopamine. In: *Interactions Between Putative Neurotransmitters in the Brain*, edited by S. Garattini, J. F. Pujol, and R. Samanin, pp. 127–149. Raven Press, New York.
10. DeVito, J. L. (1969): Projections from the cerebral cortex to intralaminar nuclei in monkey. *J. Comp. Neurol.*, 136:193–201.
11. Divac, I., Fonnum, F., and Storm-Mathisen, J. (1977): High affinity uptake of glutamate in terminals of cortico-striatal axons. *Nature*, 266:377–378.
12. Feger, J., Ohye, C., Jacquemin, J., and Martin, A. (1974): Mise en évidence chez le chat, d'activités unitaires évoquées dans la substance noire par des stimulations périphériques. *J. Physiol. (Paris)*, 69:247A.
13. Gale, K., Guidotti, A., and Costa, E. (1977): Dopamine-sensitive adenylate cyclase: Location in the substantia nigra. *Science*, 195:503–505.
14. Geffen, L. B., Jessel, T. M., Cuello, A. C., and Iversen, L. L. (1976): Release of dopamine from dendrites in rat substantia nigra. *Nature*, 260:258–260.

15. Giorguieff, M. F., Kemel, M. L., and Glowinski, J. (1977): Presynaptic effect of L-glutamic acid on dopamine release in rat striatal slices. *Neurosci. Lett.,* 6:73–77.
16. Giorguieff, M. F., Le Floc'h, M. L., Glowinski, J., and Besson, M. J. (1977): Involvement of cholinergic presynaptic receptors of nicotinic and muscarinic types in the control of the spontaneous release of dopamine from striatal dopaminergic terminals in the rat. *J. Pharmacol. Exp. Ther.,* 200:535–540.
17. Giorguieff, M. F., Le Floc'h, M. L., Westfall, T. C., Glowinski, J., and Besson, M. J. (1976): Nicotinic effect of acetylcholine on the release of newly synthesized ³H-dopamine in rat striatal slices and cat caudate nucleus. *Brain Res.,* 106:117–131.
18. Groves, P. M., Wilson, C. J., Young, S. J., and Rebec, G. V. (1975): Self inhibition by dopaminergic neurons: An alternative to the "neuronal feedback loop" hypothesis for the mode of action of certain psychotropic drugs. *Science,* 190:522–528.
19. Hadju, F., Hassler, R., and Bak, I. J. (1973): Electron microscopic study of the substantia nigra and the strio-nigral projection in the rat. *Z. Zellforsch.,* 146:207–221.
20. Kemp, J. M., and Powell, T. P. S. (1970): The cortico-striate projections in the monkey, *Brain,* 93:525–546.
21. Korf, J., Zieleman, M., and Westerink, B. H. C. (1976): Dopamine release in substantia nigra? *Nature,* 260:257–258.
22. Kunzle, H. (1975): Bilateral projections from precentral motor cortex to the putamen and other parts of the basal ganglia: An autoradiographic study in Macaca fascicularis. *Brain Res.,* 88:195–209.
23. Ljungberg, T., and Ungerstedt, U. (1976): Sensory inattention produced by 6-hydroxydopamine-induced degeneration of ascending dopamine neurons in the brain. *Exp. Neurol.,* 53:585–600.
24. Nieoullon, A., Chéramy, A., and Glowinski, J. (1977): An adaptation of the push-pull cannula method to study the in vivo release of ³H-dopamine synthesized from ³H-tyrosine in the cat caudate nucleus: Effects of various physical and pharmacological treatments. *J. Neurochem.,* 28:819–828.
25. Nieoullon, A., Chéramy, A., and Glowinski, J. (1977): Release of dopamine in vivo from cat substantia nigra. *Nature,* 266:375–377.
26. Nieoullon, A., Chéramy, A., and Glowinski, J. (1978): Release of dopamine in both caudate nuclei and both substantia nigrae in response to unilateral stimulation of cerebellar nuclei in the cat. *Brain Res. (in press).*
27. Nieoullon, A., Chéramy, A., and Glowinski, J. (1977): Interdependence of the nigrostriatal dopaminergic systems on the two sides of the brain in the cat. *Science,* 198:416–418.
28. Nieoullon, A., Chéramy, A., and Glowinski, J. (1977): Nigral and striatal dopamine release under sensory stimuli. *Nature,* 269:340–342.
29. Nieoullon, A., Chéramy, A., and Glowinski, J. (1978): Release of dopamine evoked by electrical stimulations of the motor and visual areas of the cerebral cortex, in both caudate nuclei and in the substantia nigra in the cat. *Brain Res.,* 145:69–84.
30. Petras, J. M. (1964): Some fiber connections of the precentral cortex (areas 4 and 6) with diencephalon in the monkey (Macaca mulatta) *Anat. Rec.,* 148:322.
31. Pollard, H., Llorens-Cortes, C., and Schwartz, J. C. (1977): Enkephalin receptors on dopaminergic neurons in rat striatum. *Nature,* 268:745–746.
32. Portig, P. J., and Vogt, M. (1969): Release into the cerebral ventricles of substances with possible transmitter function in the caudate nucleus. *J. Physiol. (Lond.),* 204:687–715.
33. Premont, J., Thierry, A. M., Tassin, J. P., Glowinski, J., Blanc, G., and Bockaert, J. (1976): Is the dopamine-sensitive adenylate cyclase in the rat substantia nigra coupled with "autoreceptors"? *F.E.B.S. Lett.,* 68:99–104.
34. Reubi, J. C., Iversen, L. L., and Jessel, T. M. (1977): Dopamine selectively increases ³H-GABA release from slices of rat substantia nigra in vitro. *Nature,* 268:652–654.
35. Rinvik, E. (1966): The cortico-nigral projection in the cat. *J. Comp. Neurol.,* 126:241–254.
36. Rispal-Padel, L., and Massion, J. (1970): Relations between the ventrolateral nucleus and the motor cortex in the cat. *Exp. Brain Res.,* 10:331–339.

37. Simke, J. P., and Saelens, J. K. (1977): Evidence for a cholinergic fiber tract connecting the thalamus with the head of the striatum of the rat. *Brain Res.,* 126:487–495.
38. Snider, R. S., Maiti, A., and Snider, S. R. (1976): Cerebellar pathways to ventral midbrain and nigra. *Exp. Neurol.,* 53:714–728.
39. Snider, S. R., and Snider, R. S. (1977): Alterations in forebrain catecholamine metabolism produced by cerebellar lesions in the rat. *J. Neural Transm.,* 40:115–128.
40. Spencer, H. J. (1976): Antagonism of cortical excitation of striatal neurons by glutamic acid diethyl-ester: Evidence for glutamic acid as an excitatory transmitter in the rat striatum. *Brain Res.,* 102:91–101.
41. Wagner, A., Hassler, R., and Kim, J. S. (1975): Striatal cholinergic enzyme activities following discrete centromedian nucleus lesion in cat thalamus. *Trans. Int. Soc. Neurochem. (Barcelona),* abst. 59, p. 116.
42. Webster, K. E. (1965): The cortico-striatal projection in the cat. *J. Anat.,* 99:329–337.

Advances in Biochemical Psychopharmacology, Vol. 19,
edited by P. J. Roberts et al.
Raven Press, New York © 1978.

Biochemical and Pharmacological Studies on Dopamine Receptors

G. N. Woodruff

*Pharmacology Group, School of Biochemical and Physiological Sciences, University of
Southampton, Southampton S09 3TU England*

In 1957 Blaschko (11) tentatively suggested that dopamine might have
a physiological role in its own right, in addition to its well-known function
as a precursor of norepinephrine and epinephrine. In the same year dopamine
was shown to be present in mammalian brain (19,74,99), and there has
followed a prodigious amount of research on the physiology and pharmacology of this amine. The results of electrophysiological, biochemical, histological, behavioral, and clinical studies have slotted together to build up an im-
pressive array of evidence supporting the role of dopamine as a neurotransmitter. It is not my intention to discuss these results in this chapter, since they
have been fully covered in several excellent reviews (18,54,55,62,64,110).
Instead, I shall concentrate mainly on dopamine receptors, with discussion
on the pharmacology of some drugs believed to act on dopamine receptors.
The review is not intended to be exhaustive, but the emphasis will be mainly
on work carried out at Southampton over the last 10 years.

GENERAL COMMENTS ON DOPAMINE RECEPTORS

Dopamine receptors are components of tissues with which dopamine binds
to elicit a biological response. Since a major function of dopamine appears
to be in the central nervous system, the response may be complex and difficult to quantify. If the receptor is specific for dopamine, then dopamine
should be more potent than chemically related compounds, such as norepinephrine, in eliciting the response. The apparent potency of an agonist may,
of course, be modified, particularly in *in vivo* studies, by tissue uptake or
metabolism. This may become particularly important when comparing the
potency of two compounds which differ in their affinities for uptake sites or
metabolizing enzymes.

There are several reasonably specific antagonists of dopamine available,
and these have proved useful in characterizing dopamine receptors. The
absence of antagonism of a response by a drug such as haloperidol does not,
however, prove that the response is not mediated by dopamine receptors,

89

since it is possible that there might be different types of dopamine receptors, some of which are resistant to blockade by neuroleptic drugs.

In the mammalian brain dopamine is involved as a transmitter in those regions concerned with stereotype behavior and locomotor activity. It is also involved in the regulation of the release of hormones such as prolactin and may have important cortical functions. In man dopamine is implicated in schizophrenia, and dopamine deficiency occurs in Parkinson's disease. Thus, drugs acting on dopamine receptors can be expected to have a variety of central actions and might be of great clinical value.

An ideal test system on which to study the actions of drugs affecting dopamine receptors would be an isolated tissue containing dopamine receptors, the activation of which leads to a readily quantifiable response, but lacking other types of receptors. For work in presynaptic dopamine receptors a tissue which responds to nerve stimulation is required. The absence of an uptake site for dopamine would be an advantage in studying postsynaptic dopamine receptors, since it is known that the apparent potency of catecholamines in tissues is determined not only by their affinity for the receptors but also by their affinity for neuronal uptake sites (57). In practice the ideal situation is never realized, although some progress has been made in recent years. One of the difficulties encountered in the search for dopamine receptors in mammalian peripheral tissues is that these tissues often contain α or β adrenoceptors, and it is known that dopamine will act on both of these types of receptors, although it is considerably less active than epinephrine or norepinephrine in this respect (3,85).

In recent years the existence of receptors for octopamine and phenylethanolamine has been postulated (2,4,93). The possible interaction of dopamine with these receptors and possibly with receptors for additional, related compounds should be considered.

DOPAMINE RECEPTORS IN INVERTEBRATES

Helix Neurons

Effect of Agonists

The isolated brain of the snail *Helix aspersa* is a useful preparation for pharmacological studies. It contains large neurons, some greater than 100 μm in diameter, which are readily penetrated with microelectrodes. The neurons are easily recognizable from one preparation to another, and responses can be measured in terms of membrane depolarization or hyperpolarization, or by conductance measurements. Drugs can be applied by microiontophoresis or by perfusion through the experimental bath, the latter procedure allowing an accurate determination of effective concentrations. Kerkut and Walker (60) first showed that dopamine depressed the firing of some neurons in the snail brain, and there is now good evidence that dopamine is a transmitter in the nervous system of *Helix aspersa* and in related species.

In 1969 Woodruff and Walker (106) studied the structural requirements for dopamine-like activity on specific neurons in the snail brain. The aim of the investigation was to determine whether or not specific dopamine receptors did in fact exist, and to evaluate the potential usefulness of this preparation as a model by which to study the actions of drugs which might affect the mammalian brain. At this time there were no available *in vitro* models containing dopamine receptors.

In an initial survey it was established that whereas some neurons in the snail brain are inhibited by dopamine, other cells are excited by this compound and many neurons are unaffected even by high concentrations. We worked mainly on a group of neurons in the right parietal ganglion; on these cells low concentrations of dopamine caused a powerful inhibition of firing, with hyperpolarization of the resting potential. Dopamine and dopamine analogues were applied by addition to the bath. The potency of the compounds was expressed as the equipotent molar ratio (EPMR), which is the amount of compound (moles) required to produce the same degree of inhibition as 1 mole dopamine. When the actions of potential antagonists were studied, the dopamine was usually applied iontophoretically from a second electrode positioned close to the neuron.

An example of responses produced by dopamine and epinephrine is shown in Fig. 1. It was concluded that the receptor mediating the inhibitory actions

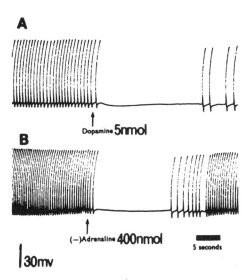

FIG. 1. Intracellular recording from a neuron in the right parietal ganglion of *Helix aspersa*. In A, addition of dopamine (5 nmoles) caused hyperpolarization and inhibition. In B, which is a recording from the same cell, epinephrine (400 nmoles) caused a similar inhibition.

of dopamine was quite unlike either an α or a β adrenoreceptor, since the α stimulant $(-)$-phenylephrine and the β stimulant isoprenaline were completely inactive in concentrations 2,000 times greater than the effective concentrations of dopamine. $(-)$-Norepinephrine and $(-)$-epinephrine were approximately 25 and 92 times less active than dopamine, respectively, on the *Helix* dopamine receptor (100,106). Further details of the structure-activity studies will be referred to in a later section. Essentially similar results on *Helix* neurons were later reported by Struyker Boudier et al. (92), who, for example, found $(-)$-norepinephrine and $(-)$-epinephrine to be, respectively, 18 and 80 times less active than dopamine. One surprising finding from our original survey was that apomorphine, which was suggested by Ernst (38) as a dopamine receptor stimulant and is now often regarded as the prototype of dopaminergic agonists, had no dopamine-like activity on the *Helix* dopamine receptor (100,106). It has more recently been shown that in fact apomorphine behaves as an antagonist in this system.

As a result of our studies on the *Helix* dopamine receptor, Woodruff (100) postulated a model of the dopamine receptor which took into account the then known structural requirements for activity at dopamine receptors (Fig. 2). It was suggested that the rigid analogue of dopamine, 2-amino-6,7-dihydroxy-1,2,3,4-tetrahydronaphthalene, would behave as a dopamine agonist on the proposed receptor (100). This compound had previously been synthesized (94) in a search for β-adrenoceptor stimulants, but had not been subjected to any detailed pharmacological analysis and had certainly not been tested on any dopaminergic systems. 2-Amino-6,7-dihydroxy-1,2,3,4-tetrahydronaphthalene was kindly synthesized for me by Dr. Roger Pinder, and more recently the compound has been generously supplied by Dr. John McDermed. In our earlier studies with 2-amino-6,7-dihydroxy-1,2,3,4-tetrahydronaphthalene we referred to the compound as ADTN. In a more recent investigation, in which we have compared the actions of a series

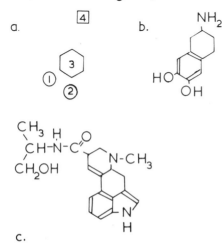

FIG. 2. A: Hypothetical model of dopamine receptor. Sites 1 and 2 represent hydroxyl binding sites. Site 3 is an aromatic ring binding site. Site 4 is a nitrogen binding site. B: The structure of 2-amino-6,7-dihydroxy-1,2,3,4-tetrahydronaphthalene, which is a dopamine agonist on the proposed receptor. Modified from Woodruff (100). C: The structure of ergometrine.

of 2-amino-1,2,3,4-tetrahydronaphthalene derivatives, we were persuaded on the good advice of the editor of the *Journal of Pharmacy and Pharmacology* to abbreviate the same compound to 6,7 diOHATN. In this chapter, for sentimental reasons, I shall refer to it as ADTN. ADTN has since been shown to act as a potent agonist at dopamine receptors in a wide range of tissues. In this section I shall simply mention that ADTN is a potent full agonist at the dopamine receptors mediating inhibition of *Helix aspersa* neurons (77).

As has already been mentioned, in addition to the neurons that are inhibited by dopamine, there are a second group of cells in *Helix* on which dopamine has an excitatory action, causing depolarization and an increase in the firing rate. The structure-activity requirements for dopamine-like activity on these cells have now been studied, and it has been claimed that the dopamine receptors mediating the excitatory actions of dopamine on these cells are different from those mediating inhibition (92). On the other hand, Swann and Carpenter (93), working with *Aplysia,* suggest that the dopamine receptors mediating inhibition are identical to those on cells excited by dopamine. ADTN is a potent agonist in mimicking both the excitatory and inhibitory actions of dopamine (77).

Effect of Antagonists

A second unpredictable finding from our studies with *Helix* was that the neuroleptic drugs haloperidol and chlorpromazine, regarded as dopamine receptor antagonists, had no blocking actions on dopamine-evoked inhibitions (100,107,108). The findings were subsequently confirmed (92), although Heiss and Hoyer (50) have reported that in *Aplysia* the inhibitory action of dopamine can be antagonized by prolonged perfusion (8 to 40 min) with haloperidol 50 μM. In our hands this concentration of haloperidol is liable to produce nonspecific membrane effects. The more potent neuroleptics such as α-flupenthixol and fluphenazine are able to antagonize the inhibitory action of dopamine in *Helix* and in *Aplysia,* although the compounds are not particularly potent in this respect (4,50), and the specificity of the antagonists has not been fully investigated.

The most potent dopamine antagonists on invertebrate dopamine receptors are derivatives of lysergic acid. The first such compound to be described was ergometrine, which in nanomolar concentrations was found to produce a long-lasting block of the dopamine inhibitory response in *Helix* (98,100, 108). An example of the blocking action of ergometrine is illustrated in Fig. 3. Although it is a potent dopamine antagonist, ergometrine has little or no α-blocking activity (14). It has subsequently been shown that ergometrinine is inactive as a dopamine antagonist (107). The ergot alkaloids ergotamine and ergotoxine are also dopamine antagonists on *Helix* neurons, although they are less active than ergometrine in this respect (98). In 1971 Woodruff

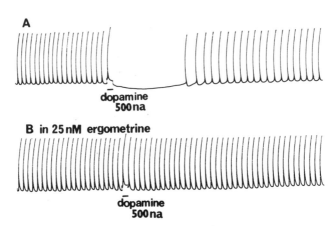

FIG. 3. Antagonism by ergometrine of the dopamine response in *Helix aspersa*. A and B are intracellular recordings from the same neuron. In A the iontophoretic application of dopamine (500 nA for 1 sec) caused hyperpolarization and inhibition. In B in the presence of 25 nM ergometrine the dopamine response was completely abolished.

et al. (107) showed that lysergic acid diethylamide (LSD) was also a potent, long-lasting antagonist of the inhibitory action of dopamine in the snail brain, a finding which raised the possibility that some of the central actions of LSD in mammals could be brought about by an action on dopamine receptors. The later finding that both LSD and ergometrine can affect mammalian central dopamine receptors strengthens support for the suggestion that the isolated brain of *Helix aspersa* is of value as a test organ on which to study the actions of drugs acting on dopamine receptors. The actions of ergometrine on mammalian dopamine receptors will be discussed in a later section. It is worth noting now, however, that both ergometrine and LSD have behavioral actions in rats which indicate that both are agonists at central dopamine receptors. On the adenylate cyclase system ergometrine and also apomorphine behave as partial agonists and thus have agonistic and antagonistic activity. It is particularly interesting, therefore, that ergometrine has been shown to have slight agonistic activity on *Aplysia* neurons (1), in addition to its powerful blocking activity. It would be of great interest to test apomorphine and LSD on *Helix* neurons under voltage clamp conditions to see whether any slight agonistic activity of these compounds could be uncovered.

Cockroach Salivary Gland

Salivary glands of the cockroach (*Nauphoeta cinerea Olivier*) have provided a useful *in vitro* preparation for the study of dopamine-like drugs (43,56). The glands can be dissected out and intracellular recordings obtained from the salivary glands. The addition of dopamine to the preparation causes a powerful hyperpolarization. The preparation has an added advantage over other available test systems in that it can be dissected out with an intact nerve input. The stimulation of the nerve results, after a delay of about 1 sec, in a frequency-dependent hyperpolarization in the salivary gland cells. There is good evidence that this evoked hyperpolarization is due to the release of dopamine. Ginsborg et al. (43) studied the actions of some dopamine-like compounds on this preparation. The only active compounds tested were those in which there were unsubstituted hydroxyl groups, a situation that is identical to that obtained on dopamine receptors in other species. Of particular interest is the finding that the dopamine agonist ADTN is equipotent with dopamine in causing hyperpolarizations in this preparation and that the neuroleptic α-flupenthixol blocks both the effects of dopamine and the hyperpolarizations induced by nerve stimulation (56).

DOPAMINE RECEPTORS IN THE MAMMALIAN PERIPHERAL SYSTEM

Dopamine-induced Vasodilatation

In addition to its known activity at α adrenoceptors, dopamine causes changes in the cardiovascular system that are quite distinct from those produced by either norepinephrine or isoprenaline. Holtz and Credner (52) showed that in the guinea pig and rabbit, dopamine caused a fall in the arterial blood pressure. A similar depressor action has been reported following the infusion of low doses of dopamine into other species (44), the effect being particularly prominent following the administration of α blockers. The depressor action of dopamine is not blocked by α or β blockers (85). We have shown that ADTN has a potent, dopamine-like depressor action on the guinea pig blood pressure (103), and that the effects of both dopamine and ADTN can be reduced by ergometrine.

Eble (34) showed that the depressor action of dopamine is due to a vasodilatation in the superior mesenteric, renal, and celiac beds, and he suggested that there might be specific dopamine receptors mediating vasodilatation. Goldberg and his colleagues (44,46) have carried out an extensive study of the receptors involved in the dopamine-induced renal and mesenteric vasodilatation and have produced good evidence for the existence of a specific dopamine receptor in these regions. Apomorphine is less active than dopamine in causing dopamine-like vasodilatation and in addition has some antagonistic activity toward dopamine, suggesting that it might be a partial agonist (45,46). ADTN, on the other hand, is more active than dopamine in causing vasodilatation in the renal and mesenteric vascular beds (30).

The vasodilator actions of dopamine can be antagonized both by neuroleptics and by ergot alkaloids. Haloperidol and spiramide have both been shown to block the depressor action of dopamine in cats treated with yohimbine (85), and haloperidol blocks the vasodilator actions of both dopamine and ADTN in the dog kidney, although the blocking action of this neuroleptic is fairly transient (30). Chlorpromazine blocks the renal vasodilatation produced by dopamine without affecting that caused by isoprenaline (13).

Bell and his colleagues have studied the vasodilator action of dopamine in the femoral and renal vasculatures. In contrast to an earlier report in which it was supposed that dopamine causes vasodilatation of the canine femoral bed by an action on β receptors (70), it has been suggested that the femoral vasculature contains specific dopamine receptors (6). Ergometrine appears to be a selective antagonist of dopamine at these receptors and at the dopamine receptors in the dog renal vasculature (5,6). Indeed, on the basis of antagonism by ergometrine it has recently been suggested that β stimulants such as isoprenaline may cause vasodilatation within the canine kidney at least in part by stimulating dopamine receptors (7). Other studies have, however, revealed little direct effect of isoprenaline on dopamine receptors.

Other Peripheral Dopamine Receptors

There is evidence that dopamine has a physiological role in other peripheral systems, for example, in the carotid body and at sympathetic ganglia. The carotid body contains appreciable amounts of dopamine (32,40) where it is present in type 1 cells (9). It has been suggested that dopamine released from cells in the carotid body functions physiologically to inhibit chemoreceptor activity (86). There is evidence that the inhibition produced by dopamine is due to a direct hyperpolarizing action on chemoreceptor afferent nerve endings (87). Details of the pharmacological receptors are not known, although the action of dopamine is reduced or abolished by droperidol (87).

Dopamine-containing neurons are present in sympathetic ganglia (10) where dopamine may be the transmitter responsible for generating the slow inhibitory postsynaptic potential (48,65). On the other hand, electrophysiological measurements have allowed Dun and Nishi (33) to conclude that the depression of ganglionic transmission produced by dopamine in the superior cervical ganglion is exerted primarily through presynaptic inhibition, causing a decrease in the amount of acetylcholine released. The postsynaptic effect of dopamine was said to play only a secondary role in the blockade of ganglionic transmission (33). The same authors reported that dopamine was less active than either epinephrine or norepinephrine in depressing the size of the excitatory postsynaptic potential (EPSP) (33). Greengard (48,66,67) and his colleagues have studied the actions of dopamine on the adenylate cyclase in sympathetic ganglia.

The effects of ADTN have not yet been studied on the above two systems.

Such a study might provide information on the possible physiological role for dopamine at these sites. We have studied the actions on ADTN on some peripheral isolated tissues. ADTN has weak α-adrenoceptor stimulating activity, and it can release norepinephrine from sympathetic nerve endings.

DOPAMINE RECEPTORS IN MAMMALIAN CNS

Iontophoretic Studies

The technique of microiontophoresis has been used to study the action of dopamine in several regions of the mammalian brain (64,110). In the striatum of rats or cats the major action of dopamine is to cause depression of firing (12,21,39,47,69,90). On the other hand, Spencer and Havlicek (91) and Bevan et al. (8) have reported a considerable proportion of striatal neurons to be excited by dopamine. In our own studies we have found that the overwhelming majority of striatal cells affected by dopamine are depressed by this compound (29,105). We have also shown that neurons in the rat nucleus accumbens are similarly depressed by dopamine (Fig. 4). Recently Kitai et al. (61) suggested that the depressant action of dopamine in the striatum might be due to dopamine causing an excitation of inhibitory interneurons. We have studied the specificity of the dopamine response in both caudate nucleus and nucleus accumbens of the rat. Extracellular recordings were made from neurons and drugs were applied microiontophoretically using standard electrophysiological techniques. Neurons were either spontaneously active or were driven by the continuous iontophoretic application of DL-homocysteic acid. The activity of neurons in both the nucleus accumbens and the striatum was consistently depressed by γ-aminobutyric acid, glycine, or dopamine. Glutamate and aspartate caused excitation of all cells onto which they were applied. Strychnine (60 nA for 4 min) antagonized the action of glycine but did not affect the responses to either γ-aminobutyric acid or dopamine. Picrotoxin blocked the inhibitory action of γ-aminobutyric acid but did not affect the responses to glycine or dopamine.

NUCLEUS ACCUMBENS

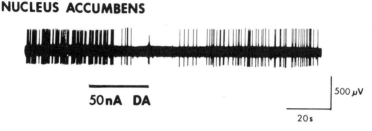

50 nA   DA

500 μV

20 s

FIG. 4. Effect of dopamine on the activity of a neuron in the nucleus accumbens of a rat anesthetized with urethane. Spikes were recorded extracellularly using a six-barrelled microelectrode. The cell was stimulated to fire by the continuous application of DL-homocysteic acid (2 nA). Figure retouched.

On the other hand, the neuroleptic α-flupenthixol selectively blocked the depressant action of dopamine on 9 out of 20 neurons in the caudate nucleus and on 12 of the 22 cells tested in the nucleus accumbens (68). These results suggest that although γ-aminobutyric acid and glycine might have a functional role in the nucleus accumbens and caudate nucleus, it is unlikely that they are involved in mediating the depressant action of dopamine in these two regions of the brain.

Whatever the mechanism by which dopamine causes depression of firing of the cells in the striatum or nucleus accumbens, this action is mimicked by the dopamine agonist ADTN and also by ergometrine (105).

Dopamine-sensitive Adenylate Cyclase

Studies on dopamine receptors in the central nervous system were greatly facilitated following the discovery that homogenates of rat striatum contain an adenylate cyclase that is stimulated by low concentrations of dopamine (59). Dopamine will also stimulate cyclic AMP production in striatal slices (76). It has been suggested that the actions of dopamine in the brain are mediated by increased synthesis of cyclic AMP, and that the dopamine receptor might be closely linked to adenylate cyclase (48,58,59). Dopamine-sensitive adenylate cyclases are present in several regions of the nervous system (15,20,53,59,78). Homogenates of striatum from rats with lesions in the substantia nigra have been reported to show enhancement of dopamine-stimulated adenylate cyclase activity, suggesting a biochemical basis for denervation supersensitivity (73). Other workers, however, have been unable to demonstrate an effect of denervation on dopamine-sensitive adenylate cyclase in striatal homogenates (63,97), although an enhanced sensitivity to dopamine was found in striatal slices (63). These studies, all at least showing no decreased adenylate cyclase activity in lesioned animals, show that the dopamine-stimulated adenylate cyclase is not located on presynaptic dopaminergic terminals and may therefore be on postsynaptic membranes. However, in a recent study, Henn et al. (51) have provided some interesting results which indicate that at least some of the dopamine-sensitive adenylate cyclase in bovine caudate nucleus, together with some haloperidol binding sites, is located on glial cells. The presence of dopamine receptors on glial cells would have fascinating physiological implications and might explain some of the differences between electrophysiological and biochemical studies on dopamine receptors.

The striatal dopamine-sensitive adenylate cyclase has been successfully used as a model on which to study the actions of drugs believed to act on dopamine receptors. We, in our laboratory, have used this model to study the structural requirements for dopamine-like activity in rat striatum and nucleus accumbens. The aim of this work was to investigate the possibility that the dopamine receptors in the nucleus accumbens might differ from those in the striatum, and also to compare the requirements for dopamine-like activity in the mammalian brain with those previously determined in invertebrates. As an extension of the structure-activity studies, we have also investigated the ability of a series of 2-amino-1,2,3,4-tetrahydronaphthalene derivatives, related to ADTN to stimulate dopamine receptors in both nucleus accumbens and striatum.

Male or female Wistar rats (about 300 g) were anesthetized with ether. The neostriatum and nucleus accumbens were dissected out using standard methods (53,59). The activity of adenylate cyclase was estimated by the method of Kebabian et al. (59). All drugs were freshly dissolved in 5 mM tartaric acid and added in a constant volume (10 μl) to the assay mixture. The reaction was started by the addition of ATP to a final concentration of 0.5 mM. The reactions were carried out for 2.5 min (striatum) or 3 min (nucleus accumbens) at 30°C. After the reaction was terminated by placing the tube in a boiling water bath for 2.5 min, the mixture was centrifuged and the cyclic AMP formed was assayed using a muscle-binding protein assay (42).

Effect of Dopamine

In the absence of dopamine the basal levels of cyclic AMP production were 40 pmoles/assay tube by homogenates of striatum and 50 pmoles/tube by homogenates of nucleus accumbens. These values were increased to about 76 and 80 pmoles/tube, respectively, in the presence of 100 μM dopamine. The dose-response relationships for dopamine-induced stimulation of cyclic AMP production are illustrated in Fig. 5. Similar effects of dopamine were obtained with homogenates of nucleus accumbens. The EC$_{50}$ values for dopamine (concentration causing 50% of maximum response) were 3.5 μM for striatal homogenates and 6.0 μM for homogenates of nucleus accumbens. Similar values have been obtained in other studies (53,59,72).

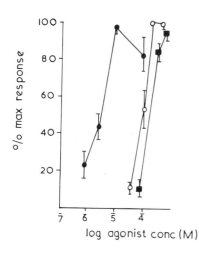

FIG. 5. Effect of drugs on dopamine-sensitive adenylate cyclase in homogenates of rat striatum. Responses are expressed as a percentage of the maximum response which was taken as that produced by 10 μM dopamine. Closed circles, dopamine; open circles, 3,4-dihydroxy-5-methoxyphenylethylamine; squares, (−)-epinephrine.

Effect of Phenylethylamine Derivatives

The dose-response relationships for $(-)$-epinephrine and for 3,4-di-hydroxy-5-methoxyphenylethylamine are shown in Fig. 5. It can be seen that whereas both compounds produced the same maximum response as dopamine, both compounds were considerably less active than dopamine. Similar results were obtained in homogenates of nucleus accumbens. The potency of the various phenylethylamine derivatives in both striatum and nucleus accumbens is summarized in Table 1. Potency is expressed as the equipotent molar ratio calculated from EC_{50} concentrations. For purposes of comparison the relative potencies of the same compounds on dopamine receptors in the snail brain are also shown. It can be seen that there is a close similarity between the relative potencies of the compounds on the three systems, indicating a similarity between the receptors.

The only active phenylethylamine derivatives on all three systems were those in which there were hydroxyl groups in both the 3 and 4 positions of the benzene ring. The importance of the hydroxyl group in the 4 position was emphasized by the demonstration that $(-)$-phenylephrine was inactive. Furthermore 3-hydroxy-4,5-dimethoxyphenylethylamine and 3,5-dihydroxy-4-methoxyphenylethylamine were both inactive, whereas 3,4-dihydroxy-5-methoxyphenylethylamine was an effective agonist on the dopamine-sensitive adenylate cyclase in both nucleus accumbens and in the striatum (Table 1). A hydroxyl group in the 3 position is also essential for dopamine-like activity, as indicated by the lack of activity of tyramine. The dopamine receptors in the nucleus accumbens and striatum are quite unlike α or β adrenoceptors, since both phenylephrine and isoprenaline are inactive. Also, in contrast to the situation at α or β receptors, the presence of a hydroxyl group on the carbon β to the terminal nitrogen reduced dopamine-like activity, norepinephrine and epinephrine being less active than dopamine and epinine.

Ergometrine and Apomorphine

In the original experiments of Kebabian et al. (59), showing that apomorphine stimulates the dopamine-sensitive adenylate cyclase in homogenates of rat striatum, the maximum response produced by apomorphine was considerably less than that produced by dopamine. Miller et al. (72) obtained similar results showing that the maximum response to apomorphine in the striatum was less than 50% of the maximum dopamine response. In our own experiments with homogenates of nucleus accumbens, the maximum response to apomorphine was similarly less than 50% of the dopamine maximum (G. N. Woodruff, K. J. Watling, and J. A. Poat, *unpublished observations*).

The action of ergometrine is similar to that of apomorphine in both

TABLE 1. *Structures and relative potencies of some compounds on dopamine receptors in 3 different systems*

Structure	Potency (EPMR) Adenylate cyclase		Helix neurons
	Nucleus accumbens	Striatum	
HO–⟨ ⟩(HO)–$CH_2 \cdot CH_2 \cdot NH_2$	2	1	1
HO–⟨ ⟩(HO)–$CH_2 \cdot CH_2 \cdot NH \cdot CH_3$	1	1	1
HO–⟨ ⟩(HO)–$\overset{OH}{CH} \cdot CH_2 \cdot NH_2$	8	24	25
HO–⟨ ⟩(HO)–$\overset{OH}{CH}CH_2 \cdot NH \cdot CH_3$	16	63	92
CH_3O–⟨ ⟩(HO)–$CH_2 \cdot CH_2 \cdot NH_2$	44	30	17
CH_3O–⟨ ⟩(HO,HO)–$CH_2 \cdot CH_2 \cdot NH_2$	In	In	In
HO–⟨ ⟩–$CH_2 \cdot CH_2 \cdot NH_2$	In	—	In
HO–⟨ ⟩(HO)–$\overset{OH}{CH} \cdot CH_2 \cdot NH \cdot CH(CH_3)_2$	In	In	In
⟨ ⟩(HO,HO)–$\overset{OH}{CH} \cdot CH_2 \cdot NH \cdot CH_3$	In	In	In
CH_3O–⟨ ⟩(HO,CH_3O)–$CH_2 \cdot CH_2 \cdot NH_2$	In	In	In

On the adenylate cyclase system potency is expressed as the EPMR relative to dopamine in the striatum. EPMR is thus the EC_{50} of agonist in either the accumbens or striatum/EC_{50} dopamine in striatum. Values are from refs. 75 and 77, and from Woodruff et al. (*unpublished observations*). Potencies on snail neurons are from ref. 106.

In, inactive.

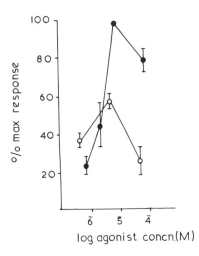

FIG. 6. Effect of ergometrine (*open circles*) and dopamine (*closed circles*) on dopamine-sensitive adenylate cyclase in homogenates of rat striatum. Responses are expressed as a percentage of the maximum which was taken as that produced by 10 μM dopamine. (From G. N. Woodruff, K. J. Watling, and J. A. Poat, *unpublished observations*.)

striatum and nucleus accumbens. In 1975 we showed (35) that ergometrine caused an increase in cyclic AMP levels in rat striatal slices. We have since shown that ergometrine behaves as a partial agonist on dopamine receptors associated with adenylate cyclase in homogenates of both striatum (77) and nucleus accumbens (Woodruff et al., *unpublished observations*). An example of the effect of ergometrine on striatal adenylate cyclase is shown in Fig. 6. Similar results with ergometrine were obtained by Schorderet (88) in the isolated retinas of the rabbit.

Conformational Studies Using 2-Amino-1,2,3,4-Tetrahydronaphthalene Derivatives and Norsalsolinol

In solution dopamine can exist in extended (anti) or folded (gauche) conformations (16,83). In the extended conformation there is the possibility of rotation about the phenyl-carbon bond, which leads to the existence of two rotameric extremes, α and β (17). We have been interested for some time in investigating the active conformation of dopamine at its receptor site. The approach we have used is to study the actions of rigid analogues of dopamine which contain the dopamine side chain locked in a fixed formation. Thus, norsalsolinol contains the dopamine skeleton in a folded conformation (Fig. 7), whereas the extended conformations of dopamine are contained in the molecules of ADTN (β rotamer) and 2-amino-5,6-dihydroxy-1,2,3,4-tetrahydronaphthalene (α rotamer) (see Fig. 7). As already mentioned, in a previous review by the present author (100) it was suggested that the active conformation of dopamine corresponds to the dopamine residue contained in the residue of ADTN, that is the extended conformation, β rotamer. Support for this hypothesis has come from studies using the INDO molecular orbital method, in which it has been shown that

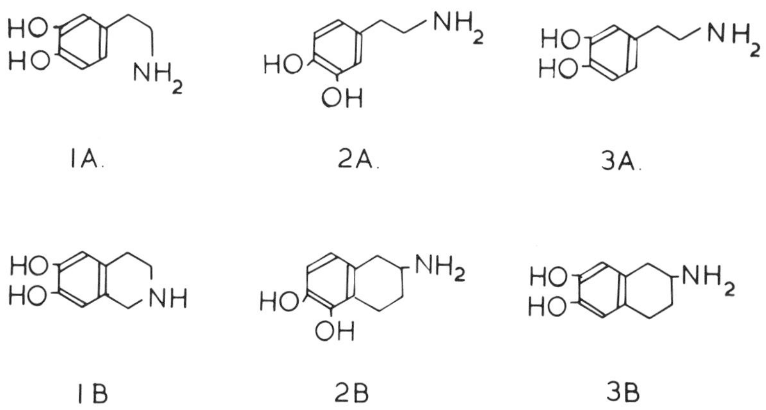

IA.   2A.   3A.

I B   2B   3B

FIG. 7. Conformations of dopamine and the structure of 3 rigid analogues. Dopamine can exist in the folded conformation (1A), which corresponds to the molecule of norsalsolinol (1B). In the extended form dopamine can exist as two rotameric extremes, α (2A) and β (3A). The dopamine residue in the extended conformations is contained in the molecules 2-amino-5,6,-dihydroxy-1,2,3,4,-tetrahydronaphthalene (2B) and ADTN (3B), respectively.

ADTN with the amino group in the equatorial position corresponds to an energetically favorable dopamine conformation (49). We have now directly tested the hypothesis by comparing the potencies of norsalsolinol, ADTN, and 2-amino-5,6-dihydroxy-1,2,3,4-tetrahydronaphthalene in the adenylate cyclase from rat striatum and nucleus accumbens. For purposes of comparison we have also tested the effects of some additional 2-amino-1,2,3,4-tetrahydronaphthalene derivatives.

TABLE 2. Potencies of dopamine and of some 2-amino-1,2,3,4-tetrahydronaphthalene derivatives on the dopamine-sensitive adenylate cyclase from rat striatum and nucleus accumbens

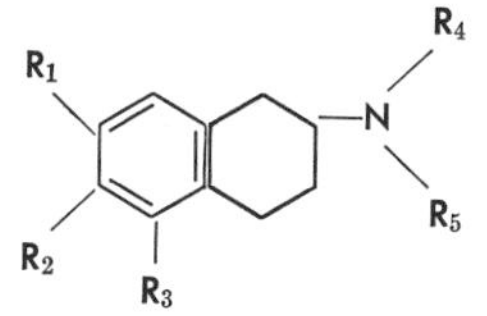

Compound	R_1	R_2	R_3	R_4	R_5	EPMR Nucleus accumbens	EPMR Striatum
1. ADTN	HO	HO	H	H	H	0.1	0.6
2.	H	HO	HO	H	H	40	33
3.	H	HO	HO	Me	Me	66	100
4.	H	HO	HO	Et	Et	18	43
5.	MeO	MeO	H	H	H	I	I
6.	H	MeO	MeO	H	H	I	I

Potencies are expressed as the equipotent molar ratios (EPMR) relative to dopamine in the nucleus accumbens. The EPMR is thus defined as EC_{50} for agonist in either striatum or nucleus accumbens/EC_{50} for dopamine in nucleus accumbens. I, inactive at 500 μM. Taken from ref. 109 and Woodruff et al. (*unpublished observations*).

Previous work in our laboratories (35,76,77) and in others (72) has shown that ADTN is equipotent with dopamine in stimulating rat striatal adenylate cyclase. Similar results have now been obtained in our latest investigation (109).

We have also extended our studies to include the dopamine-sensitive adenylate cyclase in homogenates of nucleus accumbens. ADTN mimicked the action of dopamine in homogenates of both the striatum (Table 2) and nucleus accumbens (Fig. 8), producing maximum responses that were identical to those of dopamine. On the other hand, norsalsolinol was less active, and this compound failed to produce a maximum response (Fig. 8). In terms of the EC_{50} values, ADTN was approximately equipotent with dopamine in the striatum and more potent than dopamine in homogenates of nucleus accumbens. It is of interest that the potency of ADTN in striatal adenylate cyclase (EC_{50} 3 μM) correlates well with our direct binding studies in which we have measured the binding of ^3H-ADTN to purified synaptic membranes from rat striatum (K_d 1.2 μM) (84).

In contrast to ADTN, 2-amino-5,6-dihydroxy-1,2,3,4-tetrahydronaphthalene was considerably less active than dopamine. ADTN was more than 50 times more active than 2-amino-5,6-dihydroxy-1,2,3,4-tetrahydronaphthalene in the striatum and more than 350 times more active in the nucleus accumbens. The results obtained with these and other compounds are summarized in Table 2, from which it can be seen that both 2-amino-5,6-dimethoxy-1,2,3,4-tetrahydronaphthalene and 2-amino-6,7-dimethoxy-1,2,3,4-tetrahydronaphthalene were inactive on the adenylate cyclase assays. This further emphasizes the importance of two unsubstituted hydroxyl groups for dopamine-like activity.

The effects of dopamine, ADTN, and a selection of the other agonists used were all antagonized by fluphenazine (Table 3), suggesting that the effects measured were mediated by dopamine receptors. Fluphenazine and other neuroleptics are potent antagonists of dopamine on dopamine-sensitive adenylate cyclase (20,58,71).

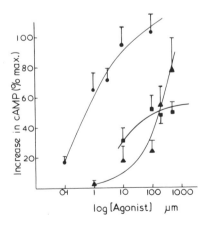

FIG. 8. Effect of rigid analogues of dopamine on the dopamine-sensitive adenylate cyclase in rat nucleus accumbens. The response is expressed as the percentage of the maximum response which was taken as that produced by 10 μM dopamine. Circles, ADTN; triangles, 2-amino-5,6-dihydroxy-1,2,3,4-tetrahydronaphthalene; squares, norsalsolinol. (From G. N. Woodruff, K. J. Watling, and J. A. Poat, *unpublished observations*.)

TABLE 3. Effect of fluphenazine (1 μM) on the response produced by some agonists on dopamine-sensitive adenylate cyclase in striatal homogenates

Compound	Response (% max) −Fluphen	+Fluphen	% Inhibition produced by fluphenazine
Dopamine	100	9.4 ± 4.9 (8)	89
ADTN (100 μM)	82.5 ± 8.5 (4)	24.7 ± 11.3 (4)	70
2 (500 μM)	44.0 ± 4.0 (4)	1.0 ± 1.0 (6)	98
4 (500 μM)	48.3 ± 16.0 (4)	10.3 ± 4.2 (6)	79

Responses are expressed as the % of the response produced by 100 μM dopamine which was tested in parallel in every experiment. The numbers in parentheses refer to the number of observations. Standard errors of mean are indicated (from ref. 109). Compound number refers to Table 2.

Behavioral Studies

Locomotor Stimulation

Following our work on the potent blocking action of ergometrine on invertebrate dopamine receptors, it was decided to study the effects of ergometrine on mammalian dopamine receptors using the technique of microinjection into dopamine-rich regions of the brain. The initial studies were carried out in Nijmegen with the excellent collaboration of A. J. J. Pijnenburg and J. M. van Rossum. Stainless steel cannulas were implanted bilaterally into regions of the rat brain under pentobarbitone anesthesia. Following a 2-week recovery period, injections were made down the cannulas using a 5-μl Hamilton syringe. The injection volume was usually 0.5 μl. The motor activity of the rats was measured using conventional activity meters of the light beam type. The bilateral injection of ergometrine into the nucleus accumbens of conscious rats caused a strong and long-lasting (up to 8 hr) stimulation of motor activity, following a delay of 30 to 60 min. This response was consistently produced by ergometrine 2 μg each side, and in some animals as little as 0.1 μg ergometrine bilaterally was effective in stimulating activity. The motor stimulation produced by ergometrine was blocked by haloperidol or pimozide but not by treatment with the tyrosine hydroxylase inhibitor α-methyl-p-tyrosine. Ergometrine injected bilaterally into the caudate nucleus of conscious rats was much less effective in producing locomotor stimulation. Injections into the septum were completely without effect. These results led us to suggest (82) that the nucleus accumbens might be important in the control of motor activity and that the locomotor stimulation caused by ergometrine might be due to a direct action of this alkaloid on dopamine receptors.

In a series of subsequent studies concerned with the injections of drugs into the nucleus of accumbens of conscious rats, it has been shown that a variety of drugs presumed to act on dopamine receptors will also cause stimulation of motor activity. These drugs include dopamine (24,80,81;

C. Andrews and G. N. Woodruff, *unpublished observations*), other phenyl-ethylamine derivatives (26,79), and isoquinoline derivatives (27). Many of these experiments were carried out in rats pretreated with a monoamine oxidase inhibitor, since dopamine, for example, is much less active in un-treated animals (81). It is of course possible that drugs causing locomotor stimulation could do so by actions other than a direct action on dopamine receptors. For example, the drugs could release dopamine from presynaptic terminals; such an action might become particularly important in rats treated with monoamine oxidase inhibitors. Thus, although such behavioral experiments are of great importance, caution should be exercised before interpreting results from such studies in terms of dopamine receptor mechanisms.

In 1975 we showed that ADTN, injected into the lateral cerebral ventricles of conscious mice, causes a long-lasting stimulation of motor activity (103). We have since reported that ADTN injected bilaterally into the nucleus accumbens of conscious rats has a similarly powerful locomotor stimulant effect, the stimulation lasting for from 15 to 20 hr after injection (36). This effect of ADTN was blocked by pretreatment with either haloperidol or pimozide. The ADTN analogue 2-amino-6,7-dimethoxy-1,2,3,4-tetra-hydronaphthalene, which has no effect on dopamine receptors, failed to enhance motor activity following bilateral injections into the nucleus ac-cumbens. ADTN injected bilaterally into the caudate nucleus was similarly ineffective as a locomotor stimulant. In an additional series of experiments we have shown that the injection of a higher dose (600 nmoles) of ADTN into the lateral ventricles of conscious rats has a potent locomotor stimulant action; this response to ADTN is much reduced in rats with bilateral electro-lytic lesions of the nucleus accumbens, but is unaffected in rats with bilateral electrolytic lesions in the caudate nucleus (104). These results support our original suggestion that the nucleus accumbens is of major importance in drug-induced locomotor stimulation. ADTN should be a useful compound in studies on the role of dopamine in the brain and in investigations of the function of the nucleus accumbens in other animal species.

Costall et al. (25) have recently reported quite different results following bilateral ADTN administration into the nucleus accumbens of rats. Although in animals pretreated with a monoamine oxidase inhibitor, ADTN, which was referred to in their paper as 2-amino-6,7-dihydroxytetralin, was a potent locomotor stimulant; in untreated rats ADTN was described as being "vir-tually inactive" (25). We can offer no suitable explanations for this dis-crepancy. Because ADTN is not a substrate for monoamine oxidase, it is not to be expected that monoamine oxidase inhibitors would potentiate the direct actions of ADTN. For this reason we have not routinely pretreated our animals with nialamide. Yet in all our experiments, involving more than 200 bilateral injections into more than 50 rats, and using samples of ADTN obtained from two independent sources, we have consistently found ADTN

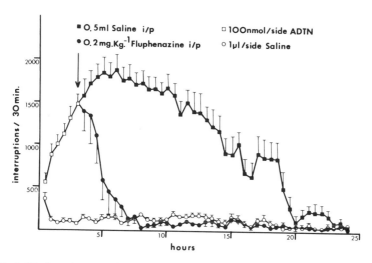

FIG. 9. Effect of fluphenazine on ADTN-induced locomotor activity in rats. Rats (15) were injected bilaterally with ADTN into the nucleus accumbens (100 nmoles each side). After 3 hr the rats were removed from the activity cages and injected intraperitoneally with either fluphenazine (*closed circles*) or 0.9% NaCl (squares) and then returned to the activity cages. Results are means, with SEM, of 7 and 8 rats, respectively. Open circles show the motor activity of rats injected bilaterally into the nucleus accumbens with saline (mean of 8 rats).

to be a potent locomotor stimulant. Our latest studies (C. Andrews and G. N. Woodruff, *unpublished observations*) have revealed that the locomotor stimulation produced by the bilateral injection of ADTN into the nucleus accumbens is blocked by a range of neuroleptic drugs, such as fluphenazine (Fig. 9). The study of the effects of drugs on ADTN-induced hyperactivity may represent a useful method of evaluating the effects of antagonists at nucleus accumbens dopamine receptors.

We have also investigated the actions of some analogues of ADTN on locomotor activity. As in previous experiments, drugs were injected bilaterally (100 nmoles on each side) into the nucleus accumbens of conscious rats. The rats were not pretreated with a monoamine oxidase inhibitor. 2-Amino-5,6-dihydroxy-1,2,3,4-tetrahydronaphthalene, which corresponds to the α rotamer of dopamine, was an effective locomotor stimulant although the duration of action of this compound (about 11 hr) was slightly less than that of ADTN. Similar injections of the same doses of 2-dimethylamino-5,6-dihydroxy-1,2,3,4-tetrahydronaphthalene caused the briefer (about 7 hr) hyperactivity response, following a delay of about 3 hr (109).

Striatal Dopamine Receptors

There have been many behavioral studies concerned with striatal dopamine receptors. Rats with unilateral 6-hydroxydopamine-induced lesions of the nigrostriatal tract have provided a convenient model by which to study the

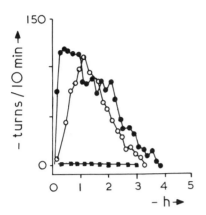

FIG. 10. Rotation produced by ergometrine in a rat with a unilateral 6-hydroxydopamine-induced lesion of the nigrostriatal tract. All turns were toward the innervated side. Open circles, turning produced by ergometrine (10 mg/kg^{-1}), injected i.p. 9 days after induction of the lesion. Squares, the same rat 2 days later, injected with haloperidol i.p. (1.0 mg/kg^{-1}) 30 min before ergometrine 10 mg/kg^{-1}; the ergometrine response was completely blocked. Closed circles, the same rat 13 days after induction of the lesion; ergometrine (10 mg/kg^{-1}) again caused strong turning. Results taken from ref. 101.

actions of directly and indirectly acting dopamine receptor stimulants. This technique was pioneered by Ungerstedt (95,96). In these animals the injection of drugs which are believed to stimulate dopamine receptors causes the rats to turn toward the innervated side; this is thought to be due to denervation supersensitivity of the dopamine receptors. Drugs such as amphetamines, which are believed to act by releasing dopamine, cause the animals to rotate toward the denervated side. We have used this technique to assess the effects of ergometrine and ADTN on striatal dopamine receptors. The technique of induction of the lesions and the measurement of drug-induced rotations were essentially as described in the papers of Ungerstedt (95,96).

Ergometrine, injected intraperitoneally in doses of 10, 25, or 50 mg/kg^{-1}, caused strong turning toward the innervated side, indicating that the drug was acting directly on dopamine receptors (101). The mean duration of

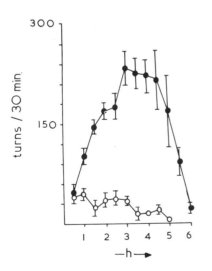

FIG. 11. Turning produced by ADTN (injected unilaterally into the lateral ventricles) in rats with unilateral 6-hydroxydopamine-induced lesions of the nigrostriatal tract. All turns were toward the innervated side. Values are the means of experiments on 6 rats. Closed circles, ADTN 150 µg; open circles, haloperidol 0.5 mg/kg^{-1}, followed by ADTN 150 µg.

action of ergometrine (25 mg/kg^{-1}) was 2.87 hr ± 0.12 (SEM) (mean of 22 injections into eight rats). This effect of ergometrine was completely abolished by haloperidol (1 mg/kg^{-1}), injected 30 min before the ergometrine (Fig. 10). Other ergot alkaloids, such as ergocornine and 2-bromoergocryptine, cause a similar turning toward the innervated side in unilaterally lesioned rats (23).

We have evidence from experiments using tritiated ADTN that this compound does not readily cross the blood-brain barrier (Woodruff et al., *unpublished observations*). In our studies with ADTN in lesioned rats the injections were therefore made into the lateral ventricle. ADTN (150 μg) was injected unilaterally on the same side as the lesion. Each animal responded to ADTN with strong and long-lasting rotations toward the lesioned side (102). The duration of ADTN was about 6 hr. The effect of ADTN is markedly reduced by pretreatment with haloperidol (Fig. 11).

Angiotensin-induced Drinking

In addition to the involvement of dopamine receptors in drug-induced rotation of lesioned rats, and in locomotor activity, dopamine may also be implicated in other behavioral responses. For example, angiotensin, when centrally administered, causes water-replete rats to drink. This response can be antagonized by haloperidol or spiroperidol, but is unaffected by phentolamine or propranolol (41). These observations suggested the involvement of dopamine in the angiotensin dipsogenic response, and we have now investigated this possibility more fully.

Stainless steel cannulas were implanted unilaterally into the lateral ventricles of male rats. The rats were used at least 1 week after surgery. Drugs were injected down the cannula in a volume of 1.5 μl, and the amount of water drunk during a 30 to 60 min test period was measured. Angiotensin induced an immediate drinking response, and the drinking was usually

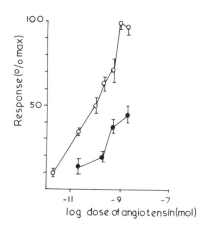

FIG. 12. Drinking induced by the unilateral injection of angiotensin into the lateral ventricles of conscious rats. Open circles, dose-response relationship for angiotensin-induced drinking. Closed circles, dose-response relationship for angiotensin-induced drinking in rats pretreated with haloperidol (39 nmoles intracerebroventricularly). Each point is the mean ± SEM of experiments on 10 to 20 rats. Data from C. Sumners, J. A. Poat, and G. N. Woodruff (*unpublished observations*).

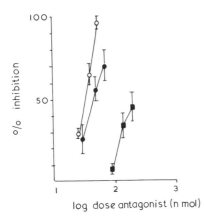

FIG. 13. Inhibition of angiotensin-induced drinking by neuroleptics. All rats received angiotensin (200 pmoles) intracerebroventricularly. Responses are expressed as percentage inhibition of the angiotensin response. Neuroleptics were injected intracerebroventricularly before the angiotensin. Open circles, haloperidol; closed circles, cis-flupenthixol; squares, clozapine. All points are the means of 5–11 observations. SEMs are indicated. Data from C. Sumners, J. A. Poat, and G. N. Woodruff (unpublished observations).

completed within 15 min of the injection. The maximum response to angiotensin was produced by a dose of 1,000 pmoles; at this dose level the amount drunk was 21.3 ± 0.9 ml (mean of 10 rats). Figure 12 shows the dose-response relationships for angiotensin-induced drinking; in this figure the response is expressed as a percentage of the maximum response. Rats which were injected into the ventricles with an equivalent volume of saline of equal osmolality always drank less than 1 ml during the 30-min test period. Also shown in Fig. 12 is the inhibition of angiotensin-induced drinking by haloperidol. This dose of haloperidol has no effect on the dipsogenic action of carbachol. We have also tested the effects of other neuroleptics on the angiotensin-induced drinking response. Figure 13 shows the inhibition of angiotensin-induced drinking produced by *cis*-flupenthixol and clozapine. The *trans*-isomer of flupenthixol had no effect on the angiotensin response in doses of up to 177 nmoles.

SUMMARY AND DISCUSSION

Our studies on the structural requirements for dopamine-like activity on the adenylate cyclase in rat nucleus accumbens, rat neostriatum, and also of *Helix* neurons show that the dopamine receptor is a very specific receptor, quite unlike the mammalian α or β adrenoceptor. The receptors differ from the α or β adrenoceptor in that for activity of phenylethylamine derivatives there is an absolute requirement for hydroxyl groups in the 3 and 4 positions of the benzene ring. Furthermore, the α-receptor agonist phenylephrine and the β-receptor agonist isoprenaline are both inactive on dopamine receptors. On the other hand, ergometrine, which has no hydroxyl groups, is able to stimulate dopamine receptors as evidenced by results from behavioral and iontophoretic studies. On the adenylate cyclase system ergometrine behaves as a partial agonist. On invertebrate dopamine receptors ergometrine is an antagonist, although it may have slight agonistic activity. It may be that in the case of compounds such as ergometrine there are additional binding sites which obviate the need for hydroxyl groups. Apomorphine resembles ergometrine in terms of its effect on mammalian adenylate cyclase, invertebrate dopamine receptors, and in its behavioral actions in rats with unilateral lesions of the nigrostriatal tract.

Cannon (17) has suggested that there might be two types of dopamine receptors, capable of accepting the two rotameric extremes of dopamine. Cools and van Rossum (22) have also invoked the presence of two dopamine receptors to explain results obtained in behavioral studies. The results reported in this study provide no support for the presence of two types of dopamine receptors associated with the adenylate cyclase in the nucleus accumbens or striatum. On the contrary, the rather close similarity between the relative potencies of the various agonists tested in the two systems suggests that the receptors are themselves similar in the two regions of the brain. Our results do not, of course, rule out the possible existence of additional dopamine receptors, the effects of which are not mediated by adenylate cyclase.

Our results further suggest that the active conformation of dopamine is in the extended rather than the folded form. Furthermore, the active conformation of dopamine appears to be closer to the β rotamer than to the α rotamer. Thus, whereas ADTN, which corresponds to the β rotamer, was equipotent with dopamine in stimulating adenylate cyclase from the striatum and more active than dopamine in homogenates of nucleus accumbens, 2-amino-5,6-dihydroxy-1,2,3,4-tetrahydronaphthalene, which corresponds to the α rotamer, was, respectively, 57 and 40 times less active than dopamine in homogenates of the two regions of the brain. ADTN is also equipotent with dopamine in causing cyclic AMP accumulation in striatal slices (76) and in homogenates of the substantia nigra (78).

ADTN has a high potency on all dopamine receptors so far examined, suggesting that the active conformation of dopamine at most mammalian and invertebrate dopamine receptors is close to the β rotamer. The actions of ADTN at a variety of mammalian and invertebrate dopamine receptors are summarized in Table 4; in all cases the potency of ADTN was similar to that of dopamine. In addition, we have shown from direct binding studies that ADTN has a high affinity for striatal dopamine receptors (84).

Our behavioral studies indicate that both ADTN and ergometrine are able to stimulate dopamine receptors in the nucleus accumbens and in the caudate nucleus. Other dopamine receptor stimulants, which are less active than ADTN when tested directly on the adenylate cyclase assay, are nevertheless quite potent behaviorally. Care must be taken, however, when attempting to interpret behavioral responses in terms of a direct action on dopamine receptors. For example, drugs injected into the nucleus accumbens might cause locomotor stimulation by acting directly on dopamine receptors, by releasing dopamine, by blocking dopamine uptake, by inhibiting phospho-

TABLE 4. *Summary of actions of ADTN and ergometrine on dopamine receptors*

System	Response to dopamine	Classification		Reference
		ADTN	Ergometrine	
Helix neurons	Hyperpolarization	Agonist	Antagonist	77, 98, 100
Helix neurons	Depolarization	Agonist	Antagonist	77, 92, 100
Cockroach salivary gland	Hyperpolarization	Agonist	Not tested	56
Guinea pig blood pressure	Hypotension	Agonist	Antagonist	103 and Woodruff et al. (*unpublished observations*)
Rat striatal neurons (iontophoresis)	Depression	Agonist	Agonist	105
Rat nucleus accumbens neurons (iontophoresis)	Depression	Agonist	Agonist	105
Adenylate cyclase striatum	Increased cAMP production	Agonist	Partial agonist	35, 76, 77, 109
Adenylate cyclase nucleus accumbens	Increased cAMP production	Agonist	Partial agonist	75, 109; Woodruff et al. (*unpublished observations*)
Dog kidney	Vasodilatation	Agonist	Antagonist	5, 30
Rats with unilateral nigrostriatal lesions	Turning	Agonist	Agonist	101, 102
Bilateral injection into rat nucleus accumbens	Locomotor stimulation	Agonist	Agonist	36, 82, 104

On all systems where it was possible to evaluate, the potency of ADTN was found to be approximately equal to that of dopamine.

diesterase, by the nonspecific activation of adenylate cyclase, or by being metabolized to an active metabolite. The stimulation or antagonism of receptors for other neurotransmitters might also initiate or modify the behavioral response. Thus the central actions of ergometrine and apomorphine might involve other mechanisms in addition to a direct action on dopamine receptors.

The locomotor stimulant action of ADTN is particularly potent and long lasting. The reason for the long duration of action is not known. ADTN is not likely to be a substrate for monoamine oxidase, although it could be methylated by catechol-O-methyltransferase. We have shown using tritiated ADTN that the compound can be taken up and released from dopaminergic nerve endings (31). It is possible that in addition to acting directly on dopamine receptors ADTN could be taken up and later released as a potent false transmitter.

ADTN has no central actions following peripheral administration, since it does not readily cross the blood-brain barrier. Some lipid-soluble analogues of ADTN should be synthesized in the search for potential antiparkinson drugs. It might also be possible to modify the ADTN molecule to obtain dopamine receptor antagonists that might have antipsychotic activity.

I have paid little attention in this chapter to the actions of neuroleptic drugs. These drugs are known from adenylate cyclase studies and from behavioral studies to block dopamine receptors (37,89). We have shown that the neuroleptics will antagonize the behavioral actions of ADTN and ergometrine and will also block the dipsogenic action of angiotensin. The latter action requires further investigation and may open up a new approach to the study of drugs affecting dopamine receptors.

ACKNOWLEDGMENTS

The author is fortunate to have received help and stimulation from a number of colleagues and students. Particular thanks are due Dr. Judith Poat who was involved in all of the biochemical studies and helped with the production of this manuscript. The following research students contributed greatly to our work on dopamine: Chris Andrews, Scarlett Batta, Abdalla El Khawad, Paul McCarthy, Colin Sumners, Keith Watling, and Alan Davis.

REFERENCES

1. Ascher, P. (1972): Inhibitory and excitatory effects of dopamine on *Aplysia* neurones. *J. Physiol. (Lond.)*, 225:173–209.
2. Axelrod, J., and Saavedra, J. M. (1977): Octopamine. *Nature*, 265:501–504.
3. Barger, G., and Dale, H. H. (1910): Chemical structure and sympathomimetic action of amines. *J. Physiol. (Lond.)*, 41:19–59.
4. Batta, S., Walker, R. J., and Woodruff, G. N. (1978): Is there a specific octopamine receptor in the brain of Helix? *J. Physiol. (Lond.)*, 270:63–64.
5. Bell, C., Conway, E. L., and Lang, W. J. (1974): Ergometrine and apomorphine as selective antagonists of dopamine in the canine renal vasculature. *Br. J. Pharmacol.*, 52:591–595.
6. Bell, C., Conway, E. L., Lang, W. J., and Padanyi, R. (1975): Vascular dopamine receptors in the canine hind limb. *Br. J. Pharmacol.*, 55:167–172.
7. Bell, C., and Mya, M. K. K. (1977): Is the renal vasodilatation induced by β-adrenoceptor stimulants in the dog mediated through dopamine receptor? *Experientia*, 33:638–639.
8. Bevan, P., Bradshaw, C. M., and Szabadi, E. (1975): Effects of desipramine on neuronal responses to dopamine, noradrenaline, 5-hydroxytryptamine and acetylcholine in the caudate nucleus of the rat. *Br. J. Pharmacol.*, 54:285–293.
9. Biscoe, T. J. (1971): Carotid body: Structure and function. *Physiol. Rev.*, 51:437–495.
10. Bjorklund, A., Cegrell, L., Falck, B., Ritzen, M., and Rosengren, E. (1970): Dopamine-containing cells in sympathetic ganglia. *Acta Physiol. Scand.*, 78:334–338.
11. Blaschko, H. (1957): Metabolism and storage of biogenic amines. *Experientia*, 13:9–12.

12. Bloom, F. E., Costa, E., and Salmoiraghi, G. E. (1965): Anaesthesia and the responsiveness of individual neurones of the caudate nucleus of the cat to acetylcholine, norepinephrine and dopamine administered by microelectrophoresis. *J. Pharmacol. Exp. Ther.,* 150:244–252.
13. Brotzu, G. (1970): Inhibition by chlorpromazine of the effects of dopamine on the dog kidney. *J. Pharm. Pharmacol.,* 22:664–667.
14. Brown, G. L., and Dale, H. H. (1936): The pharmacology of ergometrine. *Proc. R. Soc. Biol.,* 118:446–477.
15. Brown, J. H., and Makman, M. H. (1972): Stimulation by dopamine of adenylate cyclase in retinal homogenates and of adenosine-3':5'-cyclic monophosphate formation in intact retina. *Proc. Natl. Acad. Sci. U.S.A.,* 69:539–543.
16. Bustard, T. M., and Egam, R. S. (1971): The conformation of dopamine hydrochloride. *Tetrahedron,* 27:4457–4469.
17. Cannon, J. G. (1975): Chemistry of dopaminergic agonists. *Adv. Neurol.,* 9:177–183.
18. Carlsson, A. (1972): Biochemical and pharmacological aspects of parkinsonism. *Acta Neurol. Scand. [Suppl.],* 51:11–42.
19. Carlsson, A., Lindqvist, M., Magnusson, T., and Waldeck, B. (1958): On the presence of 3-hydroxytyramine in brain. *Science,* 127:471.
20. Clement-Cormier, Y. C., Kebabian, J. W., Petzold, G. L., and Greengard, P. (1974): Dopamine sensitive adenylate cyclase in mammalian brain, a possible site of action of antipsychotic drugs. *Proc. Natl. Acad. Sci. U.S.A.,* 71:1113–1117.
21. Connor, J. D. (1970): Caudate nucleus neurones: Correlation of the effects of substantia nigra stimulation with iontophoretic dopamine. *J. Physiol. (Lond.),* 208:691–703.
22. Cools, A. R., and Van Rossum, J. M. (1976): Excitation-mediating and inhibition-mediating dopamine receptors: A new concept towards a better understanding of electrophysiological, biochemical, pharmacological, functional and clinical data. *Psychopharmacologia,* 45:243–254.
23. Corrodi, H., Fuxe, K., Hökfelt, T., Lidbrink, P., and Ungerstedt, U. (1973): Effect of ergot drugs on central catecholamine neurons: Evidence for a stimulation of central dopamine neurons. *J. Pharm. Pharmacol.,* 25:409–412.
24. Costall, B., and Naylor, R. J. (1975): The behavioural effects of dopamine applied intracerebrally to areas of the mesolimbic system. *Eur. J. Pharmacol.,* 32:87–92.
25. Costall, B., Naylor, R. J., Cannon, J. G., and Lee, T. (1977): Differential activation by some 2-aminotetralin derivatives of the receptor mechanisms in the nucleus accumbens of rat which mediate hyperactivity and stereotyped biting. *Eur. J. Pharmacol.,* 41:307–319.
26. Costall, B., Naylor, R. J., and Pinder, R. M. (1976): Characterization of the mechanisms for hyperactivity induction from the nucleus accumbens by phenylethylamine derivatives. *Psychopharmacology,* 48:225–231.
27. Costall, B., Naylor, R. J., and Pinder, R. M. (1976): Hyperactivity induced by tetrahydroisoquinoline derivatives injected into the nucleus accumbens. *Eur. J. Pharmacol.,* 39:153–160.
28. Cottrell, G. A., Berry, M. S., and Macon, J. B. (1974): Synapses of a giant serotonin neurone and a giant dopamine neurone: Studies using antagonists. *Neuropharmacology,* 13:431–439.
29. Crossman, A. R., Walker, R. J., and Woodruff, G. N. (1974): Problems associated with iontophoretic studies in the caudate nucleus and substantia nigra. *Neuropharmacology,* 13:547–552.
30. Crumly, J. J., Pinder, R. M., Hinshaw, W. B., and Goldberg, L. I. (1976): Dopamine-like renal and mesenteric vasodilation caused by apomorphine 6-propylnorapomorphine and 2-amino-6,7-dihydroxy-1,2,3,4-tetrahydronaphthalene. *Nature (Lond.),* 259:584–587.
31. Davis, A., Roberts, P. J., and Woodruff, G. N. (1978): Uptake of 2-amino-6,7-dihydroxy-1,2,3,4-tetrahydronaphthalene (ADTN) into rat brain synaptosomes. *Br. J. Pharmacol.,* 61:478–479.
32. Dearnaley, D. P., Fillenz, M., and Woods, R. I. (1968): The identification of

dopamine in the rabbit's carotid body. *Proc. R. Soc. Lond.* [*Biol.*], 170:195–203.
33. Dun, N., and Nishi, S. (1974): Effects of dopamine on the superior cervical ganglion of the rabbit. *J. Physiol.* (*Lond.*), 239:155–164.
34. Eble, J. N. (1964): A proposed mechanism for the depressor action of dopamine in the anaesthetized dog. *J. Pharmacol. Exp. Ther.*, 145:64–70.
35. Elkhawad, A. O., Munday, K. A., Poat, J. A., and Woodruff, G. N. (1975): The effect of dopamine receptor stimulants on locomotor activity and cyclic AMP levels in the rat striatum. *Br. J. Pharmacol.*, 53:456–457.
36. Elkhawad, A. O., and Woodruff, G. N. (1975): Studies on the behavioural pharmacology of a cyclic analogue of dopamine following its injection into the brains of conscious rats. *Br. J. Pharmacol.*, 54:107–114.
37. Elliott, P. N. C., Jenner, P., Huizing, G., Marsden, C. D., and Miller, R. (1977): Substituted benzamides as cerebral dopamine antagonists in rodents. *Neuropharmacology*, 16:333–342.
38. Ernst, A. M. (1965): Relation between the action of dopamine and apomorphine and their o-methylated derivatives upon the CNS. *Psychopharmacologia*, 7:391–399.
39. Feltz, P., and De Champlain, J. (1972): Persistence of caudate unitary responses to nigral stimulation after destruction and functional impairment of the striatal dopaminergic terminals. *Brain Res.*, 43:596–600.
40. Fillenz, M., and Woods, R. I. (1966): Some observations on the rabbit carotid body. *J. Physiol.* (*Lond.*), 186:39–40.
41. Fitzsimons, J. T., and Setler, P. E. (1975): The relative importance of central nervous catecholaminergic and cholinergic mechanisms in drinking in response to angiotensin and other thirst stimuli. *J. Physiol.*, 250:613–631.
42. Gilman, A. G. (1970): A protein binding assay for adenosine-3':5'-cyclic monophosphate. *Proc. Natl. Acad. Sci. U.S.A.*, 67:305–312.
43. Ginsborg, B. L., Turnbull, K. W., and House, C. R. (1976): On the actions of compounds related to dopamine at a neurosecretory synapse. *Br. J. Pharmacol.*, 57:133–140.
44. Goldberg, L. I. (1972): Cardiovascular and renal actions of dopamine: Potential clinical applications. *Pharmacol. Rev.*, 24:1–29.
45. Goldberg, L. I., and Musgrave, G. (1971): Attenuation of dopamine-induced renal vasodilation by bulbocapnine and apomorphine. *Pharmacologist*, 13:227.
46. Goldberg, L. I., Sonneville, P. F., and McNay, J. L. (1968): An investigation of the structural requirements for dopamine-like renal vasodilatation: Phenylethylamines and apomorphine. *J. Pharmacol. Exp. Ther.*, 163:188–197.
47. Gonzales-Vegas, J. A. (1974): Antagonism of the dopamine-mediated inhibition in the nigro-striatal pathway: A mode of action of some catatonia-inducing drugs. *Brain Res.*, 80:219–229.
48. Greengard, P. (1976): Possible role for cyclic nucleotides and phosphorylated membrane proteins in postsynaptic actions of neurotransmitters. *Nature*, 260:101–108.
49. Grol, C. R., and Rollema, H. (1977): Conformational analysis of dopamine by the INDO molecular orbital method. *J. Pharm. Pharmacol.*, 29:153–156.
50. Heiss, W. D., and Hoyer, J. (1974): Dopamine receptor blockade by neuroleptic drugs in *Aplysia* neurones. *Experientia*, 30:1318–1320.
51. Henn, F. A., Anderson, D. J., and Sellström, A. (1977): Possible relationship between glial cells, dopamine and the effects of antipsychotic drugs. *Nature*, 266:637–638.
52. Holtz, P., and Credner, K. (1942): Die enzymatische Entstchung von Oxytyramin in Organisms und die Physiologische Bedentung der Dopadecarboxylase. *Arch. Exp. Pathol. Pharmac.*, 200:356–388.
53. Horn, A. S., Cuello, A. C., and Miller, R. J. (1974): Dopamine in the mesolimbic system of the rat brain. Endogenous levels and the effect of drugs on the uptake system and stimulation of adenylate cyclase activity. *J. Neurochem.*, 22:265–270.
54. Hornykiewicz, O. (1966): Dopamine (3-hydroxytyramine) and brain function. *Pharmacol. Rev.*, 18:925–964.
55. Hornykiewicz, O. (1971): Dopamine: Its physiology, pharmacology and patho-

logical neurochemistry. In: *The Role of Biogenic Amines and Physiological Membranes in Modern Drug Therapy, Part B*, edited by J. H. Biel and L. G. Abood, pp. 173–258. Marcel Dekker, New York.

56. House, C. R., and Ginsborg, B. L. (1976): Actions of a dopamine analogue and a neuroleptic at a neuroglandular synapse. *Nature*, 261:332–333.

57. Iversen, L. L. (1971): The uptake of biogenic amines. In: *The Role of Biogenic Amines and Physiological Membranes in Modern Drug Therapy, Part B*, edited by J. H. Biel and L. G. Abood. Marcel Dekker, New York.

58. Iversen, L. L. (1975): Dopamine receptors in the brain. *Science*, 188:1084–1089.

59. Kebabian, J. W., Petzhold, G. L., and Greengard, P. (1972): Dopamine-sensitive adenylate cyclase in caudate nucleus of rat brain and its similarity to the 'dopamine receptor.' *Proc. Natl. Acad. Sci. U.S.A.*, 69:2145–2149.

60. Kerkut, G. A., and Walker, R. J. (1961): The effects of drugs on the neurons of the snail *Helix aspersa. Comp. Biochem. Physiol.*, 3:143–160.

61. Kitai, S. T., Sugimori, M., and Kocsis, J. D. (1976): Excitatory nature of dopamine in the nigro-caudate pathway. *Exp. Brain Res.*, 24:351–363.

62. Kostowski, W. (1972): Certain aspects of the physiological role of dopamine as a synaptic transmitter in the striatum. *Acta. Physiol. Pol.*, 23:567–583.

63. Kruegar, B. K., Forn, J., Walters, J. R., Roth, R. H., and Greengard, P. (1976): Stimulation by dopamine of adenosine cyclic-3′5′-monophosphate formation in rat caudate nucleus: Effect of lesions of the nigro-neostriatal pathway. *Mol. Pharmacol.*, 12:639–648.

64. Krynjevic, K. (1974): Chemical nature of synaptic transmission in vertebrates. *Physiol. Rev.*, 54:418–539.

65. Libet, B. (1970): Generation of slow inhibitory and excitatory postsynaptic potentials. *Fed. Proc.*, 29:1945–1956.

66. McAfee, D. A., and Greengard, P. (1972): Adenosine-3′5′-monophosphate: Electrophysiological evidence for a role in synaptic transmission. *Science*, 173:310–312.

67. McAfee, D. A., Schorderet, M., and Greengard, P. (1971): Adenosine 3′5′-monophosphate in nervous tissue: Increase associated with synaptic transmission. *Science*, 171:1156–1158.

68. McCarthy, P. S., Walker, R. J., and Woodruff, G. N. (1977): On the depressant action of dopamine in rat caudate nucleus and nucleus accumbens. *Br. J. Pharmacol.*, 59:469–470.

69. McClennan, H., and York, D. H. (1967): The action of dopamine on neurones of the caudate nucleus. *J. Physiol. (Lond.)*, 189:393–402.

70. McNay, J. L., and Goldberg, L. E. (1966): Comparison of the effects of dopamine, isoproterenol, norepinephrine and bradykinin on canine renal and femoral blood flow. *J. Pharmacol. Exp. Ther.*, 151:23–31.

71. Miller, R. J., Horn, A. S., and Iversen, L. L. (1974): The action of neuroleptic drugs on dopamine-stimulated adenosine cyclic 3′5′monophosphate production in rat neostriatum and limbic forebrain. *Mol. Pharmacol.*, 10:759–766.

72. Miller, R. J., Horn, A. S., Iversen, L. L., and Pinder, R. M. (1974): Effects of dopamine-like drugs on rat striatal adenyl cyclase have implications for CNS dopamine receptor topography. *Nature*, 250:238–241.

73. Mishra, R. K., Gardner, E. L., Katzman, R., and Makman, M. H. (1974): Enhancement of dopamine-stimulated adenylate cyclase activity in rat caudate after lesions in substantia nigra: Evidence for denervation supersensitivity. *Proc. Natl. Acad. Sci. U.S.A.*, 71:3883–3887.

74. Montagu, K. A. (1957): Catechol compounds in rat tissues and in brains of different animals. *Nature*, 180:244–245.

75. Munday, K. A., Poat, J. A., Watling, K. J., and Woodruff, G. N. (1977): On the structural requirements for dopamine-like activity in homogenates of rat nucleus accumbens. *Br. J. Pharmacol.*, 61:150–151.

76. Munday, K. A., Poat, J. A., and Woodruff, G. N. (1974): Increase in the cyclic AMP content of rat striatum produced by a cyclic analogue of dopamine. *J. Physiol. (Lond.)*, 241:119–120.

77. Munday, K. A., Poat, J. A., and Woodruff, G. N. (1976): Structure activity studies

on dopamine receptors: A comparison between rat striatal adenylate cyclase and *Helix aspersa* neurones. *Br. J. Pharmacol.,* 57:452–453.

78. Phillipson, O. T., and Horn, A. S. (1976): Substantia nigra of the rat contains a dopamine sensitive adenylate cyclase. *Nature,* 261:418–420.

79. Pijnenburg, A. J. J., Honig, W. M. M., and van Rossum, J. M. (1975): Effects of antagonists upon locomotor stimulation induced by injection of dopamine and noradrenaline into the nucleus accumbens of nialamide pretreated rats. *Psychopharmacologia,* 41:175–180.

80. Pijnenburg, A. J. J., Honig, W. M. M., Van der Heyden, J. A. M., and van Rossum, J. M. (1976): Effects of chemical stimulation of the mesolimbic dopamine system upon locomotor activity. *Eur. J. Pharmacol.,* 35:45–58.

81. Pijnenburg, A. J. J., and van Rossum, J. M. (1973): Stimulation of locomotor activity following injection of dopamine into the nucleus accumbens. *J. Pharm. Pharmacol.,* 25:1003–1005.

82. Pijnenburg, A. J. J., Woodruff, G. N., and van Rossum, J. M. (1973): Ergometrine induced locomotor activity following intracerebral injection into the nucleus accumbens. *Brain Res.,* 59:289–302.

83. Rekker, R. F., Engel, D. J. C., and Nys, G. G. (1972): Apomorphine and its dopamine-like actions. *J. Pharm. Pharmacol.,* 24:589–591.

84. Roberts, P. J., Woodruff, G. N., and Poat, J. A. (1977): Binding of a conformationally restricted dopamine analogue, 2-amino-6,7-dihydroxy-1,2,3,4-tetrahydronaphthalene, to receptors on rat brain synaptic membranes. *Mol. Pharmacol.,* 13:541–547.

85. van Rossum, J. M. (1966): The significance of dopamine receptor blockade for the mechanism of action of neuroleptic drugs. *Arch. Int. Pharmacodyn. Ther.,* 160:492–494.

86. Sampson, S. R., Aminoff, M. J., Jaffe, R. A., and Vidruk, E. H. (1976): Analysis of inhibitory effect of dopamine on carotid body chemoreceptors in cats. *Am. J. Physiol.,* 230:1494–1098.

87. Sampson, S. R., and Vidruk, E. H. (1977): Hyperpolarizing effects of dopamine on chemoreceptor nerve endings from cat and rabbit carotid bodies in vitro. *J. Physiol. (Lond.),* 268:211–221.

88. Schorderet, M. (1976): Direct evidence for the stimulation of rabbit retina dopamine receptors by ergot alkaloids. *Neurosci. Lett.,* 2:87–91.

89. Seeman, P., and Lee, T. (1975): Antipsychotic drugs: Direct correlation between clinical potency and presynaptic action on dopamine neurons. *Science,* 188:1217–1219.

90. Siggins, G. R., Hoffer, B. J., and Ungerstedt, U. (1974): Electrophysiological evidence for involvement of cyclic adenosine monophosphate in dopamine responses of caudate neurones. *Life Sci.,* 15:779–792.

91. Spencer, H. J., and Havlicek, V. (1974): Alterations by anaesthetic agents of the responses of rat striatal neurones to iontophoretically applied amphetamine, acetylcholine, noradrenaline and dopamine. *Can. J. Physiol. Pharmacol.,* 52:808–813.

92. Struyker Boudier, H. A. J., Gielen, W., Cools, A. R., and van Rossum, J. M. (1974): Pharmacological analysis of dopamine-indicated inhibition and excitation of neurones of the snail *Helix aspersa. Arch. Int. Pharmacodyn. Ther.,* 209:324–331.

93. Swann, J. W., and Carpenter, D. O. (1975): Organization of receptors for neurotransmitters on *Aplysia* neurones. *Nature,* 258:751–754.

94. Thrift, R. I. (1967): Derivatives of 2-aminotetralin. *J. Chem. Sci. (C),* 288–293.

95. Ungerstedt, U. (1968): 6-Hydroxydopamine induced degeneration of central monoamine neurons. *Eur. J. Pharmacol.,* 5:107–110.

96. Ungerstedt, U. (1971): Postsynaptic supersensitivity after 6-hydroxydopamine induced degeneration of the nigro-striatal dopamine system. *Acta. Physiol. Scand. [Suppl.],* 367:69–94.

97. Von Voigtlander, P. F., Boukma, S. J., and Johnson, G. A. (1973): Dopaminergic denervation supersensitivity and dopamine stimulated adenyl cyclase activity. *Neuropharmacology,* 12:1081–1086.

98. Walker, R. J., Woodruff, G. N., Glaizner, B., Sedden, C. B., and Kerkut, G. A.

(1968): The pharmacology of *Helix* dopamine receptor of specific neurons in the snail, *Helix aspersa. Comp. Biochem. Physiol.,* 24:455–469.

99. Weil-Malherbe, H., and Bone, A. D. (1957): Intracellular distribution of catecholamines in the brain. *Nature,* 180:1050–1051.

100. Woodruff, G. N. (1971): Dopamine receptors: A review. *Comp. Gen. Pharmacol.,* 2:439–455.

101. Woodruff, G. N., Elkhawad, A. O., and Crossman, A. R. (1974): Further evidence for the stimulation of rat brain dopamine receptors by ergometrine. *J. Pharm. Pharmacol.,* 26:455–456.

102. Woodruff, G. N., Elkhawad, A. O., Crossman, A. R., and Walker, R. J. (1974): Further evidence for the stimulation of rat brain dopamine receptors by a cyclic analogue of dopamine. *J. Pharm. Pharmacol.,* 21:740–741.

103. Woodruff, G. N., Elkhawad, A. O., and Pinder, R. M. (1974): Long lasting stimulation of locomotor activity produced by the intraventricular injection of a cyclic analogue of dopamine into conscious mice. *Eur. J. Pharmacol.,* 25:80–86.

104. Woodruff, G. N., Kelly, P. H., and Elkhawad, A. O. (1976): Effects of dopamine receptor stimulants on locomotor activity of rats with electrolytic or 6-hydroxydopamine-induced lesions of the nucleus accumbens. *Psychopharmacology,* 47:195–198.

105. Woodruff, G. N., McCarthy, P. S., and Walker, R. J. (1976): Studies on the pharmacology of neurones in the nucleus accumbens of the rat. *Brain Res.,* 115:233–242.

106. Woodruff, G. N., and Walker, R. J. (1969): The effect of dopamine and other compounds on the activity of neurones of *Helix aspersa:* Structure activity relationships. *Int. J. Neuropharmacol.,* 8:279–289.

107. Woodruff, G. N., Walker, R. J., and Kerkut, G. A. (1971): Antagonism by derivatives of lysergic acid of the effect of dopamine on *Helix neurones. Eur. J. Pharmacol.,* 14:77–80.

108. Woodruff, G. N., Walker, R. J., and Kerkut, G. A. (1970): Actions of ergometrine on catecholamine receptors in the guinea pig vas deferens and in the snail brain. *Comp. Gen. Pharmacol.,* 1:54–60.

109. Woodruff, G. N., Watling, K. J., Andrews, C. D., Poat, J. A., and McDermed, J. D. (1977): Dopamine receptors in rat striatum and nucleus accumbens: Conformational studies using rigid analogues of dopamine. *J. Pharm. Pharmacol.,* 29:422–427.

110. York, D. H. (1975): Amine receptors in CNS II dopamine. In: *Handbook of Psychopharmacology, Vol. 6,* edited by L. L. Iversen, S. D. Iversen, and S. H. Snyder. Plenum Press, New York.

Advances in Biochemical Psychopharmacology, Vol. 19,
edited by P. J. Roberts et al.
Raven Press, New York © 1978.

Vascular Dopamine Receptor as a Model for Other Dopamine Receptors

Leon I. Goldberg

*Committee on Clinical Pharmacology, Departments of Pharmacological and
Physiological Sciences and Medicine, University of Chicago, Chicago, Illinois 60637*

One of the major difficulties in characterizing dopamine (DA) is the lack of an appropriate physiological model. Physiological models have proven to be extremely valuable in identifying other receptors as typified by recent studies of morphine (25). Because of this deficiency and because DA acts on many different receptors (5,7,22), it has not been possible to determine whether biochemical, behavioral, and physiological changes attributed to actions of DA are the result of action of the amine on a specific DA receptor, a family of DA receptors, or to other actions unrelated to DA receptors.

The purposes of this chapter are to describe the characteristics of the vascular DA receptor and to review the advantages and limitations of current models of this receptor as a basis for evaluating DA receptors in other areas.

IN VIVO METHODS

DA-induced renal vasodilation has been measured by essentially the same techniques by my colleagues and me for the past 15 years (13,27,42). Extensive studies of the structure-activity relationships of agonists and antagonists have convinced us that renal vasodilation produced by DA is a manifestation of the action on the amine on a specific vascular DA receptor. Because deviations in methodology have resulted in contradictory results (1,2,35), detailed description of the techniques utilized is given below.

Mongrel dogs are anesthetized with pentobarbital, 30 mg/kg intravenously, or a combination of pentobarbital, 15 mg/kg, and barbital, 20 mg/kg. Supplemental anesthetic is administered as needed to maintain light anesthesia. The kidney is exposed by flank incision and retroperitoneal dissection, and an electromagnetic flow probe is placed on the renal artery. A 23-gauge hypodermic needle, bent to an angle of approximately 80° and connected to a constant infusion system, is inserted into the artery proximal to the flow probe. The system is arranged for injection of drugs through appropriate stopcocks. Arterial blood pressure is measured from a femoral or carotid artery and blood flow and blood pressure are simultaneously recorded on an appropriate polygraph, the pens of which are carefully aligned to produce synchronized recordings. Simultaneous measurement of blood pressure and blood flow is essential to distinguish effects due to drugs on the renal vasculature from possible changes in flow resulting from alterations in arterial blood pressure. When DA is injected into the renal artery, a biphasic effect is usually observed. With smaller doses initial transient vasoconstriction is seen and then more prolonged vasodilation. With larger doses, vasoconstriction predominates. The vasoconstrictor effect can be eliminated by phenoxybenzamine (POB). Accordingly, in all studies POB is administered intra-arterially in a dose of 5 mg/kg over a 15 to 30 min period. If the vasoconstrictor effect of L-norepinephrine (1 μg) injected intra-arterially is not reversed, an additional 5 mg/kg of POB is administered. After POB, a complete dose-response curve of the increments in renal blood flow caused by DA can be recorded without interference from opposing vasoconstriction. The same methods are used for measuring mesenteric and femoral blood flow with the exception that in femoral experiments, both sciatic and femoral nerves are cut and the paw circulation is occluded to minimize neurogenic effects and cutaneous shunts.

Advantages

The advantages of this method are as follows:

1. Increase in renal blood flow occurs within 30 sec after intra-arterial administration of DA. Dose-response curves can be repeatedly demonstrated in the same animal, and thus the effects of several agonists and antagonists can be easily compared. With appropriate controls, a large number of agonists can be screened in one experiment.

2. Specific antagonism can be demonstrated by several DA antagonists in doses which do not affect other vasodilators (bradykinin or isoproterenol).

3. Opposite or identical responses due to action of DA on other receptors can be eliminated. POB eliminates the vasoconstricting effects of DA, and vasodilating actions on other receptors can be blocked by use of appropriate antagonists. Nonspecific vasodilating agents, such as nitroglycerin, can be differentiated from DA vascular agonists by study of the POB-treated, denervated femoral vascular bed.

4. DA vascular agonists do not cause similar vasodilation in the femoral bed, whereas nonspecific vasodilators are active in both femoral and renal vascular beds. Bell et al. (2) reported that DA increased femoral blood flow by action on DA vascular receptors. However, these investigators used phentolamine, rather than POB, injections into the aorta rather than the femoral artery, and did not occlude the paw circulation. It is our impression that these effects were probably related in part to neurogenic effects of DA. This conclusion was supported by recent studies by Buylaert et al. (4).

5. Neurogenic influences do not affect DA-induced renal vasodilation. The response is unchanged by administration of reserpine or by denervation provided that sufficient POB has been administered. Because reserpine and denervation accentuate the vasoconstricting actions of DA and norepinephrine, evidence of complete antagonism of norepinephrine by POB must be accomplished to prove that the vasodilation is not attenuated. Recently, inadequate administration of POB resulted in the erroneous conclusion that 2-amino-6,7-dihydroxy-1,2,3,4-tetrahydronaphthalene (A-6,7-DTN) was causing renal vasodilation by an indirect mechanism (35). Studies in our laboratory in reserpinized dogs with adequate POB pretreatment demonstrated that A-6,7-DTN is a direct-acting agonist.

6. Potency series of DA and DA vascular agonists can be compared in the renal vascular and other vascular beds to determine whether vasodilating effects are due to action on the same receptors. Identical potency series in the renal and mesenteric vascular beds indicate that vasodilation in these areas is due to action on the same receptor (10,16).

Limitations

The first limitation of this method, as in all *in vivo* systems, is that precise quantitation of agonist and antagonist ratios cannot be obtained. Concentrations of the agent at the active site may not be in equilibrium with the bathing medium, and a steady state cannot be reached. However, injections are made into the artery directly supplying blood to the responding organ, and thus the control of the agonist or antagonist dose can be fairly accurate (12). Accordingly, we have restricted our studies to rapid intra-arterial injections of agonists dissolved in small volume. This restriction causes a second limitation. Poorly soluble drugs cannot be studied. The third limitation is that drugs which affect blood pressure can influence blood flow measurements. When blood pressure and blood flow are simultaneously measured and the agonists or antagonists are administered into the renal artery, the maximal effect of a drug on renal blood flow occurs prior to changes in blood pressure which may result from recirculation of the drug. With larger doses of DA and other agonists, changes in blood pressure may be observed before the maximum effect on blood pressure is obtained, preventing inscription of a full dose-response curve. We are currently experimenting with an extracorporeal circuit from the renal vein to the jugular vein to further delay the effects of recirculating drugs on arterial blood pressure.

IN VITRO MODELS

An ideal *in vitro* model for the vascular DA receptor is needed. Present models, although confirming the existence of a DA vascular receptor, have many limitations. Most studies have been carried out with isolated canine renal (17), mesenteric (17), coronary (37), and cerebral (36) arteries. This technique is complex and expensive. In order to demonstrate DA-induced relaxation, small (less than 0.5 mm outside diameter) arteries must be used. The vessels must be bathed in a strong POB solution (10^{-5} M) for 1 hr, and they must be contracted with K^+ or prostaglandin $F_{2\alpha}$ ($PGF_{2\alpha}$). K^+ produces stable contractions, but only about 50% to 75% of K^+-treated vessels exhibit dose-related relaxation. $PGF_{2\alpha}$ is a more appropriate contracting agent, and most vessels treated by this agent relax with DA. This method has been suitable for demonstrating vascular DA receptors, but study of antagonists has been more difficult. In the initial investigation (17) phenothiazines and butyrophenones caused the contracted, isolated vessel to relax, preventing study of the response. Recently in our laboratory, DA-induced relaxation of isolated canine arteries was antagonized by metoclopramide without affecting nitroglycerin responses (*unpublished data*). Toda (*personal communication*) found that DA-induced relaxation can be specifically antagonized by droperidol without affecting relaxation produced by adenosine.

Preliminary reports have described possible use of vessels from smaller animals. DA-induced relaxation has been described in K^+ isolated rabbit renal arteries (39), but only about 50% of the vessels responded to DA. DA-induced relaxation has also been demonstrated in aortic strips cut from 2- to 6-week-old rats (30), and this response was found to be antagonized by chlorpromazine but not by propranolol. DA-induced relaxation was not observed in aortic strips obtained from older rats.

A major limitation of present *in vitro* methods is that relatively high concentrations of DA are required. Relaxation is usually initially observed with DA concentrations of 10^{-6} M and maximal effects at about 10^{-4} M. In contrast, DA-induced renal vasodilation can be demonstrated with a very small dose (1 μg), and the dose-response curve extends over a range of 4 to 5 log units. Accordingly, the present *in vitro* techniques are not suitable for screening of rare compounds, and comparisons of dose-response curves are difficult.

AGONISTS OF THE VASCULAR DA RECEPTOR

More than 200 putative DA agonists have been studied in the intact renal vascular bed. Structural requirements for action on DA vascular receptors are extraordinarily stringent (13,14,16,18,22). The only phenylethylamines found to be active thus far are N-methyl DA (which is equipotent to DA) (16) and N,N-di-n-propyl DA (which exhibits an ED_{50} approximately 1/30 that of DA) (40). Interestingly, N,N-di-n-propyl DA differs from DA in lacking beta-adrenergic activity. A large number of phenylethylamines were found to be inactive: compounds with substitutions on the benzene ring other than OH groups on the 3 and 4 positions; analogues with substitutions

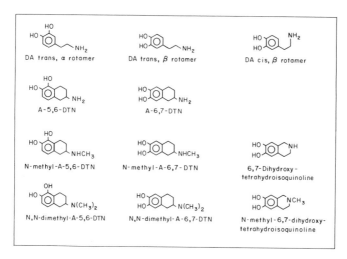

FIG. 1. Aminotetralins and isoquinolines studied on the DA vascular receptor (42).

on the alpha- or beta-carbons; 2- and 4-carbon side chain catecholamines; single nitrogen substitutions larger than CH_3 (N-ethyl, N-propyl, N-isopropyl); di-substitutions on the N-atom other than propyl (N,N-di-methyl, N,N-di-ethyl).

In view of these limitations it was surprising to find that 2-amino-6,7-dihydroxy-1,2,3,4-tetrahydronaphthalene (Fig. 1) was an active DA agonist equipotent to DA (10,42). This compound was postulated to be a DA agonist by Woodruff (44), and was subsequently synthesized by Pinder. A-6,7-DTN holds the DA molecule in the semirigid, beta-rotameric *trans* conformation. Subsequent studies in our laboratory demonstrated that the structure-activity relationships for A-6,7-DTN analogues are similar to those for the nonrigid catecholamines (14,22,42). N-methyl A-6,7-DTN is approximately equipotent to A-6,7-DTN, and N,N-n-propyl A-6,7-DTN is a much weaker agonist. N,N-di-methyl A-6,7-DTN is inactive.

Of equal importance, our studies have shown that the alpha-rotamer with a *trans* conformation, A-5,6-DTN, and its N-methyl analogue are inactive (41). Interestingly, these compounds are active as beta-adrenergic agonists, suggesting that the preferred conformation for activation of the vascular DA receptor is the beta-rotamer, whereas the preferred conformation for activation of beta$_2$-adrenergic receptors is the alpha-rotamer.

Apomorphine contains the structure of N-methyl DA with the side chain fully extended and the amino group *trans* to the catechol moiety in an alpha-rotameric conformation. Apomorphine was found to be active on the vascular DA receptor, but is much weaker than DA and appears to be a partial agonist (10,14–16,22). N-n-propyl norapomorphine is more potent than apomorphine and appears to be a full agonist with 1/30 to 1/50 the potency of DA (10,22). Interestingly, isoapomorphine, which contains the structure of N-methyl DA in a beta-rotameric conformation, is inactive as a vascular DA agonist (22). This obvious contradiction to the results with the ADTN molecule will require further study. It is possible to devise a mode of binding for apomorphine so that it would have a better fit into the postulated DA receptor than isoapomorphine. A slight distortion of the catechol binding site of apomorphine would be required (14).

In summary, the potency series of agonists active on the vascular DA receptors are as follows: DA = epinine = A-6,7-DTN = N-methyl A-6,7-DTN >> N,N-di-n-propyl DA > N,N-propyl apomorphine > apomorphine (partial agonist). Of importance for comparison with other receptors, the following compounds were found to be inactive: serotonin, histamine, lergotrile, bromocryptine, amantadine, piribedil, S-584, morphine, amphetamine, N,N-di-methyl DA, A-5,6-DTN, N-methyl A-5,6-DTN, N,N-di-methyl A-5,6-DTN, N,N-di-methyl A-6,7-DTN, and isoapomorphine (14,22).

ANTAGONISTS OF THE VASCULAR DA RECEPTOR

Several DA antagonists were found to selectively attenuate renal vasodilation produced by DA and other agonists without affecting vasodilation produced by isoproterenol or bradykinin (19,33,46). All agonists had a transient duration of action when injected into the renal artery. Studies were performed by simultaneously injecting antagonists with DA or with the other vasodilating agents. The doses of the antagonists were gradually increased until the vasodilation produced by isoproterenol and bradykinin was affected. The antagonists differed with respect to (a) doses required to shift the dose-response curve 3 to $4\times$; and (b) their range of specificity (defined as minimal dose attenuating vasodilating responses of bradykinin or isoproterenol/minimal dose attenuating vasodilating responses caused by DA). The relative potencies were as follows: sulpiride (2.9×10^{-8} M), bulbocapnine (4.7×10^{-8} M), haloperidol (1.4×10^{-7} M), chlorpromazine (2.5×10^{-7} M), prochlorperazine (2.5×10^{-7} M), trifluoperazine (2.5×10^{-7} M), fluphenazine (2.5×10^{-7} M), thioridazine (5×10^{-7} M), and metoclopramide (1.5×10^{-6}). The ranges of specificity were as follows: sulpiride > 10, metoclopramide > 10, bulbocapnine 8, and the remaining agents < 2.

COMPARISON OF THE VASCULAR DA RECEPTOR WITH OTHER DA RECEPTORS

Detailed reviews (14,18,22) describing similarities and differences of agonists and antagonists of the vascular DA receptor and other DA receptors have been presented. Comparison of the actions of the same agonists and antagonists in several models demonstrated that the chemical requirements for activation of the vascular DA receptor are more specific.

DA-sensitive Adenylate Cyclase

Pronounced similarities, both qualitative and quantitative, were noted when comparing this model with the DA vascular receptor (14,22–24, 28,38). In both systems the hydroxy groups on the catecholamine structure must be in the 3 and 4 positions, and a two-carbon side chain is required for activation. DA, epinine, and A-6,7-DTN are approximately equipotent in the two systems. A-5,6-DTN is inactive (26,45). There are, however, several discrepancies: N,N-di-methyl DA, N,N,N-tri-methyl DA, L-norepinephrine, alpha-methyl DA, 6,7-dihydroxytetrahydroisoquinoline, and S-584 increase striatal adenylate cyclase activity but are inactive as DA vascular receptor agonists.

In addition, the fluorinated phenothiazines, fluphenazine, and trifluoperazine, are more active than haloperidol in inhibiting the effects of DA on striatal adenylate cyclase (23,28), but these agents are only 50% as active as haloperidol in antagonizing renal vasodilation. Of more importance, sulpiride and metoclopramide, which are effective antagonists of the vascular DA receptor, are inactive in inhibiting the effects of DA on striatal adenylate cyclase (11,31,38).

Another possible conflict is that pimozide is active in the adenylate cyclase system, but it has been reported to be inactive as an antagonist of DA-induced renal vasodilation (21,34). We have been unable to study pimozide in our preparation because of its relative insolubility.

Receptor Binding and Striatal Homogenates

Major points of similarity in the receptor binding assays and the DA vascular model are that DA, epinine, and A-6,7-DTN are equipotent in both systems (3,32). Discrepancies are many. Apomorphine is more potent than DA in displacement of tritiated DA, whereas it is a partial agonist and much weaker than DA in the renal vascular model. More serious discrepancies are that N,N-di-methyl DA, ethyl DA, N-methyl A-5,6-DTN, N,N-di-methyl A-5,6-DTN, and N,N-di-methyl A-6,7-DTN displace tritiated DA (32) but are totally inactive as DA vascular agonists.

Autonomic Ganglion and Postganglionic Sympathetic Nerve (Presynaptic)

DA inhibits the function of autonomic ganglia and the postganglionic sympathetic nerve. Only limited structure-activity studies have been carried out with ganglionic and sympathetic nerve preparations (20,22,43). Nevertheless, major discrepancies have been found between the effects of agonists on these receptors and the DA vascular receptor. DA, epinine, and apomorphine are equipotent in inhibiting ganglionic transmission and presynaptic function, whereas DA is much more potent than apomorphine in increasing renal blood flow. A major discrepancy in comparing a vascular DA receptor with inhibition of the postganglionic sympathetic nerve is that di-methyl A-5,6-DTN and N,N-di-methyl DA are potent inhibitors of the latter system. This interesting difference is similar to that observed in receptor binding studies, suggesting the possibility that these compounds may be bound to presynaptic sites in the binding assay.

Emesis

Although L-DOPA and apomorphine induce emesis and increase renal blood flow, there are many more discrepancies since a far greater number of putative agonists cause emesis than increase renal blood flow (6). A major difference is N,N-di-methyl A-5,6-DTN, which is an extremely potent emetic. Both N,N-di-methyl and A-5,6-DTN compounds are inactive as DA vascular agonists.

Behavior

Apomorphine and L-DOPA are active in most behavioral models, but again, many compounds inactive in the DA vascular receptor have been reported to cause behavioral changes by acting on DA receptors. These include piribedil, S-584, lergotrile, bromocryptine, and several A-5,6-DTN derivatives (8,9,14,22).

Receptors Involved in Prolactin Release

DA is a potent inhibitor of prolactin release from the anterior pituitary. A-6,7-DTN is more effective than DA in this system (30a). However, many compounds inactive as DA vascular agonists are active in inhibiting prolactin release. These include A-5,6-DTN, N,N-di-methyl A-5,6-DTN, piribedil, lergotrile, and bromocryptine (41).

Neurons of *Helix aspersa*

DA and A-6,7-DTN cause excitation and inhibition in different neurons of *Helix aspersa* (29,34,44). Excitatory (DA-E) neurons have characteristics similar to the vascular DA receptor. DA-E neurons are inhibited by haloperidol, chlorpromazine, and fluphenazine, and apomorphine is a partial agonist. In contrast, haloperidol and the phenothiazines are ineffective as antagonists of the inhibitory (DA-I) neuron, and apomorphine is an antagonist. In addition, (3,4-dihydroxyphenylamino)-2-imidazoline (DPI) is active as an agonist of the DA-I neurons and is inactive as a DA renal vasodilator. Piribedil and S-584 are inactive in both DA-I and DA-E neurons. Ergometrine is an antagonist of both types of neurons, but is much more effective in inhibiting the effects of DA on DA-I neurons. Bell et al. (1)

reported that ergometrine was effective as a vascular DA antagonist when this agent was administered into the canine aorta. We did not find ergometrine to be a specific antagonist utilizing our techniques with injections into the renal artery.

CONCLUSION

Studies of the vascular DA receptor have demonstrated that the structure-activity requirements for agonists active in this receptor are extraordinarily stringent. Comparison with other DA receptors with the limited data available at this time suggests either that most DA receptors described in other areas are different from the vascular DA receptor or that models used are measuring other actions of DA.

ACKNOWLEDGMENTS

Research described in this chapter was supported by USPHS grants from NIH, GM-22220 and NS-12324.

REFERENCES

1. Bell, C., Conway, E. L., and Lang, W. J. (1974): Ergometrine and apomorphine as selective antagonists of dopamine in the canine renal vasculature. *Br. J. Pharmacol.,* 52:591–595.
2. Bell, C., Conway, E. L., Lang, W. J., and Padanyi, R. (1975): Vascular dopamine receptors in the canine hindlimb. *Br. J. Pharmacol.,* 55:167–172.
3. Burt, D. R., Enna, S. J., Creese, I., and Snyder, S. H. (1975): Dopamine receptor binding in the corpus striatum of mammalian brain. *Proc. Natl. Acad. Sci. U.S.A.,* 72:4655–4659.
4. Buylaert, W. A., Willems, J. L., and Bogaert, M. G. (1977): Vasodilation produced by apomorphine in the hindlimb of the dog. *J. Pharmacol. Exp. Ther.,* 201: 738–746.
5. Calne, D., Chase, T. N., and Barbeau, A. (editors) (1975): Dopaminergic mechanisms. *Advances in Neurology, Vol. 9:* Raven Press, New York.
6. Cannon, J. G. (1975): Chemistry of dopaminergic agonists. *Adv. Neurol.,* 9:177–184.
7. Costa, E., Gessa, G. L., editors, (1977): Nonstriatal dopaminergic neurons. In: *Advances in Biochemical Psychopharmacology, Vol. 16:* Raven Press, New York.
8. Costall, B., Naylor, R. J., Cannon, J. G., and Lee, T. (1977): Differential activation by some 2-aminotetralin derivatives of the receptor mechanisms in the nucleus accumbens of rat which mediate hyperactivity and stereotyped biting. *Eur. J. Pharmacol.,* 41:307–319.
9. Costall, B., Naylor, R. J., and Pinder, R. M. (1974): Design of agents for stimulation of neostriatal dopaminergic mechanisms. *J. Pharm. Pharmacol.,* 26:753–762.
10. Crumly, H., Hinshaw, W. B., Pinder, R., and Goldberg, L. I. (1976): Dopamine-like renal and mesenteric vasodilation caused by apomorphine, 6-propyl-norapomorphine and 2-amino-6,7-dihydroxy-1,2,3,4-tetrahydronaphthalene. *Nature,* 259: 584–587.
11. Donaldson, I. M., Jenner, P., Marsden, C. D., Miller, R., and Peringer, E. (1976): Is metoclopramide a directly acting dopamine receptor antagonist? *Br. J. Pharmacol.,* 56:373P.
12. Furchgott, R. F. (1972): The classification of adrenoceptors (adrenergic recep-

tors). An evaluation from the standpoint of receptor theory. In: *Handbook of Experimental Pharmacology*, edited by H. J. Blaschko and E. Muscholl, pp. 283–335. Springer, New York.

13. Goldberg, L. I. (1972): Cardiovascular and renal actions of dopamine: Potential clinical applications. *Pharmacol. Rev.*, 24:1–9.
14. Goldberg, L. I., Kohli, J. D., Kotake, A., and Volkman, P. H. (1977): Characteristics of the vascular dopamine receptor: Comparison with other receptors. *Fed. Proc.* (*in press*).
15. Goldberg, L. I., and Musgrave, G. (1971): Selective attenuation of dopamine-induced renal vasodilation by bulbocapnine and apomorphine. *Pharmacologist*, 13(2): 227.
16. Goldberg, L. I., Sonneville, P. F., and McNay, J. L. (1968): An investigation of the structural requirements for dopamine-like renal vasodilation: Phenylethylamines and apomorphine. *J. Pharmacol. Exp. Ther.*, 163:188–197.
17. Goldberg, L. I., and Toda, N. (1975): Dopamine-induced relaxation of isolated canine renal, mesenteric, and femoral arteries contracted with prostaglandin $F_{2\alpha}$. *Circ. Res.*, 36:I97–I102.
18. Goldberg, L. I., Volkman, P. H., and Kohli, J. D. (1978): A comparison of the vascular dopamine receptor with other dopamine receptors. *Ann. Rev. Pharmacol. Toxicol.*, 18:57–79.
19. Goldberg, L. I., and Yeh, B. K. (1971): Attenuation of dopamine-induced renal vasodilation in the dog by phenothiazines. *Eur. J. Pharmacol.*, 15:36–40.
20. Ilhan, M., Nichols, D. E., Long, J. P., and Cannon, J. G. (1975): Apomorphine-like effect of an aminotetralin on the linguomandibular reflex of the cat. *Eur. J. Pharmacol.*, 33:61–64.
21. Imbs, J. L., Schmidt, M., Velly, J., and Schwartz, J. (1976): Effects of apomorphine and of pimozide on renin secretion in the anesthetized dog. *Eur. J. Pharmacol.*, 38:175–178.
22. Iversen, L. L. (1975): Dopamine receptors in the brain. *Science*, 188:1084–1089.
23. Iversen, L. L., Horn, A. S., and Miller, R. J. (1975): Actions of dopaminergic agonists of cyclic AMP production in rat brain homogenates. *Adv. Neurol.*, 9:197–212.
24. Kebabian, J. W., Petzold, G. L., and Greengard, P. (1972): Dopamine sensitive adenylate cyclase in the caudate nucleus of rat brain and its similarity to the "dopamine receptor." *Proc. Natl. Acad. Sci. U.S.A.*, 69:2145–2149.
25. Kosterlitz, H. W., and Waterfield, A. A. (1975): In vitro models in the study of structure-activity relationships of narcotic analgesics. *Ann. Rev. Pharmacol.*, 15:29–47.
26. Kotake, C., Goldberg, L. I., Hoffmann, P. C., and Cannon, J. G. (1977): Effects of 2-aminotetralins on rat striatal adenylate cyclase. *Pharmacologist*, 19:222.
27. McNay, J. L., and Goldberg, L. I. (1966): Comparison of the effects of dopamine, isoproterenol, norepinephrine, and bradykinin on canine renal and femoral blood flow. *J. Pharmacol. Exp. Ther.*, 151:23–31.
28. Miller, R. J., Horn, A., Iversen, L. L., and Pinder, R. M. (1974): Effect of dopamine-like drugs on rat striatal adenylate cyclase: Implications for CNS dopamine receptor topography. *Nature*, 250:238.
29. Munday, K. A., Poat, J. A., and Woodruff, G. N. (1976): Structure-activity studies on dopamine receptors: A comparison between rat striatal adenylate cyclase and Helix aspersa neurones. *Br. J. Pharmacol.*, 57:452.
30. Murakami, W., and Shibata, S. (1976): Evidence for a dopamine sensitve receptor in the young rat aorta. *Chem. Pathol. Pharmacol.*, 13:349–354.
30a. Rick, J., Payne, P., Cannon, J., and Frohman, L. A. (1977): Evidence for differences in pituitary dopamine (DA) receptors from those in the kidney based on the prolactin (PRL)-suppressive effects of 2-aminotetralin analogs. *Clin. Res.*, 25(4): 566A.
31. Roufogalis, B. D., Thornton, M., and Wade, D. N. (1976): Specificity of the dopamine sensitive adenylate cyclase for antipsychotic antagonists. *Life Sci.*, 19:927–934.
32. Seeman, P., Tedesco, J. L., Lee, T., Chau-Wong, M., Muller, P., Bowles, J.,

Whitaker, P. M., McManus, C., Tittler, M., Weinrich, P., Friend, W. C., and Brown, G. M. (1978): Dopamine receptors in the central nervous system. *Fed. Proc.* (*in press*).

33. Setler, P. E., Pendleton, R. G., and Finlay, E. (1975): The cardiovascular actions of dopamine and the effects of central and peripheral catecholaminergic receptor blocking drugs. *J. Pharmacol. Exp. Ther.*, 192:702–712.

34. Struyker Boudier, H. A. J. (1975): *Catecholamine Receptors in Nervous Tissue.* Druk, Stichting Studentenpers Nijmegen.

35. Tobia, A. J., Hahn, R. A., and Wardell, J. R., Jr. (1977): Renal vasodilator responses of 2-amino-6,7-dihydroxy-1,2,3,4-tetrahydronaphthalene (ADTN). *Fed. Proc.*, 36(3):3993.

36. Toda, N. (1976): Influences of DA and noradrenaline on isolated cerebral arteries of the dog. *Br. J. Pharmacol.*, 58:121.

37. Toda, N., and Goldberg, L. I. (1975): Effects of dopamine on isloated canine coronary arteries. *Cardiovasc. Res.*, 9:384–389.

38. Trabucci, M., Longoni, R., Fresia, P., and Spano, P. F. (1976): Sulpiride: A study of the effects on dopamine receptors in rat neostriatum and limbic forebrain. *Life Sci.*, 17:1551–1556.

39. Urquilla, P. P. (1976): Effects of dopamine on the isolated rabbit renal artery partially contracted by potassium chloride. *Blood Vessels*, 13:249–252.

40. Volkman, P. H., and Goldberg, L. I. (1977): Lack of correlation between inhibition of prolactin release and stimulation of dopaminergic renal vasodilation. *Pharmacologist*, 18:130.

41. Volkman, P. H., Kohli, J. D., Goldberg, L. I., and Cannon, J. G. (1977): Dipropyldopamine, a qualitatively different dopamine (DA) agonist. *Fed. Proc.*, 36:1049.

42. Volkman, P. H., Kohli, J. D., Goldberg, L. I., Cannon, J. G., and Lee, T. (1977): Conformational requirements for dopamine-induced vasodilation. *Proc. Natl. Acad. Sci. USA*, 74:3602–3606.

43. Willems, J. L., and Bogaert, M. G. (1975): Dopamine-induced neurogenic vasodilation in isolated perfused muscle preparation of the dog. *Arch. Pharmacol.*, 286:413–428.

44. Woodruff, G. N. (1971): Dopamine receptors: A review. *Comp. Gen. Pharmacol.*, 2:439–455.

45. Woodruff, G. N., Watling, K. J., Andrews, C. D., Poat, J. A., and McDermed, J. D. (1977): Dopamine receptors in rat striatum and nucleus accumbens: Conformational studies using rigid analogues of dopamine. *J. Pharm. Pharmacol.*, 29:422–427.

46. Yeh, B. K., McNay, J. L., and Goldberg, L. I. (1969): Attenuation of dopamine renal and mesenteric vasodilation by haloperidol: Evidence for a specific dopamine receptor. *J. Pharmacol. Exp. Ther.*, 168:303–309.

Advances in Biochemical Psychopharmacology, Vol. 19,
edited by P. J. Roberts et al.
Raven Press, New York © 1978.

Dopamine-sensitive Adenylyl Cyclase: A Receptor Mechanism for Dopamine

John W. Kebabian

Experimental Therapeutics Branch, National Institute of Neurological and Communicative Disorders and Stroke, National Institutes of Health, Bethesda, Maryland 20014

The discovery of adenosine 3'5'-monophosphate (cyclic AMP) provided a single biochemical mechanism to account for the actions of numerous hormones. Thus, hormones through actions on tissue-specific receptors could affect the intracellular content of cyclic AMP and thereby initiate a tissue-specific response. Neurotransmitters have been thought of as hormones which act over a shorter distance and with a shorter time course. Indeed, a variety of substances which are identified as neurotransmitters (with varying degrees of certainty) have been shown to affect cyclic nucleotide metabolism in the brain. Dopamine is one example of a well-established neurotransmitter in both the vertebrate and the invertebrate nervous systems. Following the realization that dopamine might exert a physiological action by a mechanism involving cyclic AMP metabolism, dopamine-sensitive adenylyl cyclase has attracted considerable experimental attention. The understanding of the properties of the dopamine receptor which regulates adenylyl cyclase has provided some insight into the mechanism of actions of several medically important drugs. Furthermore, the presence of dopamine-sensitive adenylyl cyclase indicates the presence of dopamine receptors in various cellular or anatomical regions of brain. Thus, this enzyme can account for some of the effects of dopamine or dopaminergic drugs on the nervous system.

SYMPATHETIC GANGLIA

The initial understanding of the functioning of the dopamine receptor at a molecular level was gained from studies of mammalian sympathetic ganglia. In physiological studies, McAfee, Schorderet, Kalix, and Greengard (29,48) observed that physiological activity in rabbit superior cervical ganglion increased the content of cyclic AMP in this tissue. In control experiments, the electrical activity in pre- and postganglionic neurons accompanying the preganglionic stimulation was dissociated from the increase in cyclic AMP. The sensitivity of this increase in cyclic AMP to both a muscarinic cholinergic antagonist and an alpha-adrenergic antagonist suggested that the increase

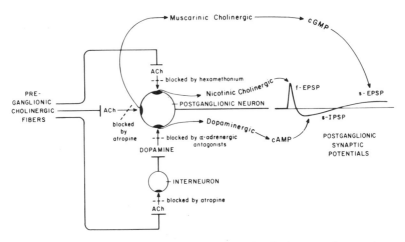

FIG. 1. A schematic diagram of the principal synaptic connections in the mammalian superior cervical ganglion, and the postulated role of cyclic nucleotides in the genesis of the postganglionic synaptic potentials. This diagram shows: the relationship between the various neuronal elements; the neurotransmitters released at the various synapses; the sensitivity of the synaptic receptors to different classes of specific antagonists; the electrical signs that accompany activation of the various postganglionic receptors following preganglionic stimulation; and the postulated involvement of cyclic nucleotides in the production of the electrophysiological responses. Abbreviations used: ACh, acetylcholine; cAMP, cyclic AMP; cGMP, cyclic GMP; F-EPSP, fast excitatory postsynaptic potential; s-IPSP, slow inhibitory postsynaptic potential; s-EPSP, slow excitatory postsynaptic potential. (Modified from 24.)

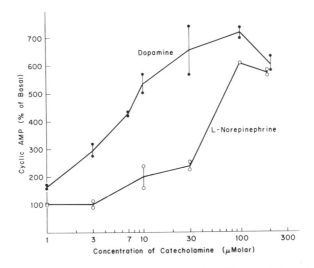

FIG. 2. Stimulation by dopamine and L-norepinephrine of cyclic AMP accumulation in blocks of bovine superior cervical ganglion. Tissue was incubated for 5 min at 37° C in oxygenated Krebs-Ringer bicarbonate buffer, pH 7.4, containing 10 mM theophylline and the indicated amount of catecholamine. Cyclic AMP accumulation during incubation in the presence of catecholamine and theophylline is expressed as the percentage of that observed during incubation in the presence of theophylline alone. The curves are drawn through the average of 2 data points; each data point represents the mean of duplicate determinations on an individual sample. (Figure modified from 34.)

occurred as a consequence of synaptic transmission within the ganglion. An adrenergic interneuron was the only cellular element within the ganglion which could account for the increase in cyclic AMP (21). The results of the combined physiological, pharmacological, and biochemical experiments support a model in which a catecholamine contained within the interneuron was released as a consequence of preganglionic stimulation (Fig. 1). In turn, this catecholamine stimulated a receptor on the postganglionic neurons and caused an accumulation of cyclic AMP within these cells. According to this model, exogenous catecholamine should mimic the effect of the endogenous catecholamine found within the ganglionic interneuron.

Since dopamine had been identified as the catecholamine within the interneuron by Björklund and his co-workers (2), it was logical to test the effects of this amine on a preparation of superior cervical ganglion (31,34). Dopamine caused a substantial accumulation of cyclic AMP in the bovine superior cervical ganglion (Fig. 2). The maximal effect of dopamine was a sevenfold increase in the level of cyclic AMP. Half-maximal accumulation of cyclic AMP occurred with a concentration of 7×10^{-6} M dopamine. The dopamine receptor was blocked by phentolamine, an alpha-adrenergic antagonist (Fig. 3), but was unaffected by the beta-adrenergic antagonist propranolol (Fig. 4) (25,34). Several lines of evidence indicated that this increase in cyclic AMP was a direct effect of dopamine: first, dopamine increases adenylyl cyclase activity in homogenates of bovine ganglion (34). Second, pretreatment with a dopamine beta-hydroxylase inhibitor did not diminish the effect of dopamine (63). Third, although a beta-adrenergic receptor also regulates gangli-

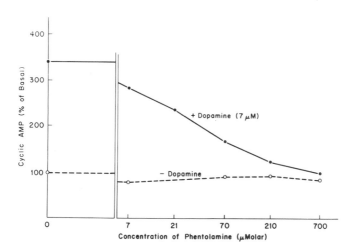

FIG. 3. Effect of the α blocker phentolamine on cyclic AMP accumulation, in the presence and absence of 7 μM dopamine, in blocks of bovine superior cervical ganglion. Tissue was incubated as in Fig. 1 with the indicated amounts of dopamine and phentolamine. Cyclic AMP accumulation is expressed as the percentage of that observed in the presence of theophylline alone. Each point represents the mean of determinations on 2–4 samples analyzed in duplicate. (Modified from 34.)

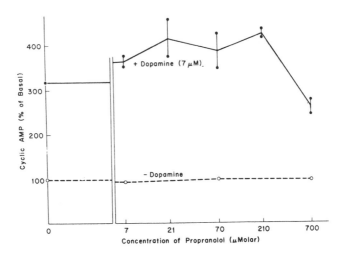

FIG. 4. Effect of the β blocker propranolol on cyclic AMP accumulation in the presence and absence of 7 μM dopamine in blocks of bovine superior cervical ganglion. Tissue was incubated as in Fig. 1 with the indicated amounts of dopamine and propranolol. Cyclic AMP accumulation is expressed as the percentage of that observed in the presence of theophylline alone. The curves are drawn through the average of 2 data points; each point represents the mean of duplicate determinations on an individual sample. (Modified from 25.)

onic cyclic AMP, the sensitivity of this receptor to a beta-adrenergic antagonist distinguishes it from the dopamine receptor (31). Thus, the response to the beta-adrenergic agonist L-isoproterenol is abolished by low concentrations of propranolol, a beta-adrenergic antagonist (Fig. 5). The postganglionic neurons are the cellular element of the bovine superior cervical ganglion which respond to dopamine with a increase of cyclic AMP (32). Utilizing a specific histochemical procedure to visualize cyclic nucleotides, dopamine was shown to increase the content of histochemically demonstrable cyclic AMP within the postganglionic neurons (Fig. 6). The beta-adrenergic receptor within the *bovine* ganglion appeared to be associated with glial elements and blood vessels within the ganglion.

The dopamine-stimulated accumulation of cyclic AMP within the bovine superior cervical ganglion has been confirmed repeatedly (63,73,78). However, attempts to produce a similar phenomenon in sympathetic ganglia of other species have demonstrated interspecies variations in responsiveness to catecholamines (79). A beta-adrenergic receptor controls the cyclic AMP content of the postganglionic neurons of the rat superior cervical ganglion; dopamine has little or no effect on this tissue (15,57). Results similar to those in the rat ganglion have been obtained from the guinea pig superior cervical ganglion (79). In the cat and rabbit superior cervical ganglion, dopamine causes accumulations of cyclic AMP (29,78,79). This degree of interspecies variability is unanticipated in view of the relative anatomical, biochemical, and physiological simplicity of the sympathetic ganglia. How-

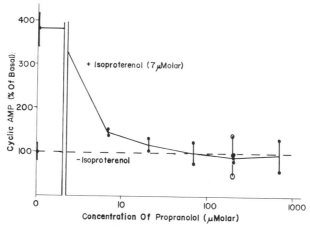

FIG. 5. Effect of the β blocker propranolol on cyclic AMP accumulation in the presence and absence of 7 µM L-isoproterenol in blocks of bovine superior cervical ganglion. Tissue was incubated as in Fig. 1 with the indicated amounts of L-isoproterenol and propranolol. Cyclic AMP accumulation is expressed as the percentage of that observed in the presence of theophylline alone. Each point represents mean ± SD (control and 7 µM L-isoproterenol) or mean and range for 2 observations, each assayed in duplicate.

ever, interspecies variations in the effectiveness of neurotransmitters on the content of cyclic AMP in neural tissue are common phenomena; the recent monograph of Daly (16) presents an encyclopedic summary of such interspecies variations.

The physiological significance of the dopamine-stimulated accumulation of cyclic AMP in sympathetic ganglia has received considerable attention. There is agreement that the dopamine-containing interneuron is the only cellular element within the rabbit ganglion which can account for the accumulation of cyclic AMP following preganglionic stimulation. However, the nature of the subsequent physiological event(s) which is initiated by the accumulation of cyclic AMP remains controversial. The electrophysiological data of McAfee and Greengard (47) support the contention that cyclic AMP initiates physiological events which are ultimately manifested as the slow inhibitory postsynaptic potential which follows preganglionic stimulation (Fig. 1). This model is based on the model developed by Eccles and Libet (20). Recently, certain aspects of the electrophysiological evidence underlying this hypothesis have been questioned by Dun and Karczmar (18,19). Although these latter investigators could confirm the work of McAfee and Greengard, they obtained apparently contradictory results from experiments designed to extend the initial observations. A second possible physiological action of dopamine and cyclic AMP involves the potentiation of a slow muscarinic depolarization of the postganglionic neurons. This second possibility is based on the recent (and as yet unconfirmed) observations of Libet and his co-workers (41–44). The controversy which surrounds the physiological role of dopamine in the

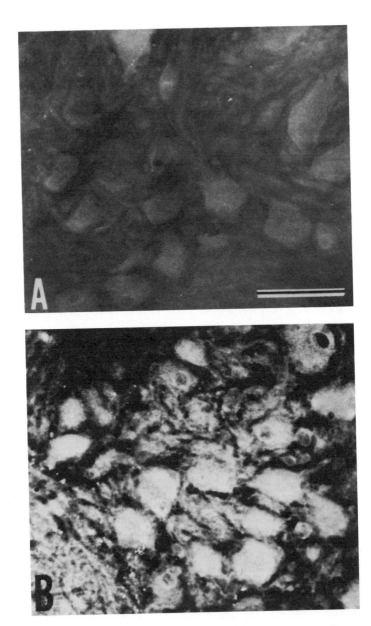

FIG. 6. Dark-field fluorescence micrographs illustrating the relative intensity of immunofluorescence staining for cyclic AMP in cryostat sections of bovine superior cervical ganglion. Blocks of ganglion tissue were incubated for 5 min in oxygenated Krebs-Ringer bicarbonate buffer containing 1 mM SQ 20,006 in the absence (A) or presence (B) of 100 μM dopamine. The histochemically demonstrable cyclic AMP was visualized with the immunohistochemical procedure of Wedne, et al. (77). The time, exposure, and development of the photomicrographs were identical, so that the relative brightness of the staining in the two micrographs is directly comparable. Tissue treated identically to that shown in A and B contained 8.3 pmoles of cyclic AMP per mg of protein and 39.6 pmoles of cyclic AMP per mg of protein, respectively. Bar in A represents 100 μM and applies to both sections. (Modified from 32.)

sympathetic ganglion indicates the difficulty which may be anticipated in identifying the physiological role of dopamine in the central nervous system.

CENTRAL NERVOUS SYSTEM

Our success in demonstrating that dopamine increases cyclic AMP levels in sympathetic ganglia prompted a search for a dopamine-sensitive adenylyl cyclase in the corpus striatum of the mammalian brain. At approximately the same time, a dopamine-sensitive adenylyl cyclase was demonstrated in the retina (7). In a collaborative effort with Gary Petzold and Paul Greengard, the dopamine receptor from the caudate-putamen of the rat brain was shown to be intimately involved in the regulation of adenylyl cyclase activity (35). The three experimental pharmacological approaches used to characterize the dopamine receptor in the original report of this enzyme activity in the striatum were: (a) structure-activity studies among the catecholamines; (b) the use of synthetic dopaminergic agonists; and (c) the use of antagonists to block the response to dopamine. Each of these experimental approaches has been extensively exploited in numerous other studies. In the initial report (Fig. 7), both dopamine and L-norepinephrine, the beta-hydroxylated ana-logue of dopamine, were shown to produce maximal stimulation of enzyme activity. Norepinephrine was less potent than dopamine. L-Isoproterenol, N-isopropyl norepinephrine, was inactive as an agonist. Subsequent studies (summarized in Table 1) have characterized the structural requirements of

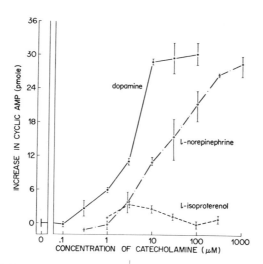

FIG. 7. Effect of catecholamines on adenylyl cyclase activity in a homogenate of rat caudate nucleus. In the absence of added catecholamine, 27.1 ± 1.0 pmoles (mean ± SEM, N = 6) of cyclic AMP was formed. The increase in cyclic AMP above this basal level is plotted as a function of catecholamine concentration. The data give mean values and ranges for duplicate determinations on each of 2–5 replicate samples. (Modified from 35.)

TABLE 1. *Structural specificity of the striatal dopamine receptor*

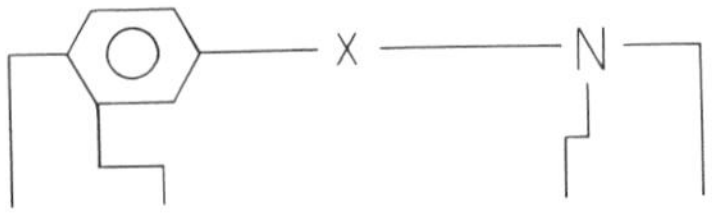

Name	Structure					% of maximal response[a]	Affinity[b] (μM)
Dopamine	OH	OH	CH$_2$—CH$_2$	H	H	100	4
Epinine	OH	OH	CH$_2$—CH$_2$	H	CH$_3$	100	7
N,N'-dimethyl dopamine	OH	OH	CH$_2$—CH$_2$	CH$_3$	CH$_3$	60	20
Norepinephrine	OH	OH	CH—CH$_2$ | OH	H	H	100	30
Alpha-methyl dopamine	OH	OH	CH$_2$—CH$_2$ | CH$_3$	H	H	58	100
Phenethylamine	H	H	CH$_2$—CH$_2$	H	H	—	—
m-Methoxytyramine	OH	OCH$_3$	CH$_2$—CH$_2$	H	H	—	—

[a] Response to 100 μM dopamine is taken as 100%.
[b] Affinity represents the concentration of compound producing a half-maximal increase in enzyme activity.
Based on data from refs. 35, 51, and 65.

agonists at this receptor. Thus, the catechol moiety was necessary for maximal agonist activity; phenethylamine (dopamine without hydroxyl groups) was devoid of agonist activity. Furthermore, the addition of more than one methyl group to the amine caused a loss of agonist activity. Thus, epinine

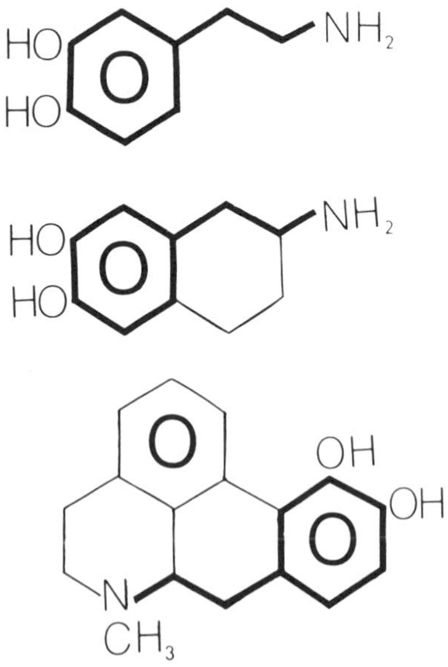

FIG. 8. The structure of compounds which stimulate dopamine-sensitive adenylyl cyclase. The structural similarities between dopamine (*top*) and either 2-amino-6,7-dihydroxyl-1,2,3,4 tetrahydronaphthalene (*middle*) or apomorphine (*bottom*) are indicated by heavy lines. These structural similarities between the latter two compounds and dopamine are thought to underlie the dopamine-like effects of the latter two compounds on the dopamine-sensitive adenylyl cyclase.

(N-methyl dopamine) was equipotent with dopamine; however, dimethyl dopamine was less potent as an agonist than was dopamine. Finally, substitution of hydroxyl or methyl groups on the two-carbon bridge caused a loss of agonist activity. Thus, norepinephrine or alpha methyl dopamine were less potent than was dopamine. In summary, no catecholamine was more potent or produced a larger-fold stimulation of the adenylyl cyclase activity of the corpus striatum than did dopamine.

The dopamine receptor regulating adenylyl cyclase can recognize several molecules which contain the structure of dopamine within a rigid molecular framework. Apomorphine is an example of such a molecule (Fig. 8). The nonpolar nature of apomorphine at physiological pH permits the molecule to rapidly cross the blood-brain barrier. This fact has been exploited in a variety of *in vivo* behavioral and biochemical experiments which suggest that apomorphine is an agonist on both presynaptic and postsynaptic dopamine receptors. When tested in the striatal adenylyl cyclase system, apomorphine at low concentrations increased enzyme activity; higher concentrations blocked this effect and lowered enzyme level to basal values (Fig. 9). The antagonist action of apomorphine on the striatal enzyme was unanticipated. Indeed, it has not been determined if any of the actions of apomorphine on the extrapyramidal nervous system are the result of its antagonist activity toward dopamine receptors. Interestingly, apomorphine functions as a pure antagonist of the dopamine receptor in the bovine parathyroid (6). Another rigid analogue of dopamine is 2-amino-6,7-dihydroxyl-1,2,3,4

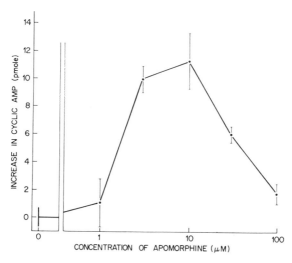

FIG. 9. Effect of apomorphine on adenylyl cyclase activity in a homogenate of rat caudate nucleus. In the absence of added apomorphine, 26.5 ± 0.7 pmoles (mean ± SEM, N = 4) of cyclic AMP was formed. The increase in cyclic AMP above this basal level is plotted as a function of apomorphine concentration. The data give mean values and ranges for duplicate determinations on each of 2–4 replicate samples. (Modified from 35.)

tetrahydronaphthalene (Fig. 8). This molecule, which contains the fully extended structure of dopamine, is as potent an agonist as is dopamine itself
both *in vivo* and *in vitro* (52,55). The tetrahydroisoquinolines, which contain a folded structure of dopamine, are weak agonists on the adenylyl
cyclase from the striatum (52,68). Based on the potency of these rigid,
synthetic compounds, it has been postulated that the preferred conformation
of dopamine which interacts with the receptor regulating adenylyl cyclase
is the fully extended *trans* form of the molecule (52,67,68).

LERGOTRILE AND RELATED ERGOT DERIVATIVES

Lergotrile (2-chloro-6-methylergoline-8β-acetonitrile) mesylate mimics
the dopaminergic inhibition of the release of prolactin from the pituitary
gland (9). The structural similarity between lergotrile and dopamine is
shown in Fig. 10; the molecule contains the structure of phenethylamine; the
hydroxy groups, which are essential for agonist activity in the catecholamines,
are not present. Nonetheless, the efficacy of the drug both in the treatment
of parkinsonism (45) and in animal behavioral models (69) suggested that
this compound functions as an agonist on the postsynaptic dopamine receptor in the corpus striatum. Therefore, it was surprising that lergotrile did
not increase adenylyl cyclase activity of striatal homogenates. Figure 11A
shows that dopamine caused an approximate doubling of the activity of the
striatal enzyme and that lergotrile diminished this stimulatory effect in a dose-
dependent manner (33). A sufficiently high concentration of lergotrile could
completely abolish the increase in enzyme activity due to dopamine. Thus,
lergotrile did function as a weak antagonist of the stimulation of this enzyme
activity by dopamine. Since such an antagonistic action of lergotrile on the
striatal dopamine receptors was unanticipated, it seemed desirable to test the
drug on the beta-adrenergic receptor which regulates the adenylyl cyclase
activity in homogenates of the rabbit cerebellar cortex (Fig. 11B). Both in
the presence and the absence of lergotrile, L-epinephrine caused an approxi-

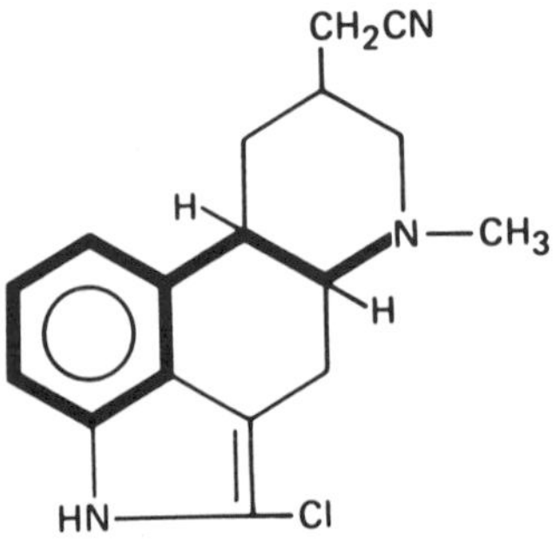

FIG. 10. Structure of lergotrile (2-chloro-6-methylergoline-8β-acetonitrile). The structural similarity between dopamine and lergotrile is indicated by the heavier lines.

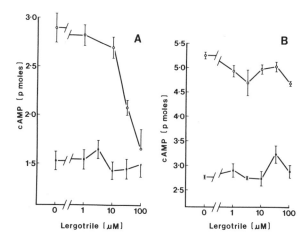

FIG. 11. Effects of lergotrile on dopamine receptors and beta-adrenergic receptors. A: Blockade by lergotrile of the dopamine-stimulated adenylyl cyclase activity of rat caudate nucleus. Adenylyl cyclase activity was measured in homogenates of rat caudate nucleus either in the absence (circles) or in the presence (squares) of 100 μM dopamine. Data represent mean ± SEM for 6 (no lergotrile) or 3 (added lergotrile) determinations of enzyme activity in replicate aliquots of a single striatal homogenate. B: Effect of lergotrile on the epinephrine-stimulated adenylyl cyclase activity of rabbit cerebellar cortex. Adenylyl cyclase activity was measured in a homogenate of rabbit cerebellar cortex either in the absence (circles) or in the presence (squares) of 100 μM L-epinephrine. Data represent mean ± SEM for 12 (no lergotrile no epinephrine), 6 (no lergotrile, plus epinephrine), or 3 (added lergotrile) determinations of enzyme activity in replicate aliquots of a single homogenate. (Modified from 33.)

mate doubling of enzyme activity. In contrast with its effect on the striatal enzyme, lergotrile did not antagonize the stimulation of the cerebellar enzyme by L-epinephrine. Thus, lergotrile functioned as a specific, although weak, dopaminergic antagonist rather than as a dopaminergic agonist.

The kinetic mechanism underlying the dopaminergic antagonism of lergotrile is complex (Fig. 12). In the presence of a single low concentration of lergotrile (0.01 mM), the response of the striatal adenylyl cyclase to dopamine was significantly altered. The maximal response to dopamine was diminished approximately 30%; in addition, considerably higher concentrations of dopamine were required to stimulate the activity of the lergotrile-treated homogenate. This type of inhibition contrasts with the competitive kinetics between dopamine and a variety of antipsychotic drugs (see below).

The ability of lergotrile to block the striatal dopamine receptor is unanticipated in view of the agonist activity of this compound in other assay systems (9,45,69). Thus, although lergotrile is a potent dopaminergic agonist *in vivo,* this compound is only a weak dopamine antagonist *in vitro.* Similarly, bromocriptine, another ergot which mimics dopamine *in vivo,* is a noncompetitive dopamine antagonist *in vitro* (74). A variety of other ergot derivatives, including LSD, are both agonists and antagonists of the striatal dopamine-sensitive adenylyl cyclase (4,65,75). However, lergotrile presents

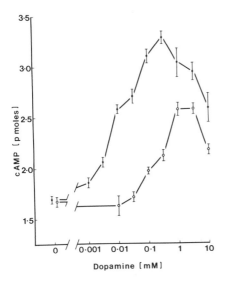

FIG. 12. The noncompetitive blockade by lergotrile of the striatal dopamine receptor. Dopamine-stimulated adenylyl cyclase activity in a homogenate of rat caudate nucleus was measured in the presence (*circle*) or in the absence (*squares*) of 10 μM lergotrile. Data represent mean $\pm$ SEM of enzyme activity determined in 5 replicate aliquots of a single tissue homogenate. (Modified from 33.)

the most striking dichotomy between *in vivo* and *in vitro* effects of such compounds. This dichotomy raises the possibility that additional classes of postsynaptic dopamine receptors may exist which are not associated with the dopamine-sensitive adenylyl cyclase. Thus, these additional postsynaptic dopamine receptors would be analogous to the presynaptic dopamine receptors on the terminals of the nigroneostriatal neurons which cannot be associated with dopamine-sensitive adenylyl cyclase activity.

A variety of drugs used to treat the symptoms of psychosis are also potent antagonists of the dopamine receptor which regulates adenylyl cyclase activity. Both the potency and the kinetic mechanism of action of these compounds as antagonists of the dopamine receptor can be determined utilizing the dopamine-sensitive adenylyl cyclase as an assay system (11,30,35,50). The kinetic mechanism of action of the antipsychotic compounds is that they function as competitive antagonists of dopamine. In the presence of antipsychotic drugs, substantially higher concentrations of dopamine are required to achieve stimulation of the enzyme activity; however, the maximal response to dopamine is not diminished. Thus, the effect of these drugs is to shift the dose-response relationship between dopamine and enzyme stimulation to the right (Fig. 13). From the concentration of drug used and the magnitude of this shift, it is possible to calculate the affinity of the dopamine receptor for these various drugs (8). The potency of a variety of the antipsychotic drugs is summarized in Table 2. Fluphenazine, which is among the most potent of the antipsychotic drugs, is the most potent ($K_i = 8$ nM) dopamine antagonist among the phenothiazine derivatives. The classic antipsychotic drug, chlorpromazine, which is less potent as an antipsychotic drug than is fluphenazine, is also a less potent dopamine antagonist ($K_i = 66$ nM). Diethazine, a phenothiazine which has little or no antipsychotic activity, is approximately 1,300-

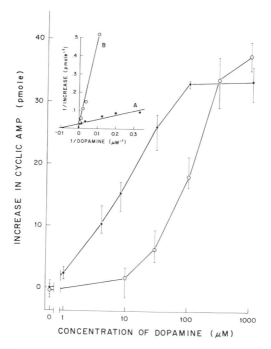

FIG. 13. Effect of various concentrations of dopamine, alone (*closed circle*) or in combination with 0.1 μM fluphenazine (*dotted circle*), on adenylate cyclase activity in a homogenate of rat caudate nucleus. In the absence of added dopamine and fluphenazine, 46.0 ± 2.0 pmoles (mean $\pm$ SEM, $N = 6$) of cyclic AMP was formed. The increase in cyclic AMP above the basal level (i.e., the level in the absence of both dopamine and fluphenazine) is plotted as a function of dopamine concentration. The data give mean values and ranges for duplicate determinations on each of three replicate samples. Inset: Double-reciprocal plot of cyclic AMP increase as a function of dopamine concentration from 3 to 300 μM. A, Control; B, 1×10^{-7} M fluphenazine. (Modified from 11.)

fold less potent than fluphenazine. The butyrophenones are another class of potent antipsychotic drugs. In contrast with the phenothiazines, the butyrophenones are relatively weaker dopamine antagonists in the adenylyl cyclase assay than might be predicted on the basis of their *in vivo* potency (Table 2, Fig. 14). The reasons for this discrepancy have not been conclusively determined; however, the accumulation of neuroleptic drugs in various regions of the brain is a well-documented phenomenon which could contribute to their apparent potency *in vivo* (40,70). The dopamine receptors from various brain regions have approximately equal affinities for the various antagonists; although some slight, but reproducible, variations have been reported (5,59). It has not been determined if these variations are of significance to the *in vivo* actions of these drugs.

Several antipsychotic compounds exist as stereoisomers; in each case, only one of the stereoisomers is biologically active. Two examples of such compounds are the *cis* and *trans* forms of flupenthixol and the enantiomers of butaclamol (46,54). In bothof these cases, the biologically active compound

TABLE 2. *Calculated inhibition constant* (K_i) *of several phenothiazine derivatives and related compounds for dopamine-sensitive adenylate cyclase of rat caudate nucleus*

	Caudate nucleus enzyme	
Drug	I_{50} (μM)	K_i (μM)
Phenothiazines and related compounds		
Fluphenazine	0.07	0.008
Trifluoperazine	0.10	0.011
Promazine	0.35	0.039
Triflupromazine	0.40	0.044
Prochlorperazine	0.50	0.055
Thioridazine	0.50	0.055
Chlorpromazine	0.60	0.066
Promethazine	15.0	1.67
Imipramine	27.0	3.00
Desmethylimipramine	28.0	3.11
Ethoproperazine	37.0	4.11
Diethazine	100.0	11.11
Butyrophenone and related compounds		
Haloperidol	2.0	0.22
Pimozide	11.0	1.22
Dibenzodiazepine		
Clozapine	0.55	0.061

Data from experiments in which the concentration of dopamine was held constant, and the concentration of the test substance was varied. The K_i value was calculated from the relationship $I_{50} = K_i(1 + S/K_m)$, where I_{50} is the concentration of drug required to give 50% inhibition of the dopamine-stimulated increase in enzyme activity, and S is the concentration (40 μM) of dopamine. K_m is the concentration of dopamine required to give half-maximal activation of the enzyme. The mean value for K_m found in this series of experiments was 5 μM.

is a potent dopamine antagonist whereas the biologically inactive form of the molecule is considerably less potent. Thus, *cis*-flupenthixol is among the most potent ($K_i = 1$ nM) dopamine antagonists whereas the *trans* form of this molecule is less potent (50). Similarly, (+)-butaclamol is approximately 500 times more potent than the (−)-enantiomer of butaclamol (46,51). The potency of the biologically active stereoisomers as *in vitro* dopamine antagonists again points to the structural specificity of the dopamine receptor regulating adenylyl cyclase.

Although other receptors regulating adenylyl cyclase are affected by phenothiazines and other antipsychotic compounds, these other receptors do not possess the structural specificity which characterizes the dopamine receptor (49). Thus, although antipsychotic compounds can block the beta-adrenergic receptor, 100-fold higher concentrations of drug are required than are necessary to block the striatal dopamine receptor. In addition, the beta-adrenergic receptor does not distinguish between the biologically active and inactive *cis*

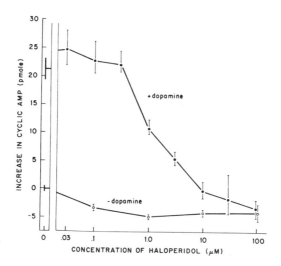

FIG. 14. Effect of haloperidol, in the absence and presence of 40 μM dopamine, on adenylate cyclase activity in a homogenate of rat caudate nucleus. In the absence of added dopamine or haloperidol, 26.43 $\pm$ 0.65 pmoles (mean $\pm$ SEM, $N = 12$) of cyclic AMP was formed; accumulation is expressed as the increase above this basal level. The data give mean values and ranges for duplicate determinations on each of 3 samples. (Modified from 35.)

and *trans* forms of flupenthixol. This contrasts with the considerable difference in the potency of *cis* and *trans* flupenthixol as dopamine antagonists. Thus, the neuroleptic drugs are most potent and most selective as antagonists of the dopamine receptor regulating adenylyl cyclase. The ability of these compounds to antagonize this striatal dopamine-sensitive adenylyl cyclase may contribute to the extrapyramidal side effects of these compounds. In addition, it is tempting to speculate that antagonism of dopamine receptors regulating adenylyl cyclase at nonstriatal loci in human brain may contribute to the antipsychotic effects of these compounds.

CELLULAR LOCATION OF DOPAMINE-SENSITIVE ADENYLYL CYCLASE

The precise cellular location of the dopamine-sensitive adenylyl cyclase in the striatum is not known. In a study utilizing subcellular fractionation, the highest specific activity of the enzyme was observed in the submitochondrial fractions enriched with nerve endings (12). As such, this observation is consistent with a synaptic location of the enzyme. The enzyme activity is not associated structurally with the dopaminergic nigroneostriatal neurons. The destruction of these dopamine-containing neurons by injection of 6-OH dopamine into the substantia nigra does not alter either the amount of properties of the dopamine-sensitive adenylyl cyclase activity in homogenates of the caudate nucleus (39). Other recent studies have attempted to selectively destroy the cellular element within the striatum which contains the dopamine-stimulated adenylyl cyclase. Local injections of kainic acid, a rigid analogue of glutamic acid, selectively destroy neurons; nerve terminals and glia are spared. In contrast with 6-OH dopamine injections, intrastriatal injections of kainic acid cause a substantial loss of the dopamine-sensitive adenylyl cyclase activity (17). Since the kainic acid injections cause considerable cellular damage within the striatum, the precise identification of the cell type(s) which contains the dopamine-sensitive adenylyl cyclase has not been achieved (17, 26). In other studies, glial cells have been identified as a cell type possessing the dopamine-sensitive adenylyl cyclase (27). However, glial cells within the striatum are not destroyed by kainic acid treatment (17,26). This apparent discrepancy between the kainic acid studies and the fractionation studies has not been resolved.

GROSS ANATOMICAL LOCATION

Dopamine is a neurotransmitter in a number of anatomical subdivisions of the mammalian brain. The possibility that the dopamine-sensitive adenylyl cyclase is a postsynaptic receptor for dopamine is reinforced by the occurrence of this enzyme activity in brain regions where dopamine has been implicated as a neurotransmitter. Thus, in addition to the caudate nucleus, dopamine-sensitive adenylyl cyclase activity occurs in preparations of the nucleus accumbens (11), the olfactory tubercule (11,28), the amygdala (62), and the frontal cerebral cortex (5). The properties of the receptor for dopamine which regulates the adenylyl cyclase activity in each of these brain regions are similar to those of the well-characterized striatal dopamine receptor. Despite considerable effort, it was not possible to observe effects of catecholamines, including dopamine, on adenylyl cyclase activity in homogenates of rat or bovine median eminence (Kebabian, Brownstein, Kizer, and Palkovits, *unpublished observations*). However, in a recent abstract, the presence of this dopamine-sensitive enzyme has been reported in the median eminence (10). It may be anticipated that this apparent discrepancy will be resolved as more investigators focus attention on the median eminence.

The zona reticulata of the substantia nigra also possess a dopamine-sensitive adenylyl cyclase (36,59,61,71). This brain region differs from the other location where this enzyme activity exists because only the cell bodies and the dendrites of the dopaminergic nigroneostriatal neurons occur within it (3). As is the case in all other brain regions studied, the properties of nigral dopamine receptor are similar to those of the striatal enzyme (Fig. 15). Thus, dopamine and N-methyl dopamine are equipotent agonists; L-norepinephrine is a weaker agonist which still provides maximal activation; the beta-adrenergic agonist L-isoproterenol is inactive (36). Neuroleptic drugs are competitive antagonists of the nigral dopamine receptor. Chlorpromazine is equipotent as an antagonist in the nigral or striatal system (K_i values are

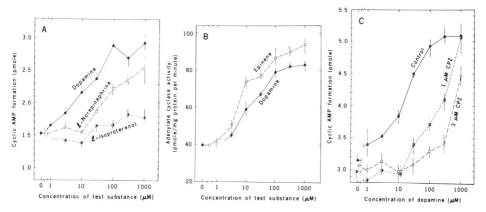

FIG. 15. A: Effects of the catecholamines dopamine (*closed circles*), L-norepinephrine (*open circles*), or L-isoproterenol (*squares*) on adenylate cyclase activity (expressed as pmoles of cyclic AMP formed per 5 min) in a homogenate of the zona reticulata of the substantia nigra. The data for no test substance addition represent mean ± SEM ($N = 18$), and the data for test substance additions represent mean and range ($N = 3$) for enzyme activity measured in replicate samples of the single homogenate. B: Effects of dopamine (*closed cirlces*) or epinine (*open circles*) on adenylate cyclase (expressed as pmoles of cyclic AMP formed per mg of protein per min) in a homogenate of the zona reticulata of the substantia nigra. The data for no test substance addition represent mean ± SEM ($N = 14$), and the data for test substance additions represent mean and range ($N = 3$) for enzyme activity measured in replicate samples of a single homogenate. C: Effects of dopamine on adenylate cyclase activity (pmoles of cyclic AMP formed per 5 min) in a homogenate of the zona reticulata and pars lateralis of the substantia nigra either in the absence (*closed circles*) or in the presence of 1 μM (*squares*) or 3 μM (*open circles*) chlorpromazine. The data represent mean ± SEM ($N = 6$) for no dopamine addition, and the data for dopamine additions represent mean and range ($N = 3$) for enzyme activity measured in replicate samples of a single homogenate. The inclusion of the pars lateralis in the tissue homogenate used for this experiment may account for both the higher enzyme activity in the absence of added dopamine and the lesser-fold stimulation of enzyme activity by dopamine in comparison with the experiment represented in A. (Modified from 36.)

67 nM and 66 nM, respectively). Thus, it was not possible to distinguish the properties of the nigral dopamine receptor regulating adenylyl cyclase from those of the striatal dopamine receptor.

These nigral dopamine receptors are not associated with the dopaminergic nigroneostriatal neurons. Although these dopaminergic neurons possess dopamine receptors (1), the destruction of these cells with 6-OH dopamine is not accompanied by any change in the activity of the nigral adenylyl cyclase activity (Fig. 16). Interestingly, either kainic acid-induced lesions of the caudate nucleus or stereotaxic lesions slightly anterior to the nigra do cause substantial losses of this enzyme (22,66). These observations suggest that the nigral dopamine-sensitive adenylyl cyclase occurs on neurons which either pass through or terminate within the substantia nigra.

The dendrites of the nigroneostriatal neurons display many similarities to the terminals of these same cells. Thus, mechanisms for the uptake, storage, synthesis, and release of dopamine have been demonstrated in preparations of substantia nigra (3,23,56). Recently, drugs have been used to differentiate several dopaminergic mechanisms in the nigra and the striatum. The first

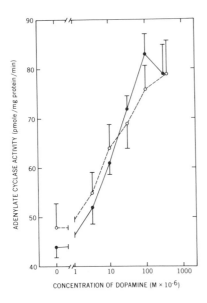

FIG. 16. Effect of 6-OH dopamine on nigral dopamine-sensitive adenylyl cyclase. Curves represent pooled results from left (*closed circles*) and right (*open circles*) zona reticulata of the substantia nigra from 5 rats. Each animal received 6-OH dopamine in the left substantia nigra. (Modified from Saavedra, Setler, and Kebabian, *in preparation.*)

drug is gamma-hydroxybutyrate, which causes a doubling of the content of dopamine in the terminals of the nigroneostriatal neurons (76). In contrast, this drug has no effect on the level of dopamine within the substantia nigra (58). The second drug is chlorpromazine, which reflexively causes an increase in the firing rate of the dopaminergic nigroneostriatal neurons. Within the striatum, the increased rate of discharge is accompanied by an increase in the content of the acidic dopamine metabolite 3,4-dihydroxyphenylacetic acid (DOPAC). No such increase in DOPAC occurs within the substantia nigra (Fig. 17), although this region of the brain contains a substantial amount of monoamine oxidase (37,64). Since electrical stimulation of the median forebrain bundle increases the level of DOPAC in both the striatum and the nigra (38), it seems probable that some class of neuron controls the release and, therefore, the metabolism of dopamine in the nigra.

At present, the physiological significance of the dopamine-sensitive adenylyl cyclase within the substantia nigra is unknown. In view of the similarities between the nigral and striatal dopamine receptors, it is possible that dopamine receptors in both anatomical regions may regulate the functioning of the extrapyramidal nervous system. Since the extensive innervation of the caudate arises from relatively few dopaminergic neurons in the nigra, effects of drugs within the nigra could profoundly affect the activity of the dopaminergic neurons in the caudate. Dopaminergic drugs are active in animals receiving kainic acid in the striatum, suggesting that the postsynaptic dopamine receptors are not essential for these effects (17). Furthermore, the recent development of a radioisotopic-enzymatic assay for apomorphine has permitted the measurement of the level of this compound in the substantia nigra following its systemic administration (Kebabian, *in preparation*). Apomorphine

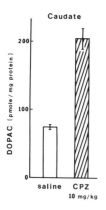
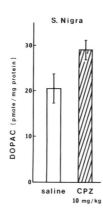

FIG. 17. Effect of chlorpromazine on the level of DOPAC in caudate nucleus and substantia nigra. Chlorpromazine (10 mg/kg) was administered by intraperitoneal injection. After 90 min the brain tissues were removed and homogenized; DOPAC was measured with a sensitive radioisotopic enzymatic assay (37). For each brain region and experimental condition, data represent mean ± SEM (N = 10)

achieves equal concentrations in nigra and striatum. These observations support the possibility that one (or more) of the nigral dopamine receptors may contribute to the inhibitory action of this drug on the dopaminergic nigro-neostriatal neurons.

ONTOGENETIC DEVELOPMENT

The dopamine-sensitive adenylyl cyclase activity, which is present in the corpus striatum of the adult brain, is also present in the striatum at birth. Spano and his colleagues (72) reported that in both neonate and adult, enzyme activities are approximately equal and the maximal effect of dopamine is an approximate doubling of the enzyme activity. These investigators noted that apomorphine was more potent as an agonist on the enzyme from the neonatal striatum than on the adult striatum; no difference in the potency of dopamine was noted. Surprisingly, in the following issue of the *Journal of Neurochemistry,* Coyle and Campochiaro (13) reported that although a dopamine-stimulated adenylyl cyclase is present in both the neonatal and the adult striatum, the activity in the neonatal striatum is only one-tenth that found in the adult. This apparent contradiction has not been resolved. Interestingly, the extensive dopaminergic innervation of the corpus striatum which is present in the adult brain is substantially less at birth (14). The adult level of dopamine is not reached until the 45th postnatal day (60). Thus, in the striatum, the presence or absence of dopaminergic nerve terminals does not appear to be obligatory for the occurrence of dopamine-sensitive adenylyl cyclase.

SUMMARY AND CONCLUSIONS

1. Dopamine causes an accumulation of cyclic AMP in a variety of mammalian tissues. This effect of dopamine occurs by virtue of its ability to stimulate adenylyl cyclase activity.

2. The properties of the dopamine receptor which regulates adenylyl cyclase activity are similar to those of the dopamine receptors which have been indirectly characterized in behavioral or biochemical experiments.

3. The dopamine-sensitive adenylyl cyclase in discrete anatomical subdivisions of mammalian brain provides a physiologically relevant postsynaptic receptor mechanism for dopamine. However, the physiological consequences of the dopamine-stimulated cyclic AMP accumulation have not been identified (53).

4. Dopamine receptors exist which are not associated with adenylyl cyclase activity. The dopaminergic "autoreceptors" on the nigroneostriatal neurons are the best example of this class of receptor. The biochemical effects of lergotrile apparently contradict its *in vivo* activity. This raises the possibility that some postsynaptic dopamine receptors may not regulate adenylyl cyclase. However, it is important to note that the *in vivo* mechanism of action of the ergots is not well understood.

ACKNOWLEDGMENT

This manuscript was prepared by Ms. E. L. Bliss.

REFERENCES

1. Aghahajanian, G. K., and Bunney, B. S. (1977): Dopamine "autoreceptors": Pharmacological characterization by microiontophoretic single cell recording studies. *N. S. Arch. Pharmacol.*, 297:1–7.
2. Björklund, A., Cegrell, L., Falck, B., Ritzen, M., and Rosengren, E. (1970): Dopamine-containing cells in sympathetic ganglia. *Acta Physiol. Scand.*, 78:334–338.
3. Björlund, A., and Lindvall, O. (1975): Dopamine in dendrites of substantia nigra neurons: Suggestions for a role in dendritic terminals. *Brain Res.*, 83:531–537.
4. Bockaert, J., Premont, J., Glowinski, J., Thierry, A. M., and Tassin, J. P. (1976): Topographical distribution of dopaminergic innervation and of dopaminergic receptors in the rat striatum. II. Distribution and characteristics of dopamine adenylate cyclase—interaction of D-LSD with dopaminergic receptors. *Brain Res.*, 107:303–315.
5. Bockaert, J., Tassin, J. P., Thierry, A. M., Glowinski, J., and Premont, J. (1977): Characteristics of dopamine and β-adrenergic sensitive adenylate cyclases in the frontal cerebral cortex of the rat. Comparative effects of neuroleptics on frontal cortex and striatal dopamine sensitive adenylate cyclases. *Brain Res.*, 122:71–86.
6. Brown, E. M., Carroll, R. J., and Aurbach, G. D. (1978): Dopaminergic stimulation of cyclic AMP accumulation and parathyroid hormone release from dispersed bovine parathyroid cells. *Proc. Natl. Acad. Sci. U.S.A.*, 74:4210–4213.
7. Brown, J. H., and Makman, M. H. (1972): Stimulation by dopamine of adenylate cyclase in retinal homogenates and of adenosine-3′:5′-cyclic monophosphate formation in intact retina. *Proc. Natl. Acad. Sci. U.S.A.*, 69:539–543.
8. Cheng, Y. C., and Prusoff, W. H. (1973): Relationship between the inhibition constant (K_i) and the concentration of inhibitor which causes 50 per cent inhibition (I_{50}) of an enzymatic reaction. *Biochem. Pharmacol.*, 22:3099–3108.
9. Clemens, J. A., Shaar, C. J., Smalstig, B., Bach, N. J., and Kornfield, E. C. (1972): Inhibition of prolactin secretion by ergolines. *Endocrinology*, 94:1171–1176.
10. Clement-Cormier, Y. C. (1977): The chemistry of dopamine receptors in the median eminence. *Pharmacologist*, 19:202.

11. Clement-Cormier, Y. C., Kebabian, J. W., Petzold, G. L., and Greengard, P. (1974): Dopamine-sensitive adenylate cyclase in mammalian brain: A possible site of action of antipsychotic drugs. *Proc. Natl. Acad. Sci. U.S.A.*, 71:1113–1117.

12. Clement-Cormier, Y. C., Parrish, R. G., Petzold, G. L., Kebabian, J. W., and Greengard, P. (1975): Characterization of a dopamine-sensitive adenylate cyclase in the rat caudate nucleus. *J. Neurochem.*, 25:143–149.

13. Coyle, J. T., and Campochiaro, P. (1976): Ontogenesis of dopaminergic-cholinergic interactions in the rat striatum: A neurochemical study. *J. Neurochem.*, 27:673–678.

14. Coyle, J. T., and Henry, D. (1973): Catecholamines in fetal and newborn rat brain. *J. Neurochem.*, 21:61–67.

15. Cramer, H., Johnson, D. G., Hanbauer, I., Silberstein, S. D., and Kopin, I. J. (1973): Accumulation of adenosine 3′,5′-monophosphate induced by catecholamines in the rat superior cervical ganglion *in vitro. Brain Res.*, 53:97–104.

16. Daly, J. W. (1977): *Cyclic Nucleotides in the Nervous System.* Plenum Press, New York.

17. DiChiara, G., Porceddu, M. L., Spano, P. F., and Gessa, G. L. (1977): Haloperidol increases and apomorphine decreases striatal dopamine metabolism after destruction of striatal dopamine-sensitive adenylate cyclase by kainic acid. *Brain Res.*, 130:374–382.

18. Dun, N. J., Kaibara, K., and Karczmar, A. G. (1977): Dopamine and adenosine 3′,5′-monophosphate responses of single mammalian sympathetic neurons. *Science*, 197:778–780.

19. Dun, N. J., and Karczmar, A. G. (1977): A comparison of the effect of theophylline and cyclic adenosine 3′,5′-monophosphate on the superior cervical ganglion of the rabbit by means of the sucrose-gap method. *J. Pharmacol. Exp. Ther.*, 202:89–96.

20. Eccles, R., and Libet, B. (1961): Origin and blockade of the synaptic responses of curarized sympathetic ganglia. *J. Physiol. (Lond.)*, 157:484–503.

21. Eranko, O. (1976): *SIF Cells: Structure and Function of the Small, Intensely Fluorescent Sympathetic Cells.* Fogarty International Center Proceeding No. 30, U.S. Government Printing Office, Washington, D.C.

22. Gale, K., Guidotti, A., and Costa, E. (1977): Dopamine-sensitive adenylate cyclase: Location in substantia nigra. *Science*, 195:503–505.

23. Geffen, L. B., Jesell, T. M., Cuello, A. C., and Iversen, L. L. (1976): Release of dopamine from dendrites in rat substantia nigra. *Nature*, 260:258–260.

24. Greengard, P., and Kebabian, J. W. (1974): Role of cyclic AMP in synaptic transmission in the mammalian peripheral nervous system. *Fed. Proc.*, 33:1059–1068.

25. Greengard, P., McAfee, D. A., and Kebabian, J. W. (1972): On the mechanism of action of cyclic AMP and its role in synaptic transmission. *Adv. Cyclic Nucleotide Res.*, 1:337–355.

26. Hattori, T., and McGeer, E. G. (1977): Fine structural changes in the rat striatum after local injections of kainic acid. *Brain Res.*, 129:174–180.

27. Henn, F. A., Anderson, D. J., and Sellstrom, A. (1977): Possible relationship between glial cells, dopamine and the effects of antipsychotic drugs. *Nature*, 266:637–638.

28. Horn, A. S., Cuello, A. C., and Miller, R. J. (1974): Dopamine in the mesolimbic system of the rat brain: Endogenous levels and the effect of drugs on the uptake mechanism and stimulation of adenylate cyclase activity. *J. Neurochem.*, 22:265–270.

29. Kalix, P., McAfee, D. A., Schorderet, M., and Greengard, P. (1974): Pharmacological analysis of synaptically mediated increase in cyclic adenosine monophosphate in rabbit superior cervical ganglion. *J. Pharmacol. Exp. Ther.*, 188:676–687.

30. Karobath, M., and Leitich, H. (1974): Antipsychotic drugs and dopamine-stimulated adenylate cyclase prepared from corpus striatum of rat brain. *Proc. Natl. Acad. Sci. U.S.A.*, 71:2915–2918.

31. Kebabian, J. W. (1973): Dopamine-sensitive adenylate cyclase: The "dopamine-receptor" in the mammalian nervous system. Ph.D. thesis, Yale University.

32. Kebabian, J. W., Bloom, F. E., Steiner, A. L., and Greengard, P. (1975): Neuro-

transmitters increase cyclic nucleotides in postganglionic neurons: Immunocyto-chemical demonstration. *Science,* 190:157–159.

33. Kebabian, J. W., Calne, D. B., and Kebabian, P. R. (1977): Lergotrile mesylate: An *in vivo* dopamine agonist which blocks dopamine receptors *in vitro. Commun. Psychopharm.,* 1:311–318.

34. Kebabian, J. W., and Greengard, P. (1971): Dopamine-sensitive adenyl cyclase: Possible role in synaptic transmission. *Science,* 174:1346–1349.

35. Kebabian, J. W., Petzold, G. L., and Greengard, P. (1972): Dopamine-sensitive adenylate cyclase in caudate nucleus of rat brain, and its similarity to the "dopamine receptor." *Proc. Natl. Acad. Sci. U.S.A.,* 69:2145–2149.

36. Kebabian, J. W., and Saavedra, J. M. (1976): Dopamine-sensitive adenylate cyclase occurs in a region of substantia nigra containing dopaminergic dendrites. *Science,* 193:683–685.

37. Kebabian, J. W., Saavedra, J. M., and Axelrod, J. (1977): A sensitive enzymatic-radioisotopic assay for 3,4-dihydroxyphenylacetic acid. *J. Neurochem.,* 28:795–801.

38. Korf, J., Zieleman, M., and Westerink, B. H. C. (1977): Metabolism of dopamine in the substantia nigra after antidromic activation. *Brain Res.,* 120:184–187.

39. Krueger, B. K., Forn, J., Walters, J. R., Roth, R. H., and Greengard, P. (1976): Dopamine stimulation of adenosine 3′,5′-monophosphate formation in rat caudate nucleus: Effect of lesions of the nigro-neostriatal pathway. *Mol. Pharmacol.,* 12: 639–648.

40. Laduron, P., and Leysen, J. (1977): Specific *in vivo* binding of neuroleptic drugs in rat brain. *Biochem. Pharmacol.,* 26:1003–1007.

41. Libet, B. (1977): The role SIF cells play in ganglionic transmission. In: *Adv. Biochem. Psychopharmacol.,* 16:541–546.

42. Libet, B., Kobayashi, H., and Tanaka, T. (1975): Synaptic coupling into the pro-duction and storage of a neuronal memory trace. *Nature,* 258:155–157.

43. Libet, B., Tanaka, T., and Tosaka, T. (1977): Different sensitivities of acetyl-choline-induced "after-hyperpolarization" compared to dopamine-induced hyper-polarization to ouabain or to lithium replacement of sodium, in rabbit sympathetic ganglia. *Life Sci.,* 20:1863–1870.

44. Libet, B., and Tosaka, T. (1970): Dopamine as a synaptic transmitter and modu-lator in sympathetic ganglia: A different mode of synaptic action. *Proc. Natl. Acad. Sci. U.S.A.,* 67:667–673.

45. Lieberman, A., Miyamoto, T., Battista, A. F., and Goldstein, M. (1975): Studies on the antiparkinsonian efficacy of lergotrile. *Neurology (Minneap.),* 25:459–462.

46. Lippmann, W., Pugsley, T., and Merker, J. (1975): Effect of butaclamol and its enantiomers upon striatal homovanillic acid and adenyl cyclase of olfactory tuber-cule in rats. *Life Sci.,* 16:213–224.

47. McAfee, D. A., and Greengard, P. (1972): Adenosine 3′,5′-monophosphate: Elec-trophysiological evidence for a role in synaptic transmission. *Science,* 178:310–312.

48. McAfee, D. A., Schorderet, M., and Greengard, P. (1971): Adenosine 3′,5′-mono-phosphate: Increase associated with synaptic transmission. *Science,* 171:1156–1158.

49. Miller, R. J. (1976): Comparison of the inhibitory effects of neuroleptic drugs on adenylate cyclase in rat tissues stimulated by dopamine, noradrenaline and glucagon. *Biochem. Pharmacol.,* 25:537–541.

50. Miller, R. J., Horn, A. S., and Iversen, L. L. (1974): The action of neuroleptic drugs on dopamine-stimulated adenosine cyclic 3′,5′-monophosphate production in rat neostriatum and limbic forebrain. *Mol. Pharmacol.,* 10:759–766.

51. Miller, R. J., Horn, A. S., and Iversen, L. L. (1975): Effect of butaclamol on dopamine-sensitive adenylate cyclase in the rat striatum. *J. Pharm. Pharmacol.,* 27: 212–213.

52. Miller, R., Horn, A., Iversen, L., and Pinder, R. (1974): Effects of dopamine-like drugs on rat striatal adenyl cyclase have implications for CNS dopamine receptor topography. *Nature,* 250:238–241.

53. Miller, R. J., and Kelly, P. H. (1975): Dopamine-like effects of cholera toxin in the central nervous system. *Nature,* 255:163–166.

54. Moller-Nielsen, I., Pedersen, V., Nymak, M., Franc, K. F., Boek, U., Fjallan, B., and Christiansen, A. V. (1973): The comparative pharmacology of flupenthixol

and some reference neuroleptics. *Acta Pharmacol. Toxicol. (Kbh.)*, 33:353–362.

55. Munday, K. A., Poat, J. A., and Woodruff, G. N. (1974): Increase in the cyclic AMP content of rat striatum produced by a cyclic analogue of dopamine. *J. Physiol. (Lond.)*, 241:119P–120P.

56. Nieoullon, A., Cheramy, A., and Glowinski, J. (1977): Release of dopamine *in vivo* from rat substantia nigra. *Nature*, 266:375–377.

57. Otten, U., Mueller, R. A., Oesch, F., and Thoenen, H. (1974): Location of an isoproterenol-responsive cyclic AMP pool in adrenergic nerve cell bodies and its relationship to tyrosine 3-monooxygenase induction. *Proc. Natl. Acad. Sci. U.S.A.*, 71:2217–2221.

58. Pericic, D., and Walters, J. R. (1976): Dopamine in substantia nigra and cortex after gamma-butyrolactone treatment. *J. Pharm. Pharmacol.*, 28:527–529.

59. Phillipson, O. T., and Horn, A. S. (1976): Substantia nigra of the rat contains a dopamine sensitive adenylate cyclase. *Nature*, 261:418–420.

60. Porcher, W., and Heller, A. (1972): Regional development of catecholamine biosynthesis in rat brain. *J. Neurochem.*, 19:1917–1930.

61. Premont, J., Thierry, A. M., Tassin, J. P., Glowinski, J., Blanc, G., and Bockaert, J. (1976): Is the dopamine sensitive cyclase in the rat substantia nigra coupled with 'autoreceptors'? *FEBS Lett.*, 68:99–104.

62. Racagni, G., and Carenzi, A. (1976): The anterior amygdala dopamine-sensitive adenylate cyclase: Point of action of antipsychotic drugs. *Pharmacol. Res. Commun.*, 8:149–158.

63. Roch, P., and Kalix, P. (1975): Effects of biogenic amines on the concentration of adenosine 3′,5′-monophosphate in bovine superior cervical ganglion. *Neuropharmacology*, 14:21–29.

64. Saavedra, J. M., Brownstein, M. J., and Palkovits, M. (1976): Distribution of catechol-O-methyl transferase, histamine N-methyl transferase and monoamine oxidase in specific areas of the rat brain. *Brain Res.*, 118:152–156.

65. Schmidt, M. J., and Hill, L. E. (1977): Effects of ergots on adenylate cyclase activity in the corpus striatum and pituitary. *Life Sci.*, 20:789–798.

66. Schwarcz, R., and Coyle, J. T. (1977): Neurochemical sequelae of kainate injections in corpus striatum and substantia nigra of the rat. *Life Sci.*, 20:431–436.

67. Sheppard, H., and Burghardt, C. R. (1974): The dopamine-sensitive adenylate cyclase of rat caudate nucleus. I. Comparison with the isoproterenol-sensitive adenylate cyclase (beta receptor system) of rat erythrocytes in responses to dopamine derivatives. *Mol. Pharmacol.*, 10:721–726.

68. Sheppard, H., and Burghardt, C. R. (1974): Effect of tetrahydroisoquinoline derivatives on the adenylate cyclases of the caudate nucleus (dopamine-type) and erythrocyte (β-type) of the rat. *Res. Commun. Pathol. Pharmacol.*, 8:527–534.

69. Silbergeld, E. K., and Pfeiffer, R. F. (1977): Differential effects of three dopamine agonists: Apomorphine, bromocriptine and lergotrile. *J. Neurochem.*, 28:1323–1326.

70. Soudijn, W., and Van Wijngaarden, I. (1972): Localization of [³H] pimozide in the rat brain in relation to its anti-amphetamine potency. *J. Pharm. Pharmacol.*, 24:773–780.

71. Spano, P. F., DiChiara, G., Tonon, G., and Trabucchi, M. (1976): A dopamine-sensitive adenylate cyclase in rat substantia nigra. *J. Neurochem.*, 27:1565–1568.

72. Spano, P. F., Kumakura, K., Govoni, S., and Trabucchi, M. (1976): Ontogenetic development of neostriatal dopamine receptors in the rat. *J. Neurochem.*, 27:621–624.

73. Tomasi, V., Biondi, C., Trevisani, A., Martini, M., and Perri, V. (1977): Modulation of cyclic AMP levels in the bovine superior cervical ganglion by prostaglandin E_1 and dopamine. *J. Neurochem.*, 28:1289–1297.

74. Trabucchi, M., Spano, P. F., Tonon, G. C., and Frattola, L. (1976): Effects of bromocriptine on central dopaminergic receptors. *Life Sci.*, 19:225–231.

75. Von Hungen, K., Roberts, S., and Hill, D. (1974): LSD as an agonist and antagonist at central dopamine receptors. *Nature*, 252:588–589.

76. Walters, J. R., and Roth, R. H. (1972): Effect of gamma-hydroxybutyrate on dopamine and dopamine metabolites in the rat striatum. *Biochem. Pharmacol.*, 21:2111–2121.

77. Wedner, H. J., Hoffer, B. J., Battenberg, E., Steiner, A. L., Parker, C. W., and Bloom, F. E. (1972): A method for detecting intracellular cyclic adenosine monophosphate by immunofluorescence. *J. Histochem. Cytochem.*, 20:293–295.
78. Williams, T. H., Black, A. C., Jr., Chiba, T., and Bhalla, R. C. (1975): Morphology and biochemistry of small, intensely fluorescent cells of sympathetic ganglia. *Nature,* 256:315–317.
79. Williams, T. H., Black, A. C., Chiba, T., and Jew, J. (1976): Species differences in mammalian SIF cells. *Adv. Biochem. Psychopharmacol.,* 16:505–511.

Advances in Biochemical Psychopharmacology, Vol. 19,
edited by P. J. Roberts et al.
Raven Press, New York © 1978.

Studies on the Pharmacological Properties of Dopamine Receptors in Various Areas of the Central Nervous System

P. F. Spano, S. Govoni, and M. Trabucchi

Institutes of Pharmacology and Pharmacognosy, University of Cagliari and University of Milan, 20129 Milan, Italy

The hypothesis of a unique physiological role of dopamine as a neurotransmitter in the mammalian brain was first put forth by Carlsson and associates in 1958 (6). The involvement of dopamine-specific receptors in the behavioral mode of action of different drugs was proposed in 1965 (13,33).

van Rossum (33), on one hand, suggested that several neuroleptic drugs may act as antagonists at central dopamine receptors. On the other hand, Ernst (13) suggested that apomorphine may bring about its behavioral effects by an agonistic interaction at the central dopamine receptors. However, the direct demonstration and the molecular pharmacological characterization of the central dopamine receptors were hampered by the approach used by these authors. Their studies in fact were based on behavioral phenomena induced by drugs injected peripherally.

Over the last years new findings have offered more direct approaches to study dopamine receptor pharmacology. An adenylate cyclase, preferentially stimulated by dopamine, has been described in homogenates of bovine superior cervical ganglia (24), calf and rat retinas (1), rat caudate nucleus (25), and nucleus accumbens and tuberculum olfactorium in the mesolimbic system (20). These findings have led to the suggestion that in these areas the dopamine-stimulated adenylate cyclase and the dopamine receptor may be related, and that the physiological effects of dopamine could be mediated by cyclic adenosine monophosphate (cyclic AMP). On the other hand, with the recently developed technique of radioreceptor binding it has been possible to label apparent postsynaptic dopamine receptor sites with [³H]dopamine or with [³H]haloperidol (2,3,9,36) and with [³H]spiroperidol (14). This technique, in addition to providing evidence for a specific binding in those brain regions rich in dopaminergic synapses, offered a new approach to investigating the affinity of drugs for the dopamine receptor (10,35,36).

The aim of this chapter is to present some data on the presence and characterization of dopamine-stimulated adenylate cyclase in various brain areas, and on the effects of various classes of recently characterized dopaminergic drugs on the activity of this enzyme and on the radioreceptor binding model. The implications of our data are that not all of the cerebral dopamine receptors are associated with an adenylate cyclase system.

LOCALIZATION OF DOPAMINE-STIMULATED ADENYLATE CYCLASE IN DOPAMINERGIC AREAS

As we stated above, pioneering studies have demonstrated the presence of an adenylate cyclase preferentially stimulated by dopamine in mammalian nucleus caudatus, nucleus accumbens, tuberculum olfactorium, and retina. In our laboratories we have extended these studies to other brain areas with dopaminergic innervation. The results of our experiments have shown the presence of a dopamine-stimulated adenylate cyclase, which is selectively inhibited by phenothiazines and butyrophenones, in the rat entorhinal cortex (41), substantia nigra (37,40), and median eminence (Table 1). This last result has also been reported recently by Clement-Cormier and Robison (7). However, we have not been able to identify a dopamine-stimulated adenylate cyclase in the pituitary gland (Table 2), in either the anterior or the posterior part. This negative finding is apparently in contrast with the data reported by MacLeod and co-workers (29), showing the presence of dopamine receptor in the anterior part of the pituitary, a finding fully confirmed in our laboratories (see Table 2). Moreover, the functional demonstration of dopamine receptor in the pituitary has also been given by MacLeod et al. (29)

TABLE 1. *Dopamine-stimulated adenylate cyclase activity in various areas of the CNS*

Brain area	Adenylate cyclase activity (pmoles cAMP/min/mg protein)		
	Basal	DA (50 μM)	DA (50 μM) +haloperidol
Striatum	204 ± 14	398 ± 19[a]	212 ± 12
Substantia nigra	198 ± 13	410 ± 22[a]	221 ± 16
Tuberculum olfactorium	141 ± 9	275 ± 15[a]	150 ± 11
Nucleus accumbens	186 ± 10	359 ± 18[a]	194 ± 12
Entorhinal cortex	65 ± 2	106 ± 6[a]	71 ± 3
Pituitary	78 ± 6	81 ± 5	74 ± 4
Median eminence	88 ± 2	116 ± 3[a]	85 ± 2
Retina	15 ± 1	31 ± 2[a]	16 ± 1

Values are the mean ± SEM of at least 10 separate determinations run in triplicate. Haloperidol was added at a concentration of 5μM. Dopamine-stimulated adenylate cyclase was determined in all the experiments following the method described by Carenzi et al. (5).

[a] $p < 0.001$ in comparison with basal values.

TABLE 2. *Stereospecific binding of ³H-haloperidol and ³H-dopamine and dopamine-stimulated adenylate cyclase activity in rat striatum and pituitary*

Brain area	³H-haloperidol (fmoles bound/mg protein)	³H-dopamine (fmoles bound/mg protein)	Dopamine-stimulated adenylate cyclase activity (pmoles cAMP/min/mg protein)
Striatum	184 ± 19	53 ± 4	196 ± 13[a]
Pituitary	81 ± 11	46 ± 2	Not detectable

³H-haloperidol and ³H-dopamine were added at a concentration of 2 nM and 4 nM, respectively, and the binding determined following the method of Burt et al. (2). Values represent the mean ± SEM of at least 10 separate determinations run in triplicate.

[a] pmoles of cAMP formed above basal activity (dopamine 5×10^{-5} M) (basal activity: 184 ± 11 pmoles cAMP/min/mg protein.

and Gräf et al. (19) since dopamine agonists and dopamine itself are able to control prolactin release either in the gland incubated *in vitro* (29) or in the gland severed *in vivo* from basal hypothalamus (19).

On the other hand, of particular relevance is the finding of a dopamine-stimulated adenylate cyclase in the substantia nigra (26,31,32,37,40). This cyclase appears to be stimulated by dopamine released from dendrites of dopaminergic cell bodies (16) and to be located on terminals of neurons which have their cell bodies in the corpus striatum (40), as suggested by experiments using brain lesions. This view has been recently confirmed using the kainic acid approach. Kainic acid injected into the striatum destroys selectively the cell bodies of neurons present in the nucleus, leaving intact nerve terminals (34). In these experimental conditions the stimulation induced by dopamine on striatal and nigral adenylate cyclase activity is virtually totally abolished (Table 3). These data strongly support the hypothesis of

TABLE 3. *Effect of striatal injection of kainic acid on striatal and nigral dopamine-stimulated adenylate cyclase*

		Adenylate cyclase activity (pmoles cAMP/min/mg protein)		
		Control side	Lesioned side	(%)
Striatum	Basal	186 ± 13	110 ± 8	−42
	DA 5×10^{-5} M	371 ± 18	125 ± 9	−66
	DA stimulated	192 ± 14	12 ± 1	−94
Substantia nigra	Basal	198 ± 13	93 ± 6	−53
	DA 5×10^{-5} M	426 ± 22	112 ± 9	−74
	DA stimulated	221 ± 14	18 ± 2	−80

Rats were injected with 3 μg of kainic acid in the right and with saline in the left striatum and were sacrificed 9 days later. The striatum of each side was homogenized and assayed individually for adenylate cyclase activity. Values are the mean ± SEM of 6 determinations in triplicate.

a localization of dopamine-stimulated adenylate cyclase at postsynaptic level in the striatum and at presynaptic level in the substantia nigra.

EFFECTS OF DOPAMINERGIC ERGOT DERIVATIVES ON DOPAMINE RECEPTORS

In addition to the anatomical localization of dopamine-stimulated adenylate cyclase in various brain areas, we have investigated the pharmacological properties of dopamine receptors in order to test the hypothesis of different classes of dopamine receptors. This hypothesis is first suggested by the finding that in the pituitary gland it is possible to demonstrate the presence of dopamine receptor probably not coupled to a specific dopamine-stimulated adenylate cyclase (Table 2). In particular, we shall report the data obtained with newly pharmacologically characterized dopamine agonists (ergot derivatives) and dopamine antagonists (benzamides, of which sulpiride is the prototype).

The effect of a number of ergot derivatives on adenylate cyclase activity in striatum and pituitary gland preparations is reported in Table 4. Bromocryptine, lisuride, and lergotrile, which have been reported in behavioral and pharmacological models to exert a strong stimulation of different dopamine functions (4,11,15,21–23,28,30,37), and metergoline do not stimulate the

TABLE 4. Comparison of the effects of various dopamine agonists on adenylate cyclase activity in rat striatum and pituitary gland homogenates

Drug	Adenylate cyclase activity (pmoles/min/mg protein)	
	Striatum	Pituitary
Basal	196 ± 11	78 ± 6
Dopamine	392 ± 20^a	81 ± 5
Apomorphine	311 ± 16^a	82 ± 5
Lergotrile	194 ± 11	84 ± 7
LSD	265 ± 14^b	79 ± 4
Ergometrine	241 ± 14^b	79 ± 5
Bromocryptine	189 ± 10	77 ± 6
Lisuride	182 ± 9	71 ± 4
Metergoline	189 ± 10	80 ± 4
DH-Ergotamine	191 ± 9	74 ± 5
DH-Ergotoxine	184 ± 10	81 ± 5

Drugs were added at a concentration of 50 μM. Norepinephrine, epinephrine, isoproterenol, serotonin, histamine, and epinine do not stimulate the adenylate cyclase activity of pituitary gland when added at a concentration of 100 μM. Values are the mean ± SEM of at least 4 separate determinations run in triplicate.
^{a} $p < 0.001$ in comparison with basal value.
^{b} $p < 0.01$ in comparison with basal value.

TABLE 5. Inhibition of dopamine-stimulated adenylate cyclase in rat striatum by various ergot derivatives

Drug	IC_{50} (M)
LSD	7×10^{-7}
Ergometrine	9×10^{-7}
Bromocriptine	3×10^{-7}
Lisuride	1×10^{-7}
Metergoline	2×10^{-7}
Lergotrile	3×10^{-7}
Ergotamine	7×10^{-7}
DH-Ergotamine	5×10^{-7}
DH-Ergotoxine	3.3×10^{-6}
DH-Ergocornine	4.5×10^{-6}
DH-Ergocryptine	3×10^{-6}
DH-Ergocristine	3×10^{-6}

The values listed are the mean concentrations of each drug required to inhibit the stimulation induced by dopamine (10 M) by 50%. Each IC_{50} value was determined from a log-probit using 3 or more concentrations of drug. Numbers are mean of at least 4 separate determinations run in triplicate. The SEM for each IC_{50} is less than 10% of the IC_{50}.

activity of striatal or pituitary adenylate cyclase. Only LSD and ergometrine, among the several ergot derivatives tested, appear to behave as weak dopamine agonists, and only in striatal preparations. On the contrary, at micromolar concentrations, all these compounds inhibited striatal dopamine-stimulated adenylate cyclase activity. The inhibitory concentration 50 (IC_{50}) on the enzyme activity obtained with concentration-response studies for the various ergot derivatives is shown in Table 5. These surprising results which appear to be in apparent contradiction with all previously reported behavioral, pharmacological, and clinical data are in agreement with some of our previous data (18,38,39,43) and raise a number of questions on the mode of action of dopaminergic ergot derivatives and on the hypothesis of the coupling between the dopamine receptor recognition sites and the dopamine-stimulated adenylate cyclase. It may be pertinent in this regard to recall that data obtained with the radioreceptor binding technique seem to indicate for some ergot derivatives, such as bromocriptine, a prevailing antagonistic action at central dopamine receptors rather than an agonistic effect (2,17).

EFFECTS OF BENZAMIDES (SULPIRIDE) ON DOPAMINE RECEPTORS

In another set of experiments we have extended our studies on the pharmacological characterization of cerebral dopamine receptors, testing the effect

TABLE 6. Effect of sulpiride on dopamine-sensitive adenylate cyclase activity in rat striatal homogenates

	With preincubation (pmoles cAMP/min/mg protein)	%	Without preincubation (pmoles cAMP/min/mg protein)	%
Control	252 ± 7	—	268 ± 15	—
DA	587 ± 26^a	133	669 ± 22^a	149
Sulpiride	262 ± 17	—	308 ± 14	—
Sulpiride + DA	542 ± 25^a	115	643 ± 17^a	140

Some samples were preincubated at 30°C for 10 min in absence of ATP and dopamine. Dopamine and sulpiride were added at a concentration of 50 μM. Values are the mean ± SEM of 4 separate determinations run in triplicate.
[a] $p < 0.001$ when compared to control.

of sulpiride on dopamine-stimulated adenylate cyclase and on the radio-receptor model. Sulpiride belongs to the class of benzamides, and has been classified as a putative dopamine antagonist with a weak cataleptogenic activity in animals, antipsychotic activity, and strong prolactin-stimulatory effects (42). As we already reported in 1975 (42) sulpiride, contrary to other cataleptogenic and noncataleptogenic neuroleptics, does not inhibit the cyclic AMP accumulation induced by dopamine in striatal and limbic area homogenates. After several periods of preincubation, sulpiride does not show any inhibitory effect. These data are summarized in Table 6. Furthermore, sulpiride, unlike haloperidol, does not block the accumulation of cyclic AMP induced *in vivo* by apomorphine (42), a result which fully substantiates the finding obtained *in vitro*.

However, the hypothesis of a specific interaction of sulpiride with cerebral dopamine receptors is supported by some findings reported below. Sulpiride,

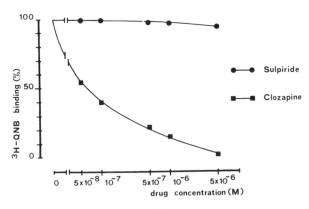

FIG. 1. Competition by sulpiride and clozapine for specific [³H]QNB binding in membranes of rat striatum. [³H]QNB binding was measured following the method of Yamamura and Snyder (44). For each curve specific binding of multiple experiments was averaged on a percentage basis, taking binding in the presence of 10^{-6} M unlabeled QNB as a blank. The ordinate refers to specific binding values.

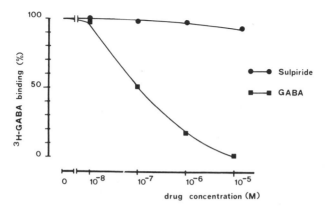

FIG. 2. Competition by sulpiride and GABA for specific [³H]GABA binding in membranes of rat striatum. [³H]GABA binding was measured following the method of Enna et al. (12). For each curve specific binding of multiple experiments was averaged on a percentage basis, taking binding in the presence of 10⁻³ M unlabeled GABA as a blank. The ordinate refers to specific binding values.

for instance, is completely devoid of antimuscarinic central activity, as is shown by the lack of interaction with [³H]-3-quinuclidinylbenzilate (³H-QNB)-binding in membranes of rat striatum (Fig. 1). This finding differentiates sulpiride from clozapine, another neuroleptic whose weak cataleptogenic activity has been ascribed to the strong interaction with muscarinic central receptors. On the other hand, sulpiride has no direct activity on GABA central receptors, as demonstrated by the lack of displacement of [³H]GABA from rat striatal membrane preparations (Fig. 2).

These data, taken together, have led us to investigate whether or not sulpiride interacts with a population of cerberal dopamine receptors not associated

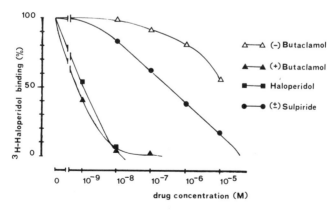

FIG. 3. Competition by sulpiride, haloperidol, (+)-butaclamol, and (−)-butaclamol for specific [³H]haloperidol binding in membranes of rat striatum. [³H]haloperidol binding was measured following the method of Burt et al. (2). For each curve specific binding of multiple experiments was averaged on a percentage basis, taking binding in the presence of 10⁻⁴ M dopamine as a blank. The ordinate refers to specific binding values.

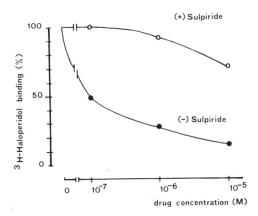

FIG. 4. Competition by (+)-sulpiride and (−)-sulpiride for specific [³H]haloperidol binding in membranes of rat striatum. [³H]haloperidol binding was measured as indicated in Fig. 3. For each curve specific binding of multiple experiments was averaged on a percentage basis, taking binding in the presence of 10⁻⁴ M dopamine as a blank. The ordinate refers to specific binding values.

with an adenylate cyclase system. Therefore, we have studied the effect of the drug on the stereospecific binding of [³H]haloperidol to rat cerebral membrane preparations. Figure 3 shows that sulpiride can displace [³H]haloperidol from putative dopamine binding sites in membranes prepared from rat striatum. The potency of sulpiride is lower than that of (+)-butaclamol and haloperidol, which correlates with clinical observations, but significantly more pronounced than that of (−)-butaclamol. The specificity of the action of sulpiride at the level of dopamine central receptors has been confirmed in our laboratories by the observation that only the (−)-enantiomer of the drug shows the property of displacing [³H]haloperidol from its stereospecific binding sites in rat striatal membranes (Fig. 4). The calculated IC_{50} of this effect is about 100 nM for (−)-sulpiride and more than 10,000 nM for (+)-sulpiride.

CONCLUDING REMARKS

One of the main conclusions that can be drawn from our observations and from the data obtained in other laboratories is that dopamine-stimulated adenylate cyclase is a unique tool to map dopamine receptors in the mammalian brain.

On the other hand, available evidence accumulated over the past few years suggests that whereas the traditional methods of measuring dopamine receptor activity involve behavioral tests which are often imprecise, the evaluation of dopamine-stimulated adenylate cyclase activity provides a reliable approach to establish whether a drug either blocks or activates dopamine receptors. However, this does not appear to be the case with the drug studied in our laboratories. Sulpiride, which shows a rather specific interaction with dopamine receptors in radioreceptor binding studies, does not block dopamine-stimulated adenylate cyclase either *in vitro* or *in vivo*. On the other hand, ergot derivatives, which are supposed to have potent stimulatory effects on dopamine receptors, do not stimulate cyclic AMP accumulation in striatal homogenates but show blocking properties on the enzyme activity stimulated by dopamine.

It has been stressed that we still do not know whether the effects of any particular neurotransmitter are coupled directly with the activation of adenylate cyclase. Available evidence indicates that different receptor populations of the same transmitter are either associated or not with a cyclic AMP system. Beta-adrenergic receptors, for instance, appear to be associated with an adenylate cyclase, although alpha-adrenergic receptors are not. The same applies to histamine-2 and histamine-1 receptors, respectively. It might well be also that dopamine receptors are two different populations of which only one is directly coupled to the activation of adenylate cyclase. Although more experiments are necessary before definite conclusions can be drawn, our results support this contention.

ACKNOWLEDGMENTS

We thank Ravizza S.p.A., Muggiò (Milan) for the generous gift of sulpiride enantiomers.

REFERENCES

1. Brown, J. N., and Makman, M. H. (1972): Stimulation by dopamine of adenylate cyclase in retinal homogenates and of adenosine 3′,5′-cyclic AMP formation in intact retina. *Proc. Natl. Acad. Sci. U.S.A.*, 69:539–543.
2. Burt, D. R., Creese, I., and Snyder, S. H. (1976): Properties of (^{3}H)-haloperidol and (^{3}H)-dopamine binding associated with dopamine receptors in calf brain membranes. *Mol. Pharmacol.*, 12:800–812.
3. Burt, D. R., Creese, I., and Snyder, S. H. (1977): Antischizophrenic drugs: Chronic treatment elevates dopamine receptor binding in brain. *Science*, 196:326–328.
4. Calne, D. B., Kartzinel, B., and Shoulson, I. (1976): An ergot derivative in the treatment of Parkinson's disease. *Postgrad. Med. J. (Suppl. 1)*, 52:81–83.
5. Carenzi, A., Gillin, C., Guidotti, A., Schwartz, M., Trabucchi, M., and Wyatt, J. (1975): Dopamine-sensitive adenyl cyclase in human caudate nucleus: A study in control subjects and schizophrenic patients. *Arch. Gen. Psychiatry*, 32:1056–1059.
6. Carlsson, A., Lindqvist, M., Magnusson, M., and Waldeck, B. (1958): On the presence of 3-hydroxytyramine in brain. *Science*, 127:471.
7. Clement-Cormier, Y., and Robison, G. A. (1977): Adenylate cyclase from various dopaminergic areas of the brain and the action of psychotic drugs. *Biochem. Pharmacol.*, 26:1719–1722.
8. Corrodi, H., Fuxe, K., Hökfelt, T., Lindbrink, P., and Ungerstedt, U. (1973): Effect of ergot drugs on central catecholamine neurons: Evidence for a stimulation of central dopamine. *J. Pharm. Pharmacol.*, 25:409–412.
9. Creese, I., Burt, D. R., and Snyder, S. H. (1975): Dopamine receptor binding: Differentiation of agonist-antagonist states with ^{3}H-dopamine and ^{3}H-haloperidol. *Life Sci.*, 17:993–1002.

10. Creese, I., Burt, D. R., and Snyder, S. H. (1976): Dopamine receptor binding predicts clinical and pharmacological potencies of antischizophrenic drugs. *Science,* 192:481–483.
11. Del Pozo, E., Brun del Re, R., Varga, L., and Friesen, H. (1972): The inhibition of prolactin secretion in man by CB 154 (2-Br-α-ergocryptine). *J. Clin. Endocrinol. Metab.,* 35:768–771.
12. Enna, S. J., Collins, J. F., and Snyder, S. H. (1977): Stereospecificity and structure-activity requirements of GABA receptor binding in rat brain. *Brain Res.,* 124: 185–190.
13. Ernst, A. M. (1965): Relation between the action of dopamine and apomorphine and their O-methylated derivatives upon the CNS. *Psychopharmacology,* 7:391–399.
14. Fields, J. Z., Reisine, I. D., and Yamamura, H. (1977): Biochemical demonstration of dopaminergic receptors in rat and human brain using (^{3}H)-spiroperidol. *Brain Res.,* 136:578–584.
15. Fuxe, K., Agnati, L. F., Corrodi, H., Everitt, B. J., Hökfelt, T., Lofstrom, A., and Ungerstedt, U. (1975): Action of dopamine receptor agonists in forebrain and hypothalamus: Rotational behavior, ovulation, and dopamine turnover. *Adv. Neurol.,* 9:223–242.
16. Geffen, L. B., Jessel, T. M., Cuello, A. C., and Iversen, L. L. (1976): Release of dopamine from dendrites in rat substantia nigra. *Nature,* 260:258–260.
17. Goldstein, M., Lew, J. Y., Hata, F., and Lieberman, A. (1978): Binding interactions of ergot alkaloids with monoaminergic receptors in the brain. *Gerontology* [*Suppl. 1*], 24:76–85.
18. Govoni, S., Iuliano, E., Spano, P. F., and Trabucchi, M. (1977): Effect of ergotamine and dihydroergotamine on dopamine-stimulated adenylate cyclase in rat caudate nucleus. *J. Pharm. Pharmacol.,* 29:45–47.
19. Gräf, K. J., Horowski, R., and El Etreby, M. F. (1977): Effect of prolactine inhibitory agents on the ectopic anterior pituitary and the mammary gland in rats. *Acta Endocrinol. (Kbh.),* 85:267–278.
20. Horn, A. S., Cuello, A. C., and Miller, R. J. (1974): Dopamine in the mesolimbic system of the rat brain: Endogenous levels and the effect of drugs on the uptake mechanism and stimulation of adenylate cyclase. *J. Neurochem.,* 22:265–270.
21. Horowski, R., and Wachtel, H. (1976): Direct dopaminergic action of lisuride hydrogen maleate, an ergot derivative, in mice. *Eur. J. Pharmacol.,* 36:373–383.
22. Johnson, A. M., Vigouret, J. M., and Loew, D. M. (1974): Central dopaminergic action of ergotoxine alkaloids and some derivatives. *Experientia,* 29:763.
23. Johnson, A. M., Vigouret, J. M., and Loew, D. M. (1976): Stimulant properties of bromocriptine on central dopamine receptors in comparison to apomorphine, (+)-amphetamine and L-DOPA. *Br. J. Pharmacol.,* 56:59–68.
24. Kebabian, J. W., and Greengard, P. (1971): Dopamine-sensitive adenyl cyclase: Possible role in synaptic transmission. *Science,* 174:1346–1349.
25. Kebabian, J. W., Petzold, G. L., and Greengard, P. (1972): Dopamine-sensitive adenylate cyclase in caudate nucleus of rat brain and its similarity to the dopamine receptor. *Proc. Natl. Acad. Sci. U.S.A.,* 69:2145–2149.
26. Kebabian, J. W., and Saavedra, J. M. (1977): Dopamine-sensitive adenylate cyclase occurs in a region of substantia nigra containing dopaminergic dendrites. *Science,* 193:683–685.
27. Lieberman, A., Kupersmith, M., Estey, E., and Goldstein, M. (1976): Lergotrile in Parkinson's disease. *Lancet,* ii:515–516.
28. Liuzzi, A., Chiodini, P. G., Botalla, L., Cremascoli, G., Müller, E. E., and Silvestrini, F. (1974): Decreased plasma growth hormone (GH) levels in acromegalic patients following CB 154 (2-Br-α-ergocryptine) administration. *J. Clin. Endocrinol. Metab.,* 38:910–919.
29. MacLeod, R. M., Kimura, H., and Login, I. (1976): Inhibition of prolactin secretion by dopamine and piribedil (ET-495). In: *Growth Hormone and Related Peptides,* edited by A. Pecile and E. E. Müller, pp. 443–453. Exerpta Medica, Amsterdam.
30. Miyamoto, T., Battista, A. F., Goldstein, M., and Fuxe, K. (1974): Long-lasting tremor activity induced by 2-Br-α-ergocryptine in monkeys. *J. Pharm. Pharmacol.,* 26:452–454.

31. Phillipson, O. T., and Horn, A. S. (1976): Substantia nigra of the rat contains a dopamine sensitive adenylate cyclase. *Nature,* 261:418–420.
32. Premont, J., Thierry, A. M., Tamin, J. P., Glowinski, J., Blanc, G., and Bockaert, J. (1976): Is the dopamine-sensitive adenylate cyclase in the rat substantia nigra coupled with "autoreceptors"? *FEBS Lett.,* 68:99–104.
33. van Rossum, J. M. (1965): Different types of sympathomimetic α-receptors. *J. Pharm. Pharmacol.,* 17:202–216.
34. Schwartz, R., and Coyle, J. (1977): Striatal lesions with kainic acid: Neurochemical characteristics. *Brain Res.,* 127:235–249.
35. Seeman, P., Chau Wong, M., Tedesco, J., and Wong, K. (1975): Brain receptors for antipsychotic drugs and dopamine: Direct binding assays. *Proc. Natl. Acad. Sci. U.S.A.,* 72:4376–4380.
36. Seeman, P., Lee, T., Chau Wong, M., and Wong, K. (1976): Antipsychotic drug doses and neuroleptic dopamine receptors. *Nature,* 261:717–719.
37. Spano, P. F., Di Chiara, G., Tonon, G. C., and Trabucchi, M. (1976): A dopamine-stimulated adenylate cyclase in rat substantia nigra. *J. Neurochem.,* 27:1565–1568.
38. Spano, P. F., Kumakura, K., Tonon, G. C., Govoni, S., and Trabucchi, M. (1975): LSD and dopamine-sensitive adenylate cyclase in various brain areas. *Brain Res.,* 93:164–167.
39. Spano, P. F., and Trabucchi, M. (1978): Interaction of ergot alkaloids with dopaminergic receptors in rat striatum and nucleus accumbens. *Gerontology [Suppl. 1],* 24:106–114.
40. Spano, P. F., Trabucchi, M., and Di Chiara, G. (1977): Localization of nigral dopamine-sensitive adenylate cyclase on neurons originating from the corpus striatum. *Science,* 196:1343–1345.
41. Trabucchi, M., Govoni, S., Tonon, G. C., and Spano, P. F. (1976): Localization of dopamine receptors in the rat cerebral cortex. *J. Pharm. Pharmacol.,* 28:244–245.
42. Trabucchi, M., Longoni, R., Fresia, P., and Spano, P. F. (1975): Sulpiride: A study of the effects on dopamine receptors in rat neostriatum and limbic forebrain. *Life Sci.,* 17:1551–1556.
43. Trabucchi, M., Spano, P. F., Tonon, G. C., and Frattola, L. (1976): Effect of bromocriptine on central dopaminergic receptors. *Life Sci.,* 19:225–232.
44. Yamamura, H. I., and Snyder, S. H. (1974): Muscarinic cholinergic binding in rat brain. *Proc. Natl. Acad. Sci. U.S.A.,* 71:1725–1729.

Advances in Biochemical Psychopharmacology, Vol. 19,
edited by P. J. Roberts et al.
Raven Press, New York © 1978.

Brain Receptors for Dopamine and Neuroleptics

P. Seeman, M. Titeler, J. Tedesco, P. Weinreich, and D. Sinclair

Department of Pharmacology, University of Toronto, Toronto, Canada M5S 1A8

Abnormal dopaminergic transmission occurs in Parkinson's disease (29), schizophrenia (31,36,39,58), Huntington's disease (33,63), Gilles de la Tourette's syndrome (65), neuroleptic-induced tardive dyskinesia (2,3,17), various choreas (13) and torsion dystonias (35), the Lesch-Nyhan syndrome (65), and minimal brain dysfunction in children.

Since some of these disorders may be associated with abnormalities in brain dopamine receptors, it is necessary to have a reliable assay for measuring such receptors in small amounts of human brain tissue. It is also desirable to have a simple *in vitro* receptor assay to screen new drugs for therapeutic purposes.

In the past few years four new *in vitro* radioreceptor assays for dopamine receptors have been described, using ³H-dopamine, ³H-haloperidol, ³H-dihydroergocryptine, and ³H-apomorphine.

³H-DOPAMINE RADIORECEPTOR ASSAYS

The first reports on the specific binding of ³H-dopamine to tissues appeared in early 1974 (45,46,48), and an example of this work is shown in

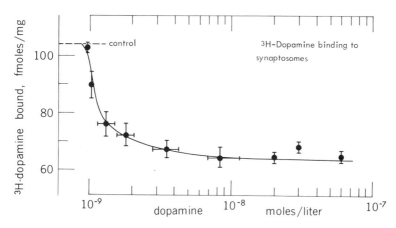

FIG. 1. Early results for the binding of ³H-dopamine to synaptosomes (rat striatum), using the centrifugation method (adapted from refs. 48 and 49). The K_d was approximately 1 nM and the total number of specific dopamine sites was about 40 fmoles/mg.

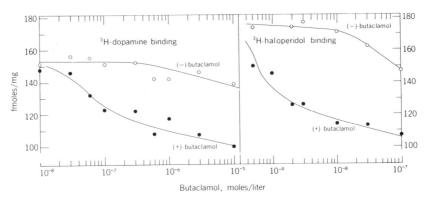

FIG. 2. Stereoselective inhibition of ³H-dopamine binding by butaclamol (adapted from ref. 49).

Fig. 1. These early experiments were done either by a centrifugation method or by a Millipore filtration method using ¹⁴C-inulin as a marker for trapped water containing ³H-dopamine. The results revealed a K_d of 6×10^{-10} M for dopamine (46,48).

In 1974 Humber and Bruderlein (30) reported the synthesis of the butaclamol enantiomers, of which only (+)-butaclamol is the active neuroleptic (5,66,67).

The butaclamol enantiomers facilitated a direct test of the 1966 hypothesis that neuroleptic drugs specifically blocked dopamine receptors (10,28,32,41, 64). In addition to having a stereospecific presynaptic action on dopamine neurons (50,51), it was soon found that (+)-butaclamol stereoselectively inhibited the binding of ³H-dopamine (8,20,49,53) (Fig. 2).

³H-HALOPERIDOL RADIORECEPTOR ASSAYS

Since neuroleptics readily adsorb to all biological cell membranes in relation to their high surface activity (47) and high fat solubility (44,55), the clear identification of specific binding sites for neuroleptics was not possible (61) until the advent of the butaclamol enantiomers, since these latter substances have identical solubilities.

When 100 nM (+)-butaclamol is used to define nonspecific ³H-haloperidol binding, the specific binding of haloperidol exhibits a K_d of between 1.3 and 3.3 nM (7,18,19,49,54,56). All clinically effective antipsychotic drugs block the stereospecific binding of ³H-haloperidol at concentrations which correlate directly with the clinical potencies (Fig. 3) and which are actually found to occur in the plasma water of patients under neuroleptic treatment (53) (see also refs. 20, 40, and 60). Although there is no simple direct proof that ³H-haloperidol is binding to the dopamine receptor site (in whatever conformation), it is true that dopamine is more effective than (−)-norepinephrine,

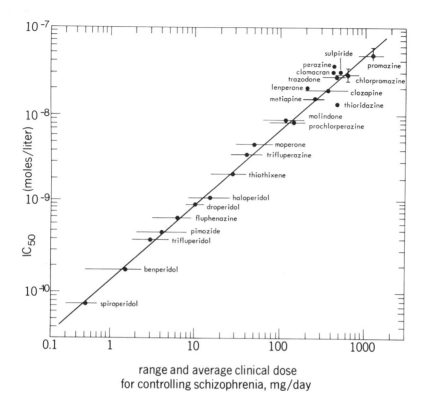

FIG. 3. Neuroleptics inhibit the binding of ^{3}H-haloperidol (to calf striatal homogenate) in direct relation to the clinical potencies (adapted from refs. 49, 52, 53).

serotonin, or other neurotransmitters in competing for ^{3}H-haloperidol binding (7,49,53).

^{3}H-LSD AND ^{3}H-DIHYDROERGOCRYPTINE AS LIGANDS FOR DOPAMINE RECEPTORS

Since D-LSD and the ergot alkaloids (ergotamine, ergocryptine, etc.) inhibit the binding of ^{3}H-dopamine at low concentrations (40 to 90 nM; ref. 6), radioligands of such drugs can be used to tag dopamine receptors (6,11,12). The binding of ^{3}H-LSD is complicated since it also attaches to serotonin receptors (4,6,34).

^{3}H-dihydroergocryptine (DHE) has been used for alpha-noradrenergic (22,26,45,68,69), serotoninergic (14), as well as dopaminergic receptors (11,12). The successful identification of ^{3}H-DHE as a valid ligand for dopamine receptors in the pituitary (11,12) was aided by the fact that the pituitary has few, if any, norepinephrine or serotonin receptors. Studies in this laboratory (M. Titeler et al.) indicate that it is also possible to use ^{3}H-DHE as a

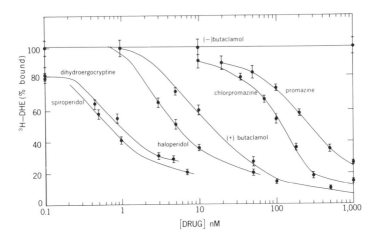

FIG. 4. In the presence of 100 nM phentolamine (to block the alpha-noradrenergic sites) it is possible to use ³H-DHE as a ligand for dopamine receptors (calf caudate homogenate; ³H-DHE concentration was 0.7 nM; adapted from ref. 62).

dopamine receptor ligand in caudate tissue if one blocks all the noradrenergic sites with 100 to 500 nM phentolamine (Fig. 4).

³H-APOMORPHINE AS A DOPAMINE RECEPTOR LIGAND

Apomorphine has been characterized as a dopamine agonist (1,23,27). In many instances, however, it acts as a partial agonist (43), and can thus an-

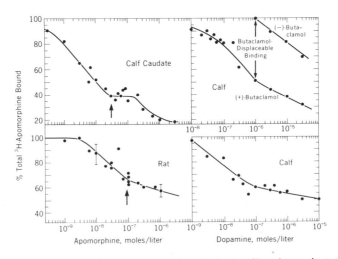

FIG. 5. The high- and low-affinity sites of ³H-apomorphine binding in calf caudate and rat striatal homogenates. Generally 40%–60% of the total binding is associated with the specific sites. (³H-apomorphine concentration = 3 nM; procedure of ref. 54.)

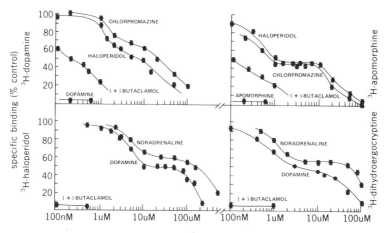

FIG. 6. An extremely detailed study of the specific binding of the 4 radioligands for dopamine/neuroleptic receptors indicates that each ligand may possibly bind to at least 2 sites. The full-scale value of 100% indicates the control amount of stereospecific binding of the ligand which is displaceable by (+)-buta-clamol. High- and low-affinity binding sites can be detected for each ligand.

tagonize the more powerful agonists such as dopamine itself (16,24,25,41).

^{3}H-apomorphine is an excellent ligand for dopamine receptors (54). In crude homogenates of the calf caudate or the rat striatum there are both high- and low-affinity sites for apomorphine; the K_d for the high-affinity site is 2 nM in the cow and 15 nM in the rat (Fig. 5). All these high-affinity sites are occupied at either 100 to 200 nM apomorphine or 1 μM (+)-butaclamol (Fig. 5).

Using ^{3}H-apomorphine as a ligand to study the structure-activity relations (SAR) of dopamine-mimetic drugs, such as the 2-aminotetralins (37,38), the aporphines (9,42), and the dopamine analogues (57), we have found (Fig. 6; J. Tedesco, J. Bowles, J. D. McDermed, and P. Seeman, *in preparation*) that the active conformation of dopamine is the beta rotamer form (15,21,70).

HIGH- AND LOW-AFFINITY SITES FOR DOPAMINE/NEUROLEPTIC RECEPTORS

We have recently reexamined in detail the competition for specific binding between various pairs of agonists and antagonists. The results in Fig. 7 indicate that high- and low-affinity specific binding sites for the radioagonist (^{3}H-dopamine or ^{3}H-apomorphine) can be detected when competing versus the antagonist (haloperidol or chlorpromazine). Conversely, high- and low-affinity sites for the radioantagonist (^{3}H-haloperidol) can be detected when competing versus the agonist (dopamine or norepinephrine).

The two types of specific sites described in Fig. 7 may provide direct evi-

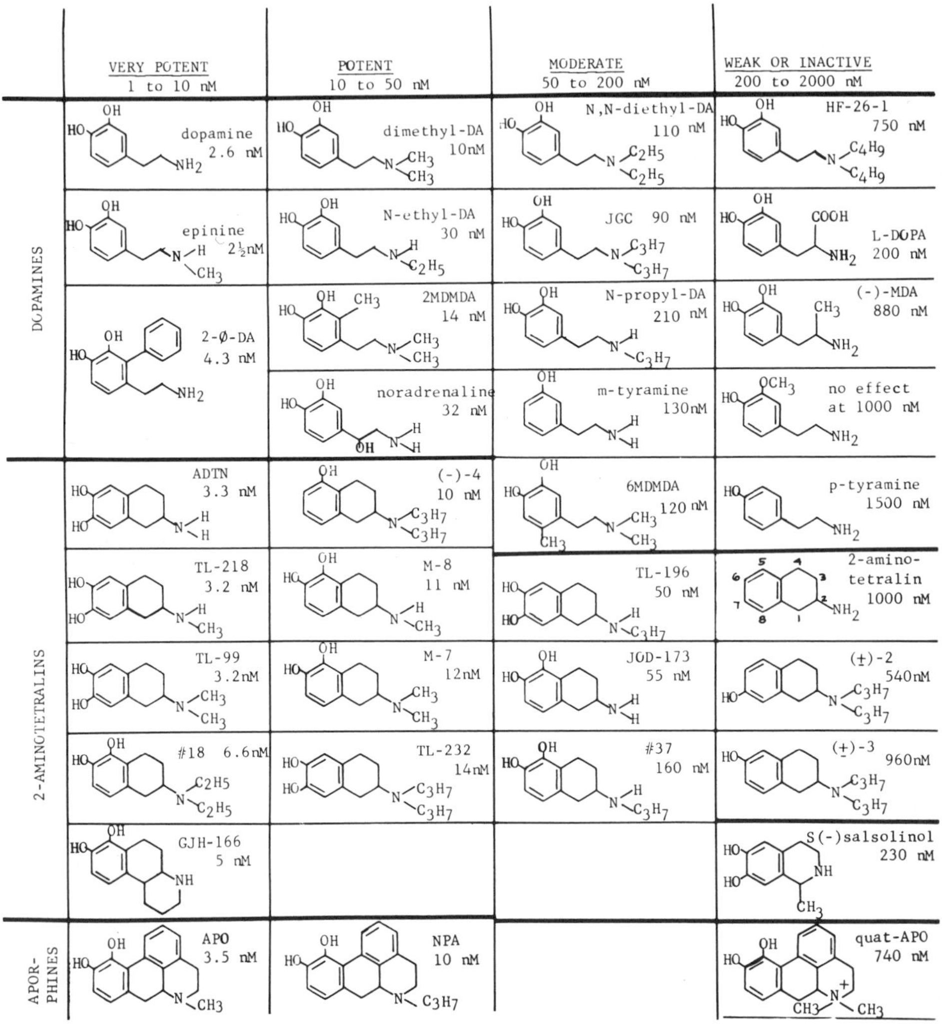

FIG. 7. The potencies (IC50 values) for various dopamine analogues, 2-aminotetralins, and apomorphines for inhibiting the specific binding of ^{3}H-apomorphine to calf caudate homogenate, defining specific binding as that which is displaceable by 200 nM apomorphine. 2-∅-DA (2-phenyl-dopamine), S(−)-salsolinol, N-ethyl-DA, 2MDMDA (or 2-methyl-N,N-dimethyl-dopamine), N,N-diethyl-DA, N-propyl-DA, 6MDMDA (or 6-methyl-N,N-dimethyl-dopamine), and (−)-MDA (or methyl-dopamine) were donated by Dr. Herbert Sheppard (Hoffman-La Roche Inc., New Jersey). Compounds #18, (−)-4, #37, (±)-2, and (±)-3 were donated by Dr. John D. McDermed (Wellcome Research Labs, North Carolina). ADTN, TL-218, TL-99, GJH-166, dimethyl-DA, M-8, M-7, TL-232, JGC, TL-196, JOD-173, HF-26-1, 2-aminotetralin, TL-68, and quat-APO (or apomorphine methoiodide) were donated by Drs. J. P. Long and J. G. Cannon (Iowa University); NPA (or N-propyl-norapomorphine) was donated by Dr. J. L. Neumeyer (Northeastern University).

dence for pre- and postsynaptic binding sites. Another possibility is that these two sites may represent different conformations of a receptor protein which can exist in two states, an agonist state and an antagonist state (see refs. 59 and 60). But this is unlikely, since at the concentration of the radiolabel used in these studies, binding should occur only to the high-affinity conformation (see ref. 62).

ACKNOWLEDGMENTS

We thank Drs. J. L. Neumeyer, J. D. McDermed, J. P. Long, J. G. Cannon, and H. Sheppard for kindly donating drug samples. This work was supported by the Ontario Mental Health Foundation and the Medical Research Council of Canada. We are grateful to Dr. W. D. Dorian (Merck Frosst Laboratories, Montreal) for generous supplies of apomorphine.

REFERENCES

1. Andén, N. E., Rubenson, A., Fuxe, F., and Hökfelt, T. (1967): Evidence for dopamine receptor stimulation by apomorphine. *J. Pharm. Pharmacol.*, 19:627–629.
2. Baldessarini, R. J. (1974): Tardive dyskinesia: An evaluation of the etiologic association with neuroleptic therapy. *Can. Psychiatr. Assoc. J.*, 19:551–554.
3. Baldessarini, R. J., and Tarsy, D. (1976): Mechanisms underlying tardive dyskinesia. In: *The Basal Ganglia,* edited by M. D. Yahr, pp. 25–36. Raven Press, New York.
4. Bennett, J. P., Jr., and Snyder, S. H. (1976): Serotonin and lysergic acid diethylamide binding in rat brain membranes. Relationship to postsynaptic serotonin receptors. *Mol. Pharmacol.*, 12:373–389.
5. Bruderlein, F. T., Humber, L. G., and Voith, K. (1975): Neuroleptic agents of the benzocycloheptapyridoisoquinoline series. 1. Synthesis and stereochemical and structural requirements for activity of butaclamol and related compounds. *J. Med. Chem.*, 18:185–188.
6. Burt, D. R., Creese, I., and Snyder, S. H. (1976): Binding interactions of lysergic acid diethylamide and related agents with dopamine receptors in the brain. *Mol. Pharmacol.*, 12:631–638.
7. Burt, D. R., Creese, I., and Snyder, S. H. (1976): Properties of ^{3}H-haloperidol and ^{3}H-dopamine binding associated with dopamine receptors in calf brain membranes. *Mol. Pharmacol.*, 12:800–812.
8. Burt, D. R., Enna, S. J., Creese, I., and Snyder, S. H. (1975): Dopamine receptor binding in the corpus striatum of mammalian brain. *Proc. Natl. Acad. Sci. USA*, 72:4655–4659.
9. Cannon, J. G. (1975): Chemistry of dopaminergic agonists. *Adv. Neurol.*, 9:177–183.
10. Carlsson, A., and Lindqvist, M. (1963): Effect of chlorpromazine or haloperidol on formation of 3-methoxytyramine and normetanephrine in mouse brain. *Acta Pharmacol. Toxicol.*, 20:140–144.
11. Caron, M. G., Drouin, J., Raymond, V., Kelly, P. A., and Labrie, F. (1976): Specificity of the catecholaminergic effect on prolactin secretion and ^{3}H-dihydroergocryptine binding. *Clin. Res.*, 24:656A.
12. Caron, M. G., Raymond, V., Lefkowitz, R. J., and Labrie, F. (1977): Identification of dopaminergic receptors in anterior pituitary: Correlation with the dopaminergic control of prolactin release. *Fed. Proc.* 36:278.

13. Chase, T. N., and Shoulson, I. (1975): Dopaminergic mechanisms in patients with extrapyramidal disease. *Adv. Neurol.,* 9:359–366.
14. Closse, A., and Hauser, D. (1976): Dihydroergotamine binding to rat brain membranes. *Life Sci.,* 19:1851–1864.
15. Colpaert, F. C., Van Bever, W. F. M., and Leysen, J. E. M. F. (1976): Apomorphine: Chemistry, pharmacology, biochemistry. *Int. Rev. Neurobiol.,* 19:225–268.
16. Costall, B., Naylor, R. J., Cannon, J. G., and Lee, T. (1977): Differential activation by some 2-aminotetralin derivatives of the receptor mechanisms in the nucleus accumbens of rat which mediate hyperactivity and stereotyped biting. *Eur. J. Pharmacol.,* 41:307–319.
17. Crane, G. E. (1973): Persistent dyskinesia. *Br. J. Psychiatr.,* 122:395–405.
18. Creese, I., Burt, D. R., and Snyder, S. H. (1975): Dopamine receptor binding: Differentiation of agonist and antagonist states with ^{3}H-dopamine and ^{3}H-haloperidol. *Life Sci.,* 17:993–1002.
19. Creese, I., Burt, D. R., and Snyder, S. H. (1975): The dopamine receptor: Differential binding of d-LSD and related agents to agonists and antagonist states. *Life Sci.,* 17:1715–1720.
20. Creese, I., Burt, D. R., and Snyder, S. H. (1976): Dopamine receptor binding predicts clinical and pharmacological potencies of antischizophrenic drugs. *Science,* 192:481–482.
21. Dandiya, P. C., Sharma, H. L., Patni, S. K., and Gambhir, R. S. (1975): An evaluation of apomorphine action on dopaminergic receptors. *Experientia,* 31:1441–1442.
22. Davis, J. N., Strittmatter, W., Hoyler, E., and Lefkowitz, R. J. (1976): ^{3}H-dihydroergocryptine (DHE) binding sites in rat brain. *Proc. Neurosci. Soc.,* 2:780.
23. Ernst, A. M. (1967): Mode of action of apomorphine and dexamphetamine on gnawing compulsion in rats. *Psychopharmacologia,* 10:316–323.
24. Goldberg, L. I. (1975): The dopamine vascular receptor. *Biochem. Pharmacol.,* 24:651–653.
25. Goldberg, L. I., Sonneville, P. F., and McNay, J. L. (1968): An investigation of the structural requirements for dopamine-like renal vasodilatation: Phenylethylamines and apomorphine. *J. Pharmacol. Exp. Ther.,* 163:188–197.
26. Greenberg, D. A., and Snyder, S. H. (1977): Selective labeling of alpha-noradrenergic receptors in rat brain with ^{3}H-dihydroergocryptine. *Life Sci.,* 20:927–932.
27. Horn, A. S., Post, M. L., and Kennard, O. (1975): Dopamine receptor blockade and the neuroleptics, a crystallographic study. *J. Pharm. Pharmacol.,* 27:553–563.
28. Horn, A. S., and Snyder, S. H. (1971): Chlorpromazine and dopamine: Conformational similarities that correlate with the antischizophrenic activity of phenothiazine drugs *Proc. Natl. Acad. Sci. U.S.A.,* 68:2325–2328.
29. Hornykiewicz, O. (editor) (1975): The pharmacology of the extrapyramidal system. Pergamon Press, Oxford.
30. Humber, L. G., and Bruderlein, F. (1974): Butaclamol hydrochloride, a novel neuroleptic agent. Synthesis and stereochemistry. *Proc. Am. Chem. Soc. Div. Med. Chem.,* 167:5.
31. Iversen, L. L. (1975): Dopamine receptors in the brain. *Science,* 188:1084–1089.
32. Janssen, P. A. J., and Allewijn, T. F. N. (1969): The distribution of the butyrophenones haloperidol, trifluperidol, moperone, and clofluperidol in rats, and its relationship with their neuroleptic activity. *Arzneim.-Forsch.,* 19:199–208.
33. Klawans, H. L., Paulson, G. W., Ringel, S. P., and Barbeau, A. (1973): The use of L-DOPA in the presynaptic detection of Huntington's chorea. *Adv. Neurol.,* 1:295–300.
34. Lovell, R. A., and Freedman, D. X. (1976): Stereospecific receptor sites for d-lysergic acid diethylamide in rat brain: Effects of neurotransmitters, amine antagonists, and other psychotropic drugs. *Mol. Pharmacol.,* 12:620–630.
35. Marsden, G. C. (1976): Dystonia: The spectrum of the disease. In: *The Basal Ganglia,* edited by M. D. Yahr, pp. 351–367. Raven Press, New York.
36. Matthysse, S., and Lipinski, J. (1975): Biochemical aspects of schizophrenia. *Annu. Rev. Med.,* 551–565.
37. McDermed, J. D., McKenzie, G. M., and Freeman, H. S. (1976): Synthesis and

dopaminergic activity (±)-, (+)-, and (−)-2-dipropylamino-5-hydroxy-1,2,3,4-tetrahydronaphthalene. *J. Med. Chem.,* 19:547–549.

38. McDermed, J. D., McKenzie, G. M., and Phillips, A. P. (1975): Synthesis and pharmacology of some 2-aminotetralins. Dopamine receptor agonists. *J. Med. Chem.,* 18:362–367.

39. Meltzer, H. Y., Sachar, E. J., Frantz, A. G. (1974): Serum prolactin levels in unmedicated schizophrenic patients. *Arch. Gen. Psychiatr.,* 31:564–569.

40. Meltzer, H. Y. (1976): Dopamine receptors and average clinical doses. *Science,* 194:545–546.

41. Neumeyer, J. L., Dafeldecker, W. P., Costall, B., and Naylor, R. J. (1977): Apomorphines. 21. Dopaminergic activity of apomorphine and benzylisoquinoline derivatives. Synthesis of 8-hydroxyapomorphines and 1-(hydroxybenzyl)-2-n-propyl-1,2,3,4-tetrahydroisoquinolines. *J. Med. Chem.,* 20:190–196.

42. Neumeyer, J. L., Reinhard, J. F., Dafeldecker, W. P., Guarino, J., Kosersky, D. S., Fuxe, K., and Agnati, L. (1976): Apomorphines. 14. Dopaminergic and antinociceptive activity of apomorphine derivatives. Synthesis of 10-hydroxyapomorphines and 10-hydroxy-N-n-propylnorapomorphine. *J. Med. Chem.,* 19:25–29.

43. Schmidt, M. J., and Hill, L. E. (1977): Effects of ergots on adenylate cyclase activity in the corpus striatum and pituitary. *Life Sci.,* 20:789–798.

44. Seeman, P. (1972): The membrane actions of anesthetics and tranquilizers. *Pharmacol. Rev.,* 24:583–655.

45. Seeman, P. (1974): Comparison of pre-synaptic and postsynaptic theories of neuroleptic action. *Proc. IX Int. Congr. Colleg. Int. Neuropsychopharmacol.* Excerpta Medica, Paris.

46. Seeman, P. (1974): Comparison of pre-synaptic and postsynaptic theories of neuroleptic action. *J. Pharmacol.* (Paris), 5: (Suppl. 2) 91.

47. Seeman, P., and Bialy, H. S. (1963): The surface activity of tranquilizers. *Biochem. Pharmacol.,* 12:1181–1191.

48. Seeman, P., Chau-Wong, M., and Lee, T. (1974): Dopamine receptor-block and nigral fiber impulse-blockade by major tranquilizers. *Fed. Proc.,* 33:246.

49. Seeman, P., Chau-Wong, M., Tedesco, J., and Wong, K. (1975): Brain receptors for antipsychotic drugs and dopamine: Direct binding assays. *Proc. Natl. Acad. Sci. U.S.A.,* 72:4376–4380.

50. Seeman, P., and Lee, T. (1975): Correlation between clinical potency and presynaptic action of neuroleptics and dopamine neurones. In: *Antipsychotic Drugs, Pharmacodynamics and Pharmacokinetics,* edited by G. Sedvall, pp. 183–191. Pergamon Press, Oxford.

51. Seeman, P., and Lee, T. (1975): Antipsychotic drugs. Direct correlation between clinical potency and presynaptic action on dopamine neurones. *Science,* 188:1217–1219.

52. Seeman, P., Lee, T., Chau-Wong, M., and Wong, K. (1976): Correlation of antipsychotic drug potency and neuroleptic receptor block. *Neurosci. Soc. Abstr.,* 6:878.

53. Seeman, P., Lee, T., Chau-Wong, M., and Wong, K. (1976): Antipsychotic drug doses and neuroleptic/dopamine receptors. *Nature,* 261:717–719.

54. Seeman, P., Lee, T., Chau-Wong, M., Tedesco, J., and Wong, K. (1976): Dopamine receptors in human and calf brains, using ³H-apomorphine and an antipsychotic drug. *Proc. Natl. Acad. Sci. U.S.A.,* 73:4354–4358.

55. Seeman, P., Staiman, A., and Chau-Wong, M. (1974): The nerve impulse-blocking actions of tranquilizers, and the binding of neuroleptics to synaptosome membranes. *J. Pharmacol. Exp. Ther.,* 190:120–123.

56. Seeman, P., Wong, M., and Tedesco, J. (1975): Tranquilizer receptors in rat striatum. *Neurosci. Soc. Abstr.,* 5:405.

57. Sheppard, H. H., and Burghardt, C. R. (1974): The dopamine-sensitive adenylate cyclase of rat caudate nucleus. 1. Comparison with the isoproterenol-sensitive adenylate cyclase (beta receptor system) of rat erythrocytes in responses to dopamine derivatives. *Mol. Pharmacol.,* 10:721–726.

58. Snyder, S. H. (1976): The dopamine hypothesis of schizophrenia: Focus on the dopamine receptor. *Am. J. Psychiatr.,* 133:197–202.

59. Snyder, S. H., Burt, D. R., and Creese, I. (1976): The dopamine receptor of mam-

malian brain: Direct demonstration of binding to agonist and antagonist states. *Neurosci. Sympos.,* 1:28–49.

60. Snyder, S. H., Creese, I., and Burt, D. R. (1975): The brain's dopamine receptor: Labeling with ³H-dopamine and ³H-haloperidol. *Psychopharmacol. Commun.,* 1:663–673.

61. Taylor, K. M. (1974): Displacement of bound ¹⁴C-fluphenazine by biogenic amines and antipsychotic drugs in homogenates of brain tissue. *Nature,* 252:238–241.

62. Titeler, M., Weinreich, P., and Seeman, P. (1977): New detection of brain dopamine receptors with ³H-dihydroergocryptine. *Proc. Natl., Acad. Sci. U.S.A.,* 74: 3750–3753.

63. Tolosa, E. S., and Sparber, S. B. (1974): Apomorphine in Huntington's chorea: Clinical observations and theoretical considerations. *Life Sci.,* 15:1371–1380.

64. van Rossum, J. M. (1966): The significance of dopamine-receptor blockade for the action of neuroleptic drugs. In: *Neuropsychopharmacology,* 5:321–329.

65. Van Woert, M. H., Jutkowitz, R., Rosenbaum, D., and Bowers, M. B., Jr. (1976): In: *The Basal Ganglia,* edited by M. D. Yahr, pp. 459–465. Raven Press, New York.

66. Voith, K. (1974): Butaclamol hydrochloride, a novel neuroleptic agent. *Proc. Am. Chem. Soc. Div. Med. Chem.,* 167:6.

67. Voith, K., and Herr, F. (1975): The behavioural pharmacology of butaclamol hydrochloride (AY-23, 028), a new potent neuroleptic drug. *Psychopharmacologia,* 42:11–20.

68. Williams, L. T., and Lefkowitz, R. J. (1976): Alpha-adrenergic receptor identification by ³H-dihydroergocryptine binding. *Science,* 192:791–793.

69. Williams, L. T., Mullikin, D., and Lefkowitz, R. J. (1976): Identification of alpha-adrenergic receptors in uterine smooth muscle membranes by ³H-dihydroergocryptine binding. *J. Biol. Chem.,* 251:6915–6923.

70. Woodruff, G. N. (1971): Dopamine receptors: A review. *Comp. Gen. Pharmacol.,* 2:439–455.

Advances in Biochemical Psychopharmacology, Vol. 19,
edited by P. J. Roberts et al.
Raven Press, New York © 1978.

ADTN (2-Amino-6,7-Dihydroxy-1,2,3,4-Tetrahydronaphthalene): A Prototype for Possible Dopaminergic False Transmitters?

P. J. Roberts and A. Davis

Pharmacology Group, School of Biochemical and Physiological Sciences, University of Southampton, Southampton S09 3TU England

Since the description of Parkinson's disease over 150 years ago, a vast range of pharmacological agents have been administered therapeutically, often on purely empirical grounds. However, with the realization that neurochemically the disease is characterized by a "dopamine deficiency," particularly in the striatum (13), a more rational approach has been possible. A major pitfall in replacement therapy was the fact that dopamine (DA) does not cross the blood-brain barrier, and not until the introduction of its immediate precursor, L-DOPA, was significant progress made in this respect. L-DOPA, because it is metabolically highly active, requires frequent administration at high doses, which generally results in numerous, often undesirable side effects in patients. Even the simultaneous administration of peripheral dopa decarboxylase inhibitors has not removed the problems associated with L-DOPA therapy.

There is therefore a need for alternative agents with direct actions on the dopamine receptors. Both apomorphine and piribedil (partial agonists) have been tested, but they are much less effective than L-DOPA. More recently, bromocryptine and lergotrile have been introduced with some success. According to Hornykiewicz (14), the ideal chemotherapeutic agent for Parkinson's disease should possess the following attributes: (a) direct, full agonist actions, specifically on DA receptors, (b) ability to cross the blood-brain barrier, and (c) metabolic stability, enabling a prolonged effect.

A highly promising prototype for a new class of potential therapeutic agents is 2-amino-6,7-dihydroxy-1,2,3,4-tetrahydronaphthalene (ADTN), which is a semirigid analogue of DA held in the extended form (Fig. 1). Compounds such as salsolinol and norsalsolinol, which contain the folded skeleton of DA, are only weak agonists on DA receptors (28).

A variety of pharmacological studies have shown that ADTN is a potent agonist at DA receptors. It is active at both invertebrate (18) and vertebrate DA receptors (5,29). In the rat, it causes long-lasting stimulation of loco-

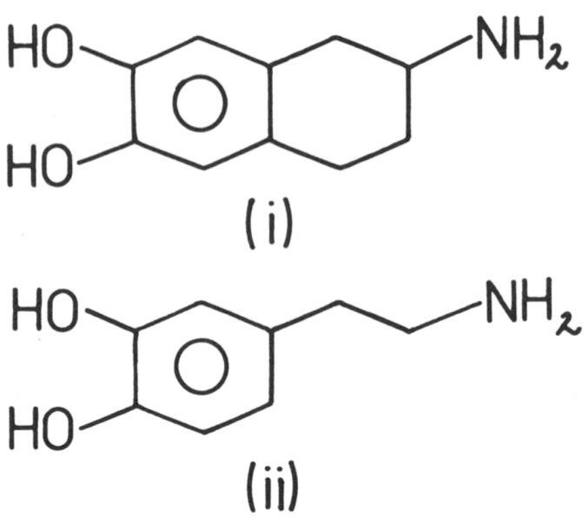

FIG. 1. Structural formulas of 2-amino-6,7-dihydroxy-1,2,3,4-tetrahydronaphthalene (ADTN) (i) and dopamine (ii).

motor activity following intraventricular injection (6), and it is equipotent with DA in its ability to activate striatal DA-sensitive adenylate cyclase (17). The outstanding problem intrinsic to ADTN itself, however, is its inability to cross the blood-brain barrier. However, a simplified four-step procedure for the synthesis of ADTN has been described recently (12), and it is likely that it will now become feasible to introduce suitable molecular modifications to circumvent this problem. *In vitro* studies with ADTN are not impeded by this problem, however, and we have therefore investigated the possibility that ADTN might be a good substrate for the neuronal DA carrier and that the molecule might be first accumulated and then be able to be released during stimulation. We have investigated also the ability of ADTN to bind to highly purified synaptic membranes prepared from rat striatum, with the aim of obtaining additional evidence for the involvement of dopamine receptors in the pharmacological actions of ADTN. In addition, because of the inconsistencies found in binding studies with a variety of ligands, the development of suitable, highly potent additional ligands to study DA receptors is essential.

UPTAKE OF [³H]ADTN

Labeled ADTN

[G-³H]ADTN was prepared by the process of catalytic exchange labeling, using 100 Ci of tritiated water. The label was stored at $-140°C$ until required. The ADTN was purified immediately before use by one-dimensional thin-layer chromatography, and following its reconstitution in distilled water containing 5 mM tartrate, the concentration of ADTN was determined by fluorometric assay with fluorescamine. The approximate specific radioactivity of the [³H]ADTN was found to be 0.105 Ci/mmole.

Time Course and Kinetics of [³H]ADTN Uptake

Although ADTN has been reported to inhibit the uptake of [³H]DA into striatal homogenates (Horn, *this volume*), there was no direct evidence in

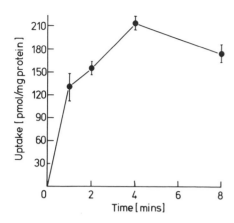

FIG. 2. Time course of [³H]ADTN uptake. Crude synaptosomes were incubated at 37°C with [³H]-ADTN (10 μM) for various periods between zero and 8 min. Results are expressed as pmoles ADTN accumulated/mg protein. Correction was made for labeled ADTN retained extracellularly. Each point is the mean ± SEM of 4 independent observations.

support of ADTN's being a substrate for the DA carrier. Hence, a study was made of the ability of a crude striatal nerve ending preparation (P₂) to accumulate [³H]ADTN. Uptake was essentially linear for the first 4 min of incubation but with a rapid decline thereafter (Fig. 2). Optimal uptake occurred at 37°C, and it was strongly inhibited by metabolic poisons such as cyanide, ouabain, p-chloromercuriphenylsulfonate, and 2,4-dinitrophenol (Fig. 3), indicating an active, energy-dependent process. The Michaelis-Menten kinetics were determined by incubating striatal synaptosomes with a wide range of [³H]ADTN concentrations. Two components could be re-

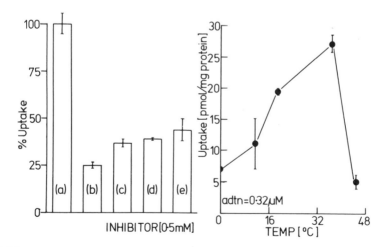

FIG. 3. Effect of temperature and metabolic inhibitors on the uptake of [³H]ADTN. Crude synaptosomes (P₂) were incubated at 37°C for 4 min with [³H]ADTN (0.32 μM) following a 5-min preincubation with metabolic inhibitors: (a) control, (b) p-chloromercuriphenylsulfonate, (c) NaCN, (d) ouabain, and (e) 2,4-dinitrophenol at a final concentration of 0.5 mM. Results are means ± SEMs of 4 observations.

Temperature dependence of uptake was studied during a 4-min incubation at temperatures ranging from 0–45°C. Results are expressed as pmoles/mg protein and are the means ± SEMs of 4 observations.

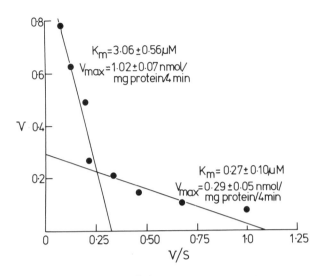

FIG. 4. Eadie-Hofstee plot of the uptake of [³H]ADTN into crude striatal synaptosomes. Synaptosomes were incubated for 4 min at 37°C in the presence of a wide range of [³H]ADTN concentrations (0.078–10.04 μM). The lines of best fit were determined by regression analysis. Each point represents the mean of at least 4 determinations. Uptake (V) is expressed as nmoles ADTN accumulated/mg protein/4 min and concentration (S) as μM.

solved, one of high affinity (apparent $K_m = 0.27 \pm 0.10$ μM) and low capacity ($V_{max} = 0.29 \pm 0.05$ nmoles/mg protein/4 min), and a second of lower affinity (apparent $K_m = 3.06 \pm 0.56$ μM) and high capacity ($V_{max} = 1.02 \pm 0.07$ nmoles/mg protein/4 min) (Fig. 4). When uptake was investigated in synaptosomes prepared from cerebellum, a region of the brain devoid of dopaminergic nerve terminals, a similar pattern emerged with both high- and low-affinity components (apparent K_ms of 0.28 ± 0.056 μM and 7.53 ± 1.53 μM, respectively). A striking difference between the two regions, however, was the much lower capacity of the two cerebellar systems (V_{max}s of 0.028 ± 0.017 and 0.126 ± 0.013 nmoles/mg protein/4 min, respectively). When uptake was studied using small (approximately $0.5 \times 0.5 \times 0.1$ mm) slices, after a 4-min incubation in the presence of [³H]ADTN (0.35 μM), a tissue:medium ratio of 172.4 was attained with the striatum, whereas with the olfactory bulbs, cerebral cortex, and medulla, ratios of only 35.7, 20.7, and 8.4, respectively, were reached, indicating a highly selective accumulation of ADTN in the striatum, which is enriched in dopaminergic terminals.

The findings on the kinetics of ADTN uptake differ from those reported by Snyder and Coyle (25) using tritiated DA, in that the uptake of DA into the striatum was mediated only by a single system with a K_m of 0.4 μM. This therefore suggests that ADTN may be a substrate for more than one carrier system in the striatum, although deviation from linearity in the Hofstee plot need not necessarily implicate different transport systems.

Inhibition of [³H]ADTN Uptake by Drugs

If ADTN is indeed a selective substrate for the high-affinity neuronal uptake mechanism for DA, then ADTN uptake should be influenced by each of those pharmacological agents with activity against DA uptake. Crude synaptosomes were incubated with [³H]ADTN and a range of concentrations of the potential inhibitory compound. Potencies of the inhibitors were expressed as IC_{50} values (Table 1). ADTN and DA were roughly equipotent in their abilities to inhibit [³H]ADTN accumulation. Benztropine and nomifensine, which are highly active inhibitors of DA uptake (15), were also potent in our system, with IC_{50}s of approximately 200 nM. Norepinephrine (NE) was five times less active than DA in inhibiting ADTN uptake, whereas the tricyclic antidepressant imipramine was almost inactive. This latter finding is consistent with the results of other workers (11,19) who found these compounds to be of very low activity against DA uptake, while being potent inhibitors of NE and 5-HT transport. The results obtained with amphetamine were also similar to those reported for the actions of this drug on DA uptake. Depletion of the tissue DA stores by pretreatment of the animal with reserpine markedly enhanced the drug's potency some 11-fold. A tricyclic imine, CDCI, has recently been reported as being a potent and specific inhibitor of DA uptake into striatal synaptosomes (10). Surprisingly, in our hands this compound was of rather low potency, but this might have been a reflection of the drug's very low solubility.

TABLE 1. *Inhibition of the uptake of [³H]ADTN into crude synaptosomes*

Drug	IC_{50} (nM)
ADTN	140
Dopamine	168
Benztropine	180
Nomifensine	200
Norepinephrine	920
Amphetamine (i)	290
Amphetamine (ii)	3,350
Imipramine	75,000

Synaptosomes were incubated with [³H]ADTN at 37°C with the drug under investigation at concentrations of generally between 0.01 and 10 μM. Log dose inhibitor concentration was plotted against [³H]ADTN uptake as a percentage of control, and the IC_{50} values were read. Each point on the plots (not shown) was the mean of 3 determinations. The results for amphetamine are derived from (i) reserpinized and (ii) control animals.

The pharmacological characteristics of ADTN uptake strongly suggest, therefore, that it is being transported into dopaminergic nerve terminals. We do not know as yet whether ADTN can be accumulated like DA into serotonergic nerve terminals. Autoradiography using more highly labeled ADTN may help to elucidate this problem.

Cellular Localization of ADTN Uptake and its Metabolic Stability

ADTN is not a substrate for monoamine oxidase, but it was thought likely that it could be metabolized by catechol-O-methyltransferase. Following a 20-min incubation of synaptosomes with [³H]ADTN, thin-layer chromatography (TLC) of tissue extracts indicated that approximately 45% of the added ADTN had been metabolized.

The subcellular localization of the uptake sites was primarily synaptosomal. This was established by studying the uptake of [³H]ADTN into purified preparations of striatal nuclei, mitochondria, myelin, and synaptosomes. This approach was found to be more satisfactory than the incubation of tissue homogenates with labeled ADTN and the subsequent application of subcellular fractionation procedures.

RELEASE OF [³H]ADTN

Hand-cut striatal slices (10 to 20 mg) were incubated with 176 μM [³H]ADTN for 20 min at 37°C and then transferred through a series of vials containing Krebs-bicarbonate medium. The released radioactivity was then determined by liquid scintillation counting. The release pattern was typically biphasic with a rapid efflux phase within the first 5 min, representing washout, followed by a slower steady efflux phase, during which approximately 4% to 5% of the total radioactivity accumulated was released in each 5-min collection period. The effects of drugs on the release of ADTN were investigated by including the agent under test during one of the collection periods.

Effect of K⁺ and Dependency of Release on Ca²⁺

The addition of 50 mM K⁺ (substituted for Na⁺) to the incubation medium produced a doubling in the rate of release of [³H]ADTN from striatal slices (Fig. 5a). The omission of Ca²⁺ ions and the supplementation of the medium with 10 mM Mg²⁺ produced a reduction in the spontaneous release, but the K⁺-evoked release was only marginally inhibited. This failure to show a clear calcium dependency probably reflects the difficulty reported by many other workers in being able to deplete sufficiently the endogenous calcium stores, particularly when using tissue slices. An alternative approach to the problem is to employ an ionophore: A23187 is a carboxylic acid antibiotic which, rather selectively, influences the movements of Ca²⁺ (7) and has been shown

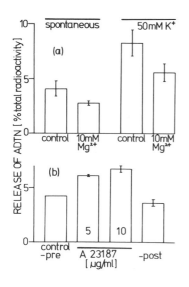

FIG. 5. Calcium dependency on the release of [³H]ADTN.

Striatal slices were incubated for 20 min with [³H]ADTN and then transferred through a series of vials containing medium, as described in the text.
a: The effects of zero calcium and added 10 mM Mg^{2+} on the spontaneous and K^+-evoked release.
b: The effect of the calcium ionophore A23187

The results are expressed as the fractional release, i.e., that percent of the total radioactivity originally in the tissue, released per collection period. Control release is the release in the period immediately prior to the test period. Results are means ± SEMs of at least 4 experiments.

to increase the release of a number of neurotransmitters (3,16). When striatal slices previously incubated with [³H]ADTN as described were exposed to a low concentration (5 to 10 μg/ml) of the ionophore, a marked enhancement of the release occurred (Fig. 5b), indicating a classic calcium dependency of release.

The cellular site from which the ADTN was being released, however, is not known apart from its being of synaptosomal origin. In order for ADTN-like compounds to serve as true false transmitters, it would be necessary for them to be accumulated by the dopaminergic nerve terminals, stored within the vesicles, and released during physiological stimulation. There is no evidence as yet to indicate whether or not ADTN equilibrates with a vesicular pool or if its location is purely cytoplasmic.

Effects of Drugs on the Release of [³H]ADTN

Although Coyle and Snyder (4) originally reported that various antiparkinsonian drugs inhibited the uptake of labeled DA into striatal synaptosomes, a number of recent reports have suggested that these pharmacological agents might be acting primarily as releasers of DA (1,9). However, the main problem which has tended to impede interpretation of experimental data is that it has not been possible to separate the components of uptake and release which may be occurring simultaneously. The elegant work of Raiteri and his colleagues (*this volume*), using a synaptosome superfusion system where reuptake is eliminated, has done much to clarify the situation. For example, nomifensine and benztropine, which were originally reported as being potent inhibitors of uptake, were essentially inactive at concentrations up to 10 μM as releasers of DA. Amphetamine, however, was found to be a

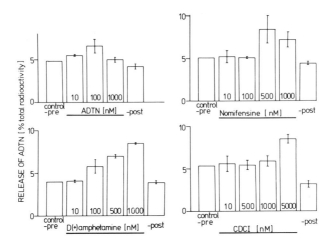

FIG. 6. Effects of drugs on the release of [³H]ADTN. The experimental procedure is as described in the text and in the legend to Fig. 5. Presence of the drug under test is indicated by the solid horizontal bars. Results are means ± SEMs of at least 4 experiments.

potent releaser at concentrations as low as 0.1 μM. In our experiments, amphetamine was found to be a potent releaser of [³H]ADTN at concentrations which were inactive against ADTN uptake (Fig. 6). The effect was dose dependent, being first apparent at 0.1 μM. ADTN itself had a slight releasing action, whereas, in contrast to the findings of Raiteri, nomifensine at concentrations of not less than 0.5 μM was an effective releasing agent. The reportedly selective DA uptake inhibitor CDCI (10) produced only a weak releasing action at 5 μM.

Neuroleptic drugs are known to increase the spontaneous release of [³H]DA and to inhibit the electrically evoked release (22). In our hands,

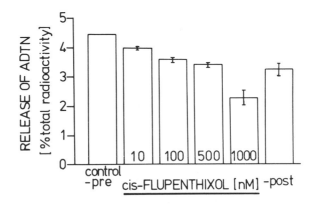

FIG. 7. Inhibition of the spontaneous release of [³H]ADTN by *cis*-flupenthixol. Procedure is as described in Fig. 6. The presence of the neuroleptic is indicated by the solid bar. Each result is the mean ± SEM of at least 4 experiments.

however, the neuroleptic *cis*-flupenthixol (10 to 1,000 nm) produced a dose-dependent decrease in the spontaneous release of [³H]ADTN (Fig. 7). The pharmacologically inactive *trans* isomer did not influence the release.

The ability of any of these agents to affect the K⁺-evoked release of ADTN was not studied.

BINDING OF [³H]ADTN TO SYNAPTIC MEMBRANES

A number of laboratories have investigated the binding of DA, haloperidol (2,21), and apomorphine (23) to crude homogenates prepared from rat, bovine, or human brain tissues, with the aim of obtaining a more direct measure of dopamine receptor sensitivity than by using the DA-sensitive adenylate cyclase (Kebabian, *this volume*). There are a number of problems associated with these binding studies, however: Seeman has commented on the rapid desorption rates of both DA and haloperidol from their binding sites (23). This can be countered only by the use of large amounts of tissue coupled with very rapid, reproducible methods for recovery of the bound ligand. Secondly, it has been reported recently (27) that hallucinogenic tryptamines selectively block haloperidol but not DA binding, suggesting that the ligand may not be specific. Although the information to date suggests a good correlation between the ability of the neuroleptic drugs to block ligand binding to the membrane receptors for DA and the clinical efficacy of these agents (24), it must be considered that the use of ligands which are not completely specific, combined with heterogeneous biological preparations, may lead to binding of the ligand to additional sites such as enzymes or transport systems, for which the ligand may have greater affinity than for the genuine receptor. [³H]apomorphine was introduced (23) in an attempt to circumvent these problems, but the evidence that apomorphine has a specific action on DA receptors is tenuous. In any event, at DA receptors apomorphine acts as a partial agonist.

There is therefore a clear need for alternate radioligands for the investigation of the dopamine receptor. It is likely that ADTN will prove to be highly valuable in this respect. Investigations to date have yielded a limited amount of information because of the low specific radioactivity of the [³H]ADTN available, which has precluded the investigation of its binding to membranes at equivalent concentrations to those used with the other ligands studied.

[³H]ADTN Binding Assay

The [³H]ADTN binding assays were performed using a rapid centrifugation method. Highly purified rat striatal synaptic membranes (20) were incubated in the absence or presence of a large molar excess (1 mm) of unlabeled ADTN or DA. The specific [³H]ADTN binding was obtained by subtraction.

Saturability of Binding Sites

The specific binding represented approximately 10% to 20% of the total radioactivity bound. It was found to be saturable with half-maximal binding at about 1 μM (Fig. 8). This contrasted with the nonspecific component which was not saturable and increased linearly with increasing radioligand concentration.

Lineweaver-Burk analysis of the specific binding of [³H]ADTN revealed a linear plot, indicating that binding occurred to a single population of sites

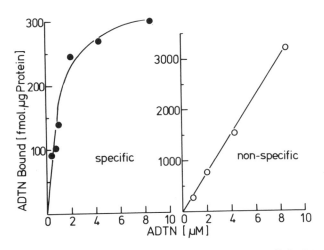

FIG. 8. Saturability of specific [³H]ADTN binding. Increasing concentrations of [³H]ADTN were incubated with striatal synaptic membranes, in the absence and presence of 1 mM unlabeled ADTN. The results obtained in the presence of the unlabeled ADTN represent nonspecific binding. Each result is the mean of at least 4 replicate assays, and the variation between individual observations was less than 15%.

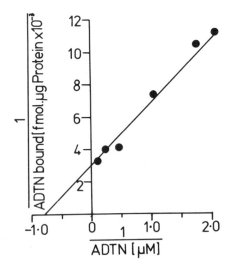

FIG. 9. Lineweaver-Burk plot of specific [³H]ADTN binding. The line of best fit was determined by regression analysis. Each point is the mean of quadruplicate determinations. ADTN bound is expressed as fmoles/mg protein.

(Fig. 9). The apparent dissociation constant (K_d) was 1.20 ± 0.29 μM, which contrasts markedly with the affinities of dopamine, haloperidol, and apomorphine reported by other workers (2,21,23). The apparent dissociation constant for DA was in the range of 10 to 25 nM, whereas that found by us for ADTN was approximately 100 times greater. The figure of 1.2 μM is, however, very close to that for the half-maximal stimulation of the striatal adenylate cyclase system by both ADTN and DA (20).

Time Course of [³H]ADTN Binding

At 27°C, binding reached equilibrium after approximately 5 min (Fig. 10), whereas at 0°C it was much slower. Nonspecific binding, however, was not time dependent and appeared to be essentially instantaneous.

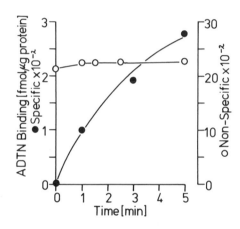

FIG. 10. Time course of [³H]ADTN binding. The rate of binding at 27°C of [³H]ADTN to striatal membranes was determined as described in the text. Each point is the mean of triplicate determinations.

Subcellular Distribution of Binding Sites

The binding of [³H]ADTN to various membrane fractions obtained by conventional subcellular fractionation techniques (8) was studied. No specific ADTN binding was detected in either the whole homogenate or the crude nuclear or mitochondrial pellets (Table 2). Specific binding was found in the P_2 fraction, and this became enriched approximately 3.5-fold in the crude synaptosomal fraction.

Effects of Drugs on Specific [³H]ADTN Binding

If [³H]ADTN binds to the same sites with which DA primarily interacts, then binding of the ligand should be inhibited both by DA and its structural analogues and by the neuroleptic drugs. In a preliminary study, the binding of [³H]ADTN (4 μM) in the presence of a large excess of the drug under investigation was measured. IC_{50} values were determined later for those agents

TABLE 2. Subcellular distribution of [³H]ADTN binding sites

Fraction	Binding (fmoles/μg protein)		
	Total	Nonspecific	Specific
Whole homogenate	368	373	—
Nuclear pellet	425	455	—
P₂	595	562	33
Myelin	564	552	12
Synaptosomes	474	373	101
Mitochondrial pellet	456	455	—

Subcellular fractions were prepared from rat striata and [³H]ADTN binding was determined. Data represent the means of 3 experiments.

which possessed demonstrable activity (Table 3). The specific binding of [³H]ADTN was totally abolished in the presence of 1 mM ADTN or DA. There were marked differences in the ability of the two isomers of flupenthixol to affect the binding; the *trans* isomer was completely ineffective, whereas the pharmacologically active *cis* form was approximately half as effective at this concentration as was ADTN itself in displacing [³H]ADTN binding. Benztropine, which has negligible affinity for dopamine receptors, produced a modest inhibition of specific binding, whereas the putative neurotransmitters histamine and glycine were inactive.

Chemical Nature of the ADTN Binding Site

The thermal stability of specific [³H]ADTN binding was examined. Preincubation of the synaptic membranes at 70°C for 10 min completely abolished the specific binding. Proteolytic enzymes such as trypsin (0.4 mg/ml) produced a 77% inhibition of binding, and concanavalin A produced a 47%

TABLE 3. Drug effects on specific [³H]ADTN binding to synaptic membranes

Compound	Specific binding (fmoles/μg protein)	Inhibition (%)	IC₅₀ (μM)
None	239 ± 28 (10)		
ADTN	26 ± 3 (6)	89	30
DA		100	9.3
cis-Flupenthixol	115 ± 33 (4)	52	178
trans-Flupenthixol	247 ± 30 (4)		
Benztropine	188 ± 66 (6)	21	
Glycine	233 ± 69 (4)	3	
Histamine	217 ± 217 (4)	9	

The binding of [³H]ADTN (4 μM) to striatal membranes was determined in the presence of 1 mM of the drug under investigation. Values are means ± SEMs for the number of experiments shown in parentheses. IC₅₀ values were determined as shown with the inihibitor at concentrations from 10–1,000 μM.

reduction. Prior treatment of the membranes with a low concentration (0.04%) of Triton X-100 enhanced ADTN binding fourfold. It is likely, therefore, that the ADTN receptor is a membrane protein or glycoprotein.

CONCLUSIONS

Pharmacologically, ADTN is at least equipotent with DA. However, its main attribute is that metabolically it is immensely more stable. If suitable molecular modifications can be introduced to circumvent the problem shared by DA, that of accessibility to the CNS, then we will be a step closer to the ideal chemotherapeutic agent for the treatment of Parkinson's disease.

ADTN is actively accumulated into nerve terminals; this occurs preferentially in the striatum and is potently inhibited by those agents which interfere with the high-affinity transport mechanism for DA. The cellular localization of accumulated ADTN has not been identified, but since it is clearly a substrate for the carrier on the neuronal membrane, it might be presumed to be capable of entering the storage vesicles.

Following accumulation, labeled ADTN can be released into the incubation medium in response to depolarizing stimuli or the presence of the calcium ionophore A23187, and by the drugs amphetamine, nomifensine, and benztropine.

The data obtained from the binding studies are the most difficult to interpret. It seems likely that ADTN is binding to specific sites which can accommodate both ADTN and DA, and that these sites are highly localized to synaptic membranes. However, because of the marked differences between our data and those obtained by different laboratories where much lower concentrations of other ligands were employed (2,21,23), coupled with the low sensitivity of the binding of ADTN to inhibition by neuroleptics (IC_{50}s in the nontherapeutic micromolar range), it seems possible that ADTN is binding to some other membrane component for which it is a substrate. Catechol-O-methyltransferase, which can exist in a membrane-bound form, was thought to be a likely candidate; however, binding was not antagonized by pyrocatechol. A study where fluphenazine was employed as the radioligand (26) found a K_d of 4 μM, with a sensitivity to inhibition by neuroleptics similar to that reported here. It is clear, therefore, that, depending on the concentrations of ligand selected, a number of distinct binding components may be detected, the individual relevance of which to the physiological DA receptor has yet to be determined.

ACKNOWLEDGMENTS

Alan Davis was supported by the M.R.C. We thank Dr. Judith A. Poat for collaborating in the binding studies, and Academic Press for permission to reproduce Figs. 8 through 10. The ionophore A23187 was the generous gift of Eli Lilly and Company, Indianapolis, and the compound CDCI was the gift of Dr. W. F. Herblin.

REFERENCES

1. Baumann, P. A., and Maitre, L. (1976): Is drug inhibition of dopamine uptake a misinterpretation of *in vitro* experiments. *Nature,* 264:789–790.
2. Burt, D. R., Creese, I., and Snyder, S. H. (1976): Properties of [³H]haloperidol and [³H]dopamine binding associated with dopamine receptors in calf brain membranes. *Mol. Pharmacol.,* 12:800–812.
3. Colburn, R. W., Thoa, N. B., and Kopin, I. J. (1975): Influence of ionophores which bind calcium on the release of norepinephrine from synaptosomes. *Life Sci.,* 17:1395–1400.
4. Coyle, J. T., and Snyder, S. H. (1969): Antiparkinsonian drugs: Inhibition of dopamine uptake in the corpus striatum as a possible mechanism of action. *Science,* 166:899–901.
5. Elkawad, A. O., Munday, K. A., Poat, J. A., and Woodruff, G. N. (1975): The effect of dopamine receptor stimulants on locomotor activity and cyclic AMP levels in rat striatum. *Br. J. Pharmacol.,* 53:456–457P.
6. Elkhawad, A. O., and Woodruff, G. N. (1975): Studies on the behavioural pharmacology of a cyclic analogue of dopamine following its injection into the brains of conscious rats. *Br. J. Pharmacol.,* 54:107–114.
7. Foreman, J. C., Mongar, J. L., and Gomperts, B. D. (1973): Calcium ionophores and movement of calcium ions following the physiological stimulus to the secretory process. *Nature,* 245:249.
8. Gray, E. G., and Whittaker, V. P. (1962): The isolation of nerve endings from brain: An electron microscopic study of cell fragments derived by homogenization and centrifugation. *J. Anat.,* 96:79–87.
9. Heikkila, R. E., Orlansky, H., and Cohen, G. (1975): Studies on the distinction between uptake inhibition and release of [³H]dopamine in rat brain tissue slices. *Biochem Pharmacol.,* 24:847–852.
10. Herblin, W. F. (1977): The selective inhibition of dopamine uptake by a tricyclic imine. *Neurochem. Res.,* 2:111–116.
11. Horn, A. S., Coyle, J. T., and Snyder, S. H. (1971): Catecholamine uptake by synaptosomes from rat brain. *Mol. Pharmacol.,* 7:66–80.
12. Horn, A. S., Grol, C. J., and Dijkstra, D. (1978): Facile synthesis of potent dopaminergic agonists. *Nature (in press).*
13. Hornykiewicz, O. (1973): Parkinson's disease: From brain homogenate to treatment. *Fed. Proc.,* 32:183–190.
14. Hornykiewicz, O. (1975): Parkinson's disease and its chemotherapy. *Biochem. Pharmacol.,* 24:1061–1065.
15. Hunt, P., Kannengiesser, M.-H., and Raynaud, J. P. (1974): Nomifensine: A new potent inhibitor of dopamine uptake into synaptosomes from rat brain corpus striatum. *J. Pharm. Pharmacol.,* 26:370–371.
16. Levi, G., Roberts, P. J., and Raiteri, M. (1976): Release and exchange of neurotransmitters in synaptosomes: Effects of the ionophore A23187 and of ouabain. *Neurochem. Res.,* 1:409–416.
17. Miller, R. J., Horn, A. S., Iversen, L. L., and Pinder, R. M. (1974): Effects of dopamine-like drugs on rat striatal adenyl cyclase have implications for CNS dopamine topography. *Nature,* 250:238–241.
18. Munday, K. A., Poat, J. A., and Woodruff, G. N. (1976): Structure activity studies on dopamine receptors; A comparison between rat striatal adenylate cyclase and Helix aspersa neurones. *Br. J. Pharmacol.,* 57:452–453P.
19. Raiteri, M., Angelini, F., and Bertollini, A. (1976): A comparative study of the effects of mianserin, a tetracyclic antidepressant, and of imipramine on uptake and release of neurotransmitters in synaptosomes. *J. Pharm. Pharmacol.,* 28:483–488.
20. Roberts, P. J., Woodruff, G. N., and Poat, J. A. (1977): Binding of a conforma-

tionally restricted dopamine analogue, 2-amino-6,7-dihydroxy-1,2,3,4-tetrahydro-naphthalene, to receptors on rat brain synaptic membranes. *Mol. Pharmacol.*, 13: 541–547.

21. Seeman, P., Chau-Wong, M., Tedesco, J., and Wong, K. (1975): Brain receptors for anti-psychotic drugs and dopamine: Direct binding assays. *Proc. Natl. Acad. Sci. U.S.A.*, 72:4376–4380.

22. Seeman, P., and Lee, T. (1975): Antipsychotic drugs: Direct correlation between clinical potency and presynaptic action on dopamine neurons. *Science*, 188:1217–1219.

23. Seeman, P., Lee, T., Chau-Wong, M., Tedesco, J., and Wong, K. (1976): Dopamine receptors in human and calf brains, using [^{3}H]apomorphine and an antipsychotic drug. *Proc. Natl. Acad. Sci. U.S.A.*, 73:4354–4358.

24. Seeman, P., Lee, T., Chau-Wong, M., and Wong, K. (1976): Antipsychotic drug doses and neuroleptic/dopamine receptors. *Nature*, 261:717–718.

25. Snyder, S. H., and Coyle, J. T. (1969): Regional differences in [^{3}H]norepinephrine and [^{3}H]dopamine uptake into rat brain homogenates. *J. Pharm. Pharmacol.*, 165: 78–86.

26. Taylor, K. M. (1974): Displacement of bound [^{14}C]fluphenazine by biogenic amines and antipsychotic drugs in homogenates of brain tissue. *Nature*, 252:238–241.

27. Whitaker, P. M., and Seeman, P. (1977): Hallucinogen binding to dopamine: Neuroleptic receptors. *J. Pharm. Pharmacol.*, 29:506–507.

28. Woodruff, G. N. (1971): Dopamine receptors: A review. *Comp. Gen. Pharmacol.*, 2:439–455.

29. Woodruff, G. N., McCarthy, P. S., and Walker, R. J. (1976): Studies on the pharmacology of neurones in the nucleus accumbens of the rat. *Brain Res.*, 115:233–242.

Advances in Biochemical Psychopharmacology, Vol. 19,
edited by P. J. Roberts et al.
Raven Press, New York © 1978.

Studies on Tuberoinfundibular Dopamine Neurons

K. E. Moore, L. Annunziato, and G. A. Gudelsky

Department of Pharmacology, Michigan State University, East Lansing, Michigan 48824

The rat brain contains several distinct dopaminergic neuronal systems (18). Three of the major systems are depicted schematically in Fig. 1. We have measured the steady-state concentrations and the turnover of dopamine in the striatum, olfactory tubercle, and median eminence, which contain the terminals of the nigrostriatal, mesolimbic, and tuberoinfundibular neurons, respectively. The results of these biochemical studies indicate that dopamine neurons in the tuberoinfundibular system respond to pharmacological and endocrinological manipulations in a manner that is qualitatively different from dopamine neurons in the other two major systems.

METHODS

Male or female Sprague-Dawley rats weighing 200 to 300 g were treated in a variety of ways, decapitated, and the brains removed. The median eminence was first dissected from the hypothalamus with the aid of a stereomicroscope and homogenized in 20 to 30 μl of 0.4 N perchloric acid containing 10% EGTA. The striata and olfactory tubercles were then dissected

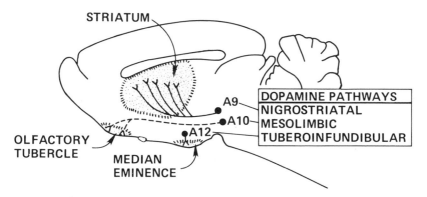

FIG. 1. Schematic diagram of major dopaminergic pathways in the rat brain (modified from Ungerstedt, 18).

and homogenized in 40 volumes of the same solution. In some experiments the hypothalamus was also removed and homogenized in 15 volumes of this solution. After centrifugation, 10 μl aliquots of the supernatants were analyzed for catecholamines by sensitive radioenzymatic methods (2,15) and the pellet was analyzed for protein (14).

RESULTS AND DISCUSSION

Changes in Steady-State Concentrations of Dopamine

Each median eminence weighs less than 0.2 mg and contains approximately 2.5 ng dopamine. The concentration of dopamine in a large number of median eminence samples was approximately 15 μg/g. This is higher than the average dopamine concentrations in striatum (10 μg/g) and olfactory tubercle (7.5 μg/g). There are qualitative differences in the manner in which drugs alter the steady-state concentrations of dopamine in these three brain regions.

γ-Butyrolactone (GBL) and baclofen increase the concentration of dopamine in the striatum, presumably as a result of the abilities of these drugs to reduce impulse flow in the nigrostriatal pathway (1,4,9,19). As illustrated in Fig. 2, a single intraperitoneal injection of GBL (750 mg/kg) significantly increased the concentration of dopamine in both the striatum and olfactory tubercle, but not in the median eminence. A similar pattern was observed after the injection of baclofen (40 mg/kg, i.p.). Muscimol, which is reported to be a potent GABA agonist (16), was also expected to reduce impulse flow in the nigrostriatal and mesolimbic pathways. An intravenous injection of

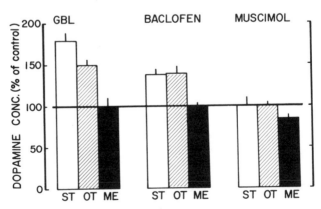

FIG. 2. Drug-induced changes of dopamine concentrations in the striatum, olfactory tubercle, and median eminence. Male rats were injected with γ-butyrolactone (GBL, 750 mg/kg, i.p.) 90 min before sacrifice, baclofen (40 mg/kg, i.p.) 60 min before sacrifice, or muscimol (2.5 mg/kg, i.v.) 60 min before sacrifice. The height of each column and the vertical line represent the mean and 1 S.E. of the dopamine concentration in the striatum (ST), olfactory tubercle (OT), and median eminence (ME) (N = 8).

TABLE 1. Concentrations of dopamine and norepinephrine in the median eminence and hypothalamus of female rats

	Dopamine		Norepinephrine	
	Median eminence	Hypothalamus	Median eminence	Hypothalamus
Diestrus 1	150 ± 16	5.4 ± 0.4	49 ± 7	22.7 ± 1.3
Diestrus 2	140 ± 10	5.4 ± 0.3	40 ± 5	22.7 ± 1.5
Proestrus	144 ± 10	5.6 ± 0.4	44 ± 2	24.7 ± 1.7
Estrus	165 ± 10	5.3 ± 0.5	48 ± 5	24.2 ± 1.7
Ovariectomy	214 ± 13[a]	5.7 ± 0.4	60 ± 5	26.8 ± 2.7
Ovariectomy + estrogen	145 ± 17[b]	5.9 ± 0.5	61 ± 10	29.0 ± 2.0

Values represent the means ± SE of the ng catecholamine/mg protein as determined in 8–11 animals. Ovariectomized rats were sacrificed 4 weeks after surgery; estradiol benzoate (25 μg/kg, s.c.) was administered daily for 7 days prior to sacrifice.

[a] Indicates a significantly greater concentration of dopamine.
[b] Indicates a significant difference from ovariectomy alone.

2.5 mg/kg of muscimol, which produced central nervous system depression similar to that observed after injections of the other two drugs, failed to alter the dopamine concentration in any of the three brain regions examined. These results indicate that all dopaminergic neuronal systems do not respond in the same manner to drugs. After GBL and baclofen the concentration of dopamine increases in the terminals of the nigrostriatal and mesolimbic neurons, but not in the terminals of tuberoinfundibular neurons. On the other hand, certain endocrinological manipulations can selectively increase the steady-state concentration of dopamine in tuberoinfundibular neurons.

There were no changes in the dopamine or norepinephrine concentrations in the median eminence or hypothalamus during the estrus cycle (Table 1). Four weeks after ovariectomy the concentration of dopamine in the median eminence, but not in the hypothalamus, was significantly increased. This increase was reversed by seven daily injections of estradiol benzoate. Ovariectomy did not alter the concentration of norepinephrine in the median eminence or hypothalamus.

Although the concentration of dopamine in the terminals of tuberoinfundibular neurons responds differently from other dopamine neurons to the actions of drugs and endocrinological manipulations, steady-state concentrations of dopamine do not provide any information on the activity of these neurons. In order to determine if differences exist in the mechanisms regulating the activity of nigrostriatal and tuberoinfundibular neurons, we estimated the turnover of dopamine in the terminal regions of these neurons.

Endocrine-induced Changes of Dopamine Turnover in the Median Eminence

There are limitations associated with all of the current procedures for estimating turnover rates of catecholamines (20). Nevertheless, these procedures are useful for comparing relative turnover rates in response to various treatments. Hökfelt and Fuxe (13), employing a semiquantitative histofluorescent procedure to estimate the decline of dopamine after inhibition of synthesis with α-methyltyrosine (αMT), noted that treatment of rats with prolactin selectively increased the turnover of dopamine in the terminals of the tuberoinfundibular neurons. The results depicted in Fig. 3, obtained by directly quantifying the αMT-induced decline of dopamine by microchemical analysis, confirmed this observation. Repeated injections of ovine prolactin to rats increased the rate of the αMT-induced decline of dopamine in the median eminence, but not in the striatum. There was a pronounced latent period before this effect was observed; no significant effect was obtained 2 and 10 hr after the start of the prolactin injections, whereas significant enhancement of dopamine turnover was observed after 26 and 74 hr. Thus, the activity of tuberoinfundibular dopaminergic neurons increases in response to elevated blood levels of prolactin, but only after a definite latent period.

In the next study, rather than administer exogenous prolactin, we examined the effects of increasing the animal's own serum prolactin concentrations with injections of estrogen. Fuxe et al. (8) noted that estrogen treatment increased the turnover of dopamine in the median eminence of the rat. The results summarized in Fig. 4 confirm this finding. Male rats were injected daily with

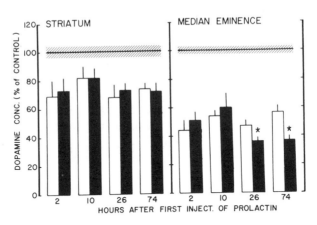

FIG. 3. Effects of prolactin on the αMT-induced reduction of dopamine concentrations in the striatum and median eminence. Female rats which were ovariectomized 4 days previously were injected with vehicle or ovine prolactin (5 mg/kg, s.c.) 1, 2, 4, or 10 times; injections were made every 8 hr and animals were sacrificed 2 hr after the last injection. One hour prior to sacrifice half of the animals at each time point were injected with saline (zero time controls) and the other half with αMT (250 mg/kg, i.p.). Since there were no significant differences in the dopamine concentrations of the brain regions of vehicle- or prolactin-pretreated zero time control animals, these values were combined, set at 100%, and represented by the horizontal lines and the SE by the shaded areas. The dopamine concentrations in animals sacrificed 60 min after the injection of αMT were calculated as a percentage of their respective zero time controls; values from vehicle-pretreated animals are represented by open bars and values from prolactin-pretreated animals are represented by solid bars; vertical lines represent 1 SE based on 6–8 determinations. * indicates values in prolactin-pretreated rats which are significantly different (p < 0.05) from vehicle-treated rats. From Gudelsky et al. (12) with permission.

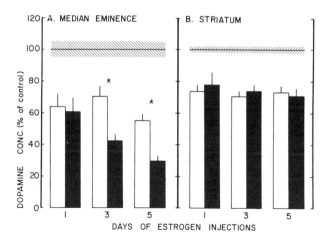

FIG. 4. Effects of estrogen on the αMT-induced reduction of dopamine concentrations in the median eminence and striatum. Male rats were injected daily with estradiol benzoate (25 μg/kg, s.c.) or corn oil vehicle for 1, 3, or 5 days, the last injection being made 24 hr prior to sacrifice. One hour prior to sacrifice half of the animals at each time point were injected with saline (zero time controls) and the other half with αMT (250 mg/kg, i.p.). Since there were no significant differences in the dopamine concentrations of median eminence and striatum of vehicle- and estrogen-pretreated rats which received saline, these values were combined, set at 100%, and represented by the horizontal lines and ± 1 SE by the shaded areas. The dopamine concentrations in the brain regions of animals sacrificed 60 min after the injection of αMT were calculated as a percentage of their respective zero time controls. Values from vehicle-pretreated animals which received αMT are represented by open bars and values from estrogen-pretreated animals which received αMT are represented by solid bars; vertical lines represent 1 SE based on 5–9 determinations. * indicates values in estrogen-pretreated rats which are significantly different from vehicle-pretreated rats (p < 0.05) as determined by Student's t-test for unpaired data. From Eikenburg et al. (6) with permission.

estradiol benzoate (25 μg/kg, s.c.) or corn oil vehicle for 1, 3, or 5 days. Rats were sacrificed 1 day after the last estradiol injection. One hour prior to sacrifice half of the rats in each group were injected with saline (zero-time values) and the other half with αMT. After 3 and 5 days of estradiol treatment the αMT-induced depletion of dopamine in the median eminence was significantly enhanced. This effect of estrogen was selective for tuberoinfundibular neurons; at no time was dopamine turnover enhanced in the striatum.

The serum concentrations of prolactin in those animals described above which were treated with estradiol for 3 days are summarized in Fig. 5. The serum prolactin concentrations in rats treated for 3 days with estradiol were significantly higher than in those animals receiving daily injections of corn oil. αMT increased the serum prolactin concentration in animals pretreated with corn oil, but produced an even greater increase in those animals pretreated for 3 days with estradiol. The enhanced ability of αMT to increase prolactin levels may be due to the removal of the increased inhibitory input by tuberoinfundibular dopamine neurons. That is, the increased activity of tuberoinfundibular neurons in response to estrogen (see Fig. 4) tends to

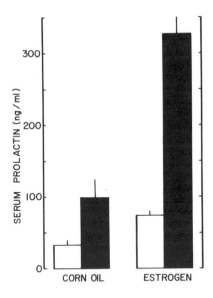

FIG. 5. Effects of estrogen and αMT on rat serum concentrations of prolactin. Male rats were injected daily with estradiol benzoate (25 μg/kg, s.c.) or corn oil vehicle for 3 days. One hour prior to sacrifice on the fourth day rats were injected i.p. with saline (*open columns*) or αMT (250 mg/kg; *solid columns*). The height of each bar and the vertical line represent the mean and 1 SE determined from 6 animals.

dampen the estrogen-stimulated rise in serum prolactin concentrations. By interrupting dopamine synthesis with αMT, this damping effect is eliminated and the prolactin levels increase markedly.

It has been reported that estrogens bind to the cell bodies of dopamine-tuberofundibular neurons in the arcuate nucleus (17), and Fuxe et al. (8) have proposed that estrogens exert a direct stimulatory effect on these neurons. In light of the ability of prolactin to increase dopamine turnover in the terminals of the tuberoinfundibular neurons, we reasoned that estrogen might increase dopamine turnover indirectly as a consequence of the elevated

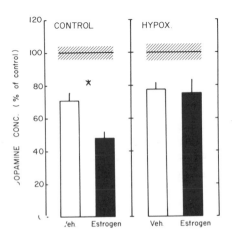

FIG. 6. Effects of estrogen on the αMT-induced reduction of dopamine concentrations in the median eminence of control and hypophysectomized rats. Male rats were injected daily with estradiol benzoate (25 μg/kg, s.c.) or corn oil vehicle for 3 days. See legend to Fig. 4 for details of drug administration. The means of zero time controls were set at 100% and represented by the horizontal lines and ± 1 SE by the shaded areas. Median eminence dopamine concentrations of animals sacrificed 60 min after the injection of αMT were calculated as a percentage of their respective zero time controls. Values from vehicle-pretreated animals which received αMT are represented by open bars, and values from estrogen-pretreated animals which received αMT are represented by solid bars; vertical lines represent 1 SE based on 10–14 determinations. * indicates the value in estrogen-pretreated rats which is significantly different from vehicle-pretreated rats (p < 0.05). From Eikenburg et al. (6) with permission.

circulating concentration of prolactin rather than through a direct action. Studies on the effects of estrogen in hypophysectomized rats support an indirect action of this hormone.

The ability of three daily injections of estradiol to enhance the αMT-induced depletion of dopamine in the median eminence of normal rats is completely abolished in hypophysectomized animals (Fig. 6). This suggests that estrogens do not act directly on dopamine neurons in the hypothalamus, but rather act indirectly by inducing changes in the release of hormones, possibly prolactin, from the anterior pituitary. Thus, endogenously released prolactin may exert a controlling influence on the activity of tuberoinfundibular dopamine neurons.

Haloperidol-induced Changes in Dopamine Turnover

We have previously reported that 2 hr after an i.p. injection of a moderate dose of haloperidol (0.5 mg/kg), the turnover of dopamine was increased in nigrostriatal and mesolimbic neurons but not in the tuberoinfundibular neurons (10). These results suggested that the latter neurons are not regulated by a neuronal feedback loop, or that they are less sensitive to the actions of drugs. It is well documented that haloperidol increases the concentration of prolactin in plasma (5). Since prolactin increases the turnover of dopamine

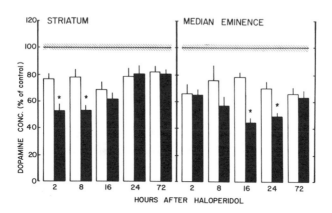

FIG. 7. Effects of haloperidol on the αMT-induced reduction of dopamine concentrations in the striatum and median eminence. Male rats were injected s.c. with vehicle (0.3% tartaric acid) or haloperidol (2.5 mg/kg) and sacrificed 2, 8, 16, 24, or 72 hr later. One hour prior to sacrifice half of the animals at each time point were injected with saline (zero time controls) and the other half with αMT (250 mg/kg, i.p.). Since there were no significant differences in the dopamine concentrations of brain regions in vehicle- or haloperidol-pretreated zero time control animals, these values were combined, set at 100%, and represented by the horizontal lines and ±1 SE by the shaded areas. The dopamine concentrations in animals sacrificed 60 min after the injection of αMT were calculated as a percentage of their respective zero time controls. Values from vehicle-pretreated animals are represented by open bars and values from haloperidol-pretreated animals are represented by solid bars; vertical lines represent 1 SE based on 6–18 determinations. * indicates values in haloperidol-pretreated rats which are significantly different (p < 0.05) from vehicle-treated rats. Modified from Gudelsky and Moore (11).

in tuberoinfundibular nerves, haloperidol should also eventually increase the activity of these neurons indirectly through the action of prolactin. Accordingly, a complete time course of the effects of a larger dose of haloperidol was determined on the turnover of dopamine in the striatum and median eminence (Fig. 7). In the striatum the αMT-induced depletion of dopamine was enhanced 2 and 8 hr after the injection of haloperidol. This is consistent with the well-known neuronal feedback loop which regulates the activity of the nigrostriatal neurons (3). At 16, 24, and 72 hr the αMT-induced depletion of dopamine was the same in the striatum of vehicle- and haloperidol-treated rats. Quite a different time course was observed in the median eminence. Haloperidol had no significant effect on the decline of dopamine after 2 and 8 hr, but by 16 and 24 hr the decline of dopamine in the haloperidol-treated animals was enhanced. Fuxe et al. (7) have reported a similar time course for changes in the dynamics of dopamine in the median eminence after injections of pimozide.

These results suggest that haloperidol influences the dynamics of dopamine in the nigrostriatal and tuberoinfundibular neuronal systems by different mechanisms (Fig. 8). The immediate effect of haloperidol in the striatum is to accelerate the turnover of dopamine. This is presumably due to blockade of dopamine receptors in the striatum which causes a compensatory increase in the activity of neurons in the nigrostriatal pathway through a neuronal feedback mechanism. Dopamine neurons in the tuberoinfundibular system do not appear to be controlled by a similar neuronal feedback mechanism. Rather, by blocking dopamine receptors on the pituitary, haloperidol disrupts the tonic inhibitory action of the tuberoinfundibular system on prolactin release. This causes the plasma concentration of this hormone to increase. The elevated circulating concentration of prolactin, in turn, may activate receptors

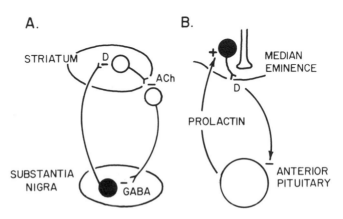

FIG. 8. Schematic diagram of (A) a possible neuronal feedback mechanism controlling the activity of nigrostriatal dopamine neurons and (B) a possible hormonal feedback mechanism controlling the activity of tuberoinfundibular dopamine neurons. D, dopamine, ACh, acetylcholine; GABA, γ-aminobutyric acid.

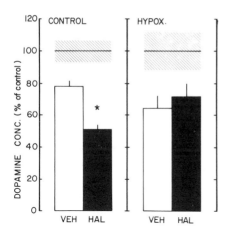

FIG. 9. Effects of haloperidol on the αMT-induced reduction of dopamine concentrations in the median eminence of control and hypophysectomized rats. Male rats were injected with haloperidol (2.5 mg/kg, s.c.) or a 0.3% tartaric acid vehicle 16 hr prior to sacrifice. One hour prior to sacrifice animals received an i.p. injection of saline (zero time controls set at 100%; *horizontal lines*) or αMT (250 mg/kg; *columns*). The height of each column represents the mean and the vertical line 1 SE determined from 7–9 animals. *, the dopamine concentration in the haloperidol-pretreated animal which is significantly different from the vehicle-pretreated animals ($p < 0.05$).

in the brain to increase the activity of tuberoinfundibular neurons. In effect, prolactin in the plasma acts to inhibit its own release by activating the tuberoinfundibular inhibitory system. If the delayed increase in the activity of tuberoinfundibular neurons in response to haloperidol is mediated by prolactin, this action of the drug should not be obtained in hypophysectomized rats.

The effects of haloperidol on the αMT-induced decline of dopamine in the median eminence of control and hypophysectomized rats are depicted in Fig. 9. Sixteen hours after the injection of haloperidol in control rats, the turnover of dopamine in the median eminence was enhanced. This acceleration was not seen in hypophysectomized animals. These results suggest, there-

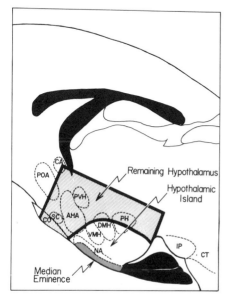

FIG. 10. Sagittal view of the rat brain depicting the regions examined after hypothalamic deafferentation. The inner curved heavy dark line represents the site of the deafferentation, and the outer straight heavy dark line indicates the borders used in dissecting the remaining hypothalamus. AHA, anterior hypothalamic area; CA, anterior commissure; CC, corpus callosum; CO, optic chiasm; CT nucleus centralis tegmenti; DMH, dorsomedial nucleus; FX, fornix; IP, interpeduncular nucleus; NA, arcuate nucleus; PH, posterior hypothalamic nucleus; PVH, paraventricular nucleus; POA, preoptic area.

fore, that the delayed increase in the activity of tuberoinfundibular neurons after haloperidol is dependent on the presence of the pituitary gland, presumably on the ability of haloperidol to increase the concentration of prolactin in plasma.

Prolactin may activate the feedback mechanism by acting directly on tuberoinfundibular or other intrahypothalamic neurons, or it might act on neurons outside the hypothalamus. A modified Halász knife was used to isolate a portion of the medial basal hypothalamus from the rest of the brain so that the hypothalamic island contained the cell bodies and terminals of the tuberoinfundibular dopaminergic neurons (i.e., arcuate nucleus and median eminence; Fig. 10). This lesion significantly reduced the norepinephrine concentration in the median eminence and hypothalamic island, but not in the remainder of the hypothalamus. The lesion did not alter the dopamine concentration in any of these brain regions. The αMT-induced decline of dopamine in the median eminence, hypothalamic island, and remaining hypothalamus are depicted in Fig. 11. Haloperidol administered 16 hr before sacrifice increased the dopamine turnover in median eminence, but not in the other two brain regions. The results illustrated in Fig. 12 indicate that the haloperidol enhancement of the αMT-induced decline of dopamine in the median eminence is essentially the same in normal and deafferented rats. Thus, the proposed hormonal-neuronal feedback mecha-

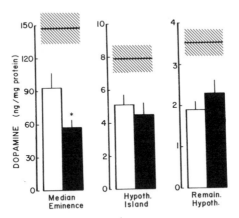

FIG. 11. Effects of haloperidol on the αMT-induced decline of the dopamine concentrations in the median eminence, hypothalamic island, and remaining hypothalamus of rats deafferented 16–33 days prior to the experiment. Rats were sacrificed 16 hr after a single injection of haloperidol (2.5 mg/kg, s.c.) or vehicle (0.3% tartaric acid). One hour before sacrifice half of the animals in each group received saline and the other half received αMT (250 mg/kg, i.p.). No significant differences were observed in the dopamine concentration in the median eminence, hypothalamic island, and remaining hypothalamus of haloperidol- and vehicle-pretreated animals which received saline. These zero time values were combined and represented by the horizontal lines; the shaded areas indicate ± 1 SE. The means of the αMT-depleted values are represented by the open (vehicle) and solid (haloperidol) columns, and are based on 7–10 determinations; vertical lines represent ± 1 SE. * indicates a significantly (p < 0.05) greater αMT-induced depletion.

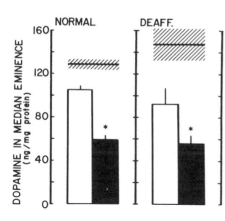

FIG. 12. Effect of haloperidol on the αMT-induced depletion of dopamine in the median eminence of normal control and deafferented rats. The experimental protocol was the same as that described in legend to Fig. 11 except that half of the animals were not deafferented (normal). The means of the αMT-depleted values are represented by the open (vehicle) and solid (haloperidol) columns; * indicates a significantly greater depletion ($p < 0.05$).

nism regulating the activity of tuberoinfundibular dopamine neurons and prolactin secretion appears to involve an action of prolactin directly on neurons within the medial basal hypothalamus, possibly on dopamine-containing cell bodies of the tuberoinfundibular neurons in the arcuate nucleus.

SUMMARY

All dopaminergic neurons in the central nervous system do not respond to pharmacological and endocrinological manipulations in the same manner. Tuberoinfundibular neurons appear to be regulated, in part, by circulating levels of prolactin. Prolactin increases the activity of these neurons by acting directly within the medial basal hypothalamus, possibly on the tuberoinfundibular neurons.

ACKNOWLEDGMENTS

Many of the studies described in this chapter were supported by USPHS Grant NS09174. G. A. Gudelsky was a predoctoral student supported by USPHS Training Grant GM 1761. Dr. L. Annunziato is a Visiting Professor at Michigan State University on leave from the Department of Pharmacology in the Second Faculty of Medicine, University of Naples; he is supported by a fellowship from NATO-CNR. The excellent technical assistance of Mrs. Sue Stahl is gratefully acknowledged.

REFERENCES

1. Andén, N.-E., and Wachtel, H. (1977): Biochemical effects of baclofen (β-parachlorophenyl-GABA) on the dopamine and the noradrenaline in the rat brain. *Acta Pharmacol. Toxicol.*, 40:310–320.
2. Ben-Jonathan, N., and Porter, J. C. (1976): A sensitive radioenzymatic assay for dopamine, norepinephrine, and epinephrine in plasma and tissue. *Endocrinology*, 98:1497–1507.
3. Carlsson, A., and Lindqvist, M. (1963): Effect of chlorpromazine or haloperidol

on formation of 3-methoxytyramine and normetanephrine in mouse brain. *Acta Pharmacol. (Kbh.),* 20:140–143.

4. Da Prada, M., and Keller, H. H. (1976): Baclofen and hydroxybutyrate: Similar effects on cerebral dopamine neurons. *Life Sci.,* 19:1253–1264.
5. Dickerman, S., Clark, J., Dickerman, E., and Meites, J. (1972): Effects of haloperidol on serum and pituitary prolactin and a hypothalamic PIF in rats. *Neuroendocrinology,* 9:332–340.
6. Eikenburg, D., Ravitz, A., Gudelsky, G. A., and Moore, K. E. (1977): Effects of estrogen on prolactin and tuberoinfundibular dopaminergic neurons. *J. Neural Transm.,* 40:235–244.
7. Fuxe, K., Agnati, L., Tsuchiya, K., Hökfelt, T., Johansson, O., Jonsson, G., Lindbrink, P., Löfström, A., and Ungerstedt, U. (1975): Effect of antipsychotic drugs on central catecholamine neurons of rat brain. In: *Antipsychotic Drugs, Pharmacodynamics and Pharmacokinetics,* edited by G. Sedvall, pp. 117–132. Pergamon Press, Oxford.
8. Fuxe, K., Hökfelt, T., and Nilsson, O. (1969): Castration, sex hormones and tuberoinfundibular dopamine neurons. *Neuroendocrinology,* 5:107–120.
9. Gianutsos, G., and Moore, K. E. (1977): Increase in mouse brain dopamine content by baclofen: Effects of apomorphine and neuroleptics. *Psychopharmacology,* 52:217–221.
10. Gudelsky, G. A., and Moore, K. E. (1976): Differential drug effects on dopamine concentrations and rates of turnover in the median eminence, olfactory tubercle and corpus striatum. *J. Neural Transm.,* 38:95–105.
11. Gudelsky, G. A., and Moore, K. E. (1977): A comparison of the effects of haloperidol on dopamine turnover in the striatum, olfactory tubercle and median eminence. *J. Pharmacol. Exp. Ther.,* 202:149–156.
12. Gudelsky, G. A., Simpkins, J., Mueller, G. P., Meites, J., and Moore, K. E. (1976): Selective actions of prolactin on catecholamine turnover in the hypothalamus and on serum LH and FSH. *Neuroendocrinology,* 22:206–215.
13. Hökfelt, T., and Fuxe, K. (1972): Effects of prolactin and ergot alkaloids on the tuberoinfundibular dopamine neurons. *Neuroendocrinology,* 9:100–122.
14. Lowry, O. H., Rosenbrough, N. J., Farr, A. L., and Randall, R. J. (1951): Protein measurement with Folin phenol reagent. *J. Biol. Chem.,* 193:265–275.
15. Moore, K. E., and Phillipson, O. T. (1975): Effects of dexamethasone on phenylethanolamine N-methyltransferase and adrenaline in the brains and superior cervical ganglia of adult and neonatal rats. *J. Neurochem.,* 25:289–294.
16. Naik, S. R., Guidotti, A., and Costa, E. (1976): Central GABA receptor agonists: Comparison of muscimol and baclofen. *Neuropharmacology,* 15:479–484.
17. Stumpf, W. E., and Sar, M. (1977): Steroid hormone target cells in the periventricular brain: Relationship to peptide hormone producing cells. *Fed. Proc.,* 36:1973–1977.
18. Ungerstedt, U. (1971): Stereotaxic mapping of the monoamine pathways in the rat brain. *Acta Physiol. Scand. [Suppl.],* 367:1–48.
19. Walters, J. R., Roth, R. H., and Aghajanian, G. K. (1973): Dopaminergic neurons: Similar biochemical and histochemical effects of γ-hydroxybutyrate and acute lesions of the nigro-neostriatal pathway. *J. Pharmacol. Exp. Ther.,* 186:630–639.
20. Weiner, N. (1974): A critical assessment of methods for the determination of monoamine synthesis turnover rates *in vivo.* In: *Neuropsychopharmacology of Monoamines and Their Regulatory Enzymes,* edited by E. Usdin, pp. 143–159. Raven Press, New York.

Advances in Biochemical Psychopharmacology, Vol. 19,
edited by P. J. Roberts et al.
Raven Press, New York © 1978.

Studies on Mesocortical Dopamine Systems

A. M. Thierry, J. P. Tassin, G. Blanc, and J. Glowinski

Groupe NB—INSERM U 114, College of France, 75231 Paris Cedex 05 France

For many years, the dopaminergic innervation of the central nervous system has been attributed to three main pathways. The nigrostriatal dopaminergic system, which has been extensively studied, plays an important role in motor coordination. Several symptoms observed in Parkinson's disease are attributed to the degeneration of this pathway. The tuberoinfundibular dopaminergic system modulates the release of some pituitary hormones and thus controls various neuroendocrine functions. The mesolimbic dopaminergic system, which innervates several limbic structures such as the nucleus accumbens, the olfactory tubercles, the amygdala, the septum, and the stria terminalis, may contribute to the regulation of emotional behavior. In fact, according to some authors (2,11) the antipsychotic effects of neuroleptics could be related to the blockade of dopamine (DA) receptors distributed in areas innervated by the mesolimbic dopaminergic system. However, since the recent discovery of the mesocortical dopaminergic system, these effects could be attributed as well to the blockade of the cortical DA receptors. The existence of DA terminals in the cerebral cortex was first revealed in biochemical studies (40,42). Then, rapidly, results obtained with the histofluorescence method confirmed the occurrence of a dopaminergic innervation in three main cortical areas: the frontal, the cingular, and the entorhinal cortices (4,14,22). The cell bodies of these DA neurons are located in the mesencephalon, both in the tegmental ventral area A10 group) and in the substantia nigra (A9 group) (12,24). The aim of this chapter is to describe the main steps which were involved in the identification and mapping of the mesocortical DA neurons and to discuss recent pharmacological and behavioral studies which provide some information about their role.

IDENTIFICATION AND MAPPING OF THE MESOCORTICAL DOPAMINERGIC SYSTEMS

Identification of Dopaminergic Terminals in the Cerebral Cortex

The discrepancy between the levels of DA in the cerebellum and the cerebral cortex, two structures innervated by noradrenergic terminals originating from neurons located in the locus coeruleus, was the first observation which led us to suspect the existence of a dopaminergic innervation in the cerebral cortex. In the cerebellum DA levels could not be detected with the classic spectrofluorimetric methods; in contrast, the concentration of DA in the cerebral cortex reached as much as 50% that of norepinephrine (NE). We thus attempted to determine whether DA was only the precursor of NE in noradrenergic terminals or was also acting as a transmitter synthesized in cortical DA nerve endings. To test this last hypothesis the contents of DA and NE as well as the synthesis of ^{3}H-catecholamine from ^{3}H-tyrosine were estimated in the cerebral cortices of rats deprived of noradrenergic innervation. Three experimental procedures were used to destroy the noradrenergic innervation: (a) bilateral electrolytic lesions of the locus coeruleus were performed (40,42); (b) 6-hydroxydopamine (6-OHDA, 2 μg/1 μl) was injected bilaterally into the lateral part of the pedonucleus cerebellaris superior (L-PCS), which contains the ascending noradrenergic bundles (40,42); (c) 6-OHDA (100 μg/g) was injected intraperitoneally into fetus or newborn rats in which the blood-brain barrier was not yet fully developed (39). These three procedures induced a significant decline in cortical levels of NE (77% to 98%) without affecting the content of DA in the cerebral cortex. Estimated *in vivo* or *in vitro,* the synthesis of ^{3}H-NE from L-3,5-^{3}H-tyrosine was markedly reduced, whereas ^{3}H-DA formation still occurred in the lesioned animals (39,40). Similar results were obtained on synaptosomes prepared from the cerebral cortices of rats deprived of noradrenergic innervation (40). These experiments demonstrated that the synthesis of ^{3}H-DA from L-3,5-^{3}H-tyrosine was occurring in dopaminergic nerve endings.

Another biochemical marker was then used to identify the cortical DA terminals. We attempted to demonstrate the existence of a specific uptake process for DA in the cerebral cortex. DA can be taken up by dopaminergic and noradrenergic nerve endings; however, each type of terminal exhibits a specific transport process. For instance, desipramine and benztropine specifically block the uptake processes of catecholamines in noradrenergic and dopaminergic neurons, respectively. The uptake of DA was affected by both drugs in homogenates of the cerebral cortex of normal animals (33,38). It was no longer inhibited by desipramine but was markedly reduced by benztropine in animals deprived of noradrenergic innervation (38). This further revealed the presence of dopaminergic terminals.

Finally, a DA-sensitive adenylate cyclase was detected in homogenates of the rat cerebral cortex (7,44,45). Added in saturating concentrations, DA and isoproterenol, a β-adrenergic agonist, induced additive effects suggesting the occurrence of two distinct populations of receptor sites. However, NE appears to be an agonist of both dopaminergic and β-adrenergic receptors (7). Electrophysiological studies have also revealed that some cortical cells are sensitive to DA, NE, or both (8).

Distribution of Dopaminergic Innervation in the Rat Cerebral Cortex

The regional distribution of the cortical dopaminergic innervation was first described in histofluorescent studies. Concordant results were obtained using different methodological approaches (4,5,14,22,24). In contrast to the noradrenergic terminals which are widespread throughout all cortical areas, the dopaminergic fibers are mainly confined to the frontal, supragenual, and entorhinal cortices. Since they are fine and sinuous, the dopaminergic fibers can be distinguished from the relatively thick and varicose noradrenergic terminals. The dopaminergic innervation is particularly rich in the deep layers (mainly V and VI) of the frontal cortex in a medial field extending to the ventral part, anterior and dorsal to the genu of the corpus callosum. In contrast, the dopaminergic fibers were scattered in all cortical layers in the foremost part of the frontal lobe (Fig. 1). Another field of dopaminergic fibers was also detected between the dorsal lip of the rhinal sulcus and the lateral cortex above it (Fig. 1). In this case numerous fibers were found in layers V and VI; they seemed to give rise to terminal aggregations in the second and third layers. In the supragenual cortex dopaminergic fibers have been described. They are close to the white matter and extend with decreasing density in the anteroposterior direction and appear to be an extension of the anteromedial frontal plexus. The ventral part of the entorhinal cortex has been shown to contain patchy networks of dopaminergic fibers mainly located in the middle layers.

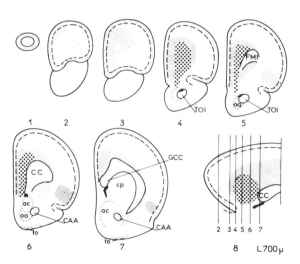

FIG. 1. Distribution and relative density of the dopaminergic innervation in the neocortex of the rat. Increasing coarseness and density of stipple represent increasing density of dopaminergic innervation. Planes 2–7, correspond, respectively, to levels 4b–7b, 9b, and 12b of the Atlas of König and Klippel. TOI, tractus olfactorius intermedius; FMI, forceps minor of corpus callosum; oa, nucleus olfactorius anterior; CC, corpus callosum; ac, nucleus accumbens; CAA, commissura anterior; to, tuberculum olfactorium; GCC, genu of corpus callosum; cp, nucleus caudatus putamen. From Berger et al. (5).

The distribution of the dopaminergic innervation in the various cortical areas has also been quantitatively estimated by means of biochemical studies. The content of DA (35,37), the specific uptake of ^{3}H-DA (37), and the DA-sensitive adenylate cyclase activity (6) were determined in cortical microdiscs punched out from frozen brain slices. The distribution of the three biochemical markers was identical and in agreement with the results obtained from histochemical studies.

Origin of the Cortical Dopaminergic Terminals

The perikarya of the dopaminergic neurons innervating the cerebral cortex are located in the complex of dopaminergic cells distributed in the ventral tegmental area (A10 group) and in the substantia nigra (A9 group). In earlier lesion studies Lindvall et al. (24) indicated that the dopaminergic innervation of the frontal and of the anterior cingulate cortices originated from the A10 group and from the lateral part of the A9 group, respectively. However, Fuxe et al. (12) found that the degeneration of dopaminergic nerve terminals of the cingulate and entorhinal cortices was better correlated with the degeneration of dopaminergic endings of the tuberculum olfactorium than with those of the nucleus caudatus. They thus concluded on a medial A9 lateral A10 origin of the cortical DA innervation. In our biochemical studies we observed that discrete lesions of the ventral tegmental area induced a decrease of ^{3}H-DA uptake activity in the frontal but not in the cingular cortex (35). Various authors (3,9,23) were able to identify labeled cells only within the A10 and medial A9 groups after small injections of horseradish peroxidase in various DA cortical areas. Cells projecting to the anteromedial frontal cortex and to the suprarhinal cortex were located within the A10 group. Those projecting to the supragenual cortex originated mainly from the ventrolateral A10 and medial A9 groups. Simon et al. (31) have used the Fink-Heimer method to follow the anterograde degeneration induced by electrolytic or 6-hydroxydopamine lesions made in the tegmental ventral area or in the substantia nigra. They observed that a lesion of the A10 group induced a degeneration of fibers in the frontal cortex and, to a lesser extent, in the cingular cortex. A lesion of the A9 group induced degenerations in the cingular and the enthorhinal cortex, but no degenerating fibers were observed in the frontal area. It is interesting to note that direct projections from the tegmental ventral area and the medial part of the substantia nigra to layer III of the cortical areas 4 and 6 had already been observed in the cat in 1967 (25). These various data suggest that the dopaminergic innervation of the frontal cortex arises mainly if not entirely from the A10 group. The limbic cortical dopaminergic innervation seems to originate mainly from cells located in the ventrolateral part of the A10 group and in the medial part of the A9 group.

EFFECTS OF DRUGS ON THE MESOCORTICAL DOPAMINERGIC SYSTEM

The effects of neuroleptics on the mesocortical dopaminergic system have been extensively studied. These drugs exert their effects by blocking dopaminergic transmission. Their extrapyramidal side effects are very likely related to the blockade of DA receptors in the striatum. As already mentioned, their antipsychotic properties could be related to their action on mesolimbic and or mesocortical dopaminergic neurons. Two biochemical approaches were used to study the effects of neuroleptics on the mesocortical dopaminergic neurons. One consisted of analyzing the changes in cortical DA metabolism, the other was based on the estimation of the drug effect on the DA-sensitive adenylate cyclase activity in cortical homogenates.

The reactivity of dopaminergic neurons to neuroleptics can be appreciated by measuring the changes in DA synthesis or turnover. These changes could be mediated by the blockade of postsynaptic DA receptors or of DA "autoreceptors." The synthesis of DA was estimated *in vitro* in the striatum, the nucleus accumbens and tuberculum olfactorium, and the frontal and anterior cingulate cortex of rats previously injected with the drugs. These structures were selected since they are, respectively, innervated by the nigrostriatal, the mesolimbic, and the mesocortical dopaminergic systems. The synthesis of DA was stimulated in the terminals of the three dopaminergic systems shortly after the administration of various neuroleptics (thioproperazine, pipotiazine, or haloperidol) (15,29,30). However, the mesocortical neurons appeared much less sensitive than the mesolimbic or nigrostriatal neurons. For example, the doses of thioproperazine required to induce a 50% rise in DA synthesis in the striatum, in the limbic structures, and in the cerebral cortex were, respectively, 0.08 mg/kg s.c., 0.9 mg/kg s.c., and 6 mg/kg s.c. Another interesting difference, which may have some clinical significance, was observed after chronic neuroleptic treatment (15,29). Moderate doses of thioproperazine, haloperidol, or pipothiazine were injected daily for 11 days. As seen after acute treatment, shortly after the last injection of neuroleptics, DA synthesis was increased in the limbic and cortical structures; however, no effect could be detected in the nigrostriatal DA terminals. The striatum was the only structure in which DA synthesis was decreased 24 hr after the last neuroleptic injection. Finally, the time course of the effects of a long-acting neuroleptic on DA synthesis in the three DA systems was also analyzed (15,28). A single injection of the palmitic ester of pipotiazine (32 mg/kg), which is slowly released from its site of injection and constantly delivered in minute quantities to the brain for several weeks, induced biphasic changes in DA synthesis in the nigrostriatal and mesolimbic systems (Fig. 2). In the striatum an initial activation of DA synthesis was followed by a sustained inhibition. In the limbic structures the initial activation was longer and the

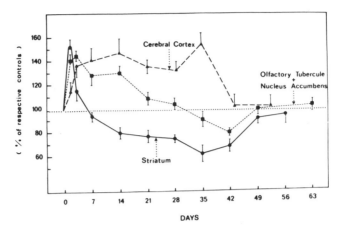

FIG. 2. Time course of the effects of the palmitic ester of pipotiazine on DA synthesis in various dopaminergic pathways. Animals were injected with either sesame oil (controls) or pipotiazine palmitate (32 mg/kg s.c.). Ten animals of each group were killed at various times after the injection, and slices from the striatum, tuberculum olfactorium and nucleus accumbens, or anterior cerebral cortex were incubated for 15 min with L-3,5-^{3}H-tyrosine. ^{3}H-H$_2$O (striatum, tuberculum olfactorium and nucleus accumbens) or ^{3}H-DA (cerebral cortex) accumulated in slices and their incubating medium were determined. Each point is the mean ± SEM of 10 determinations and is represented as a percentage of the respective control values. From Julou et al. (15).

phase of inhibition much shorter. In contrast, in the cerebral cortex a single phase of activation of the transmitter synthesis was observed; it lasted for at least 5 weeks.

As indicated in electrophysiological studies, neuroleptics selectively block the DA-inhibiting effect on cells located in deep layers of the frontal cortex (1,8). They also block the DA-induced activation of the DA-sensitive adenylate cyclase (6). The differences in the reactivity of the mesocortical and nigrostriatal systems to acute or chronic neuroleptic treatments could be explained by differences in the sensitivity of the respective DA receptors to these drugs (6,7). Haloperidol, which competitively inhibited the stimulatory effect of DA on the striatal and the cortical DA-sensitive adenylate cyclases, was slightly more potent in inhibiting the cortical ($K_i = 27$ nM) than the striatal ($K_i = 67$ mM) DA-sensitive adenylate cyclase. Fluphenazine was more potent than haloperidol in the striatum, but both drugs were equipotent in the frontal cortex. Thioproperazine was two times less potent in the frontal cortex than in the striatum. Thioridazine, chlorpromazine, and clozapine exhibited the same affinity for DA receptors within the two structures.

FUNCTIONAL ROLE OF THE MESOCORTICAL DOPAMINERGIC SYSTEM

The sites of dopaminergic innervation in the frontal lobe of the rat and other species coincide with the terminal areas of neurons originating in the mediodorsal nucleus of the thalamus (21,23). This cortical area also receives direct projections from the amygdala (16). Finally, as already discussed, the cells of origin of the frontal DA terminals are localized in the "limbic midbrain area." This anatomical organization suggests that the mesocortical frontal dopaminergic system plays an important role in complex behaviors and in the regulation of emotional states. The involvement of the mesocortical dopaminergic system in such functions can be analyzed by two different approaches which consist of studying the behavioral changes induced by their destruction of the modification of their activity in animals subjected to a perturbed environment.

Behavioral Effect of the Lesion of the Ventral Tegmental Area in the Rat

During the last few years Le Moal et al. (17,19) have shown that the electrolytic lesion of ventral tegmental area induces a complex nonvicarious syndrome. This ventral tegmental area syndrome is characterized by: "locomotor hyperactivity and hyporeactivity without change in total sleep time; difficulty in suppressing previously learned responses or in tolerating frustrating situations; disappearance of freezing reaction and improvement of conditioned response in an active avoidance conditioning; disappearance of hoarding behaviour and of the alternation behaviour in a T. maze." According to these authors, "fundamental behaviour was not quantitatively impaired but seems qualitatively disorganized." Similar behavioral disturbances were seen after electrolytic lesion of the tegmental ventral area or after local microinjection of 6-hydroxydopamine in this area (18). Thus the syndrome appeared to be due, at least in part, to the destruction of dopaminergic cells of the A10 group. Since the mesocortical and mesolimbic dopaminergic systems partly originate from the tegmental ventral area, their respective participation in the "tegmental ventral area syndrome" was analyzed by a combined biochemical and behavioral approach (36,37). The locomotor hyperactivity induced by bilateral electrolytic lesions of the tegmental ventral area was correlated with the decline in DA levels in the frontal cerebral cortex and in the nucleus accumbens, structures innervated by the mesocortical and mesolimbic dopaminergic systems, respectively (36). A correlation was found between the changes in locomotor activity and the decrease of DA levels in the nucleus accumbens ($r = -0.47$, $N = 24$, $p < 0.05$). However, a more striking correlation was observed between the increase in locomotor activity and the decrease of DA levels in the frontal cerebral cortex ($r = -0.82$, $N = 20$, $p < 0.01$). Since the ascending serotoninergic fibers run through the tegmental ventral area, the lesion could also destroy these neurons. However, no correlation has been found between the increase of locomotor activity and the decrease of serotonin content in the hippocampus, the striatum, and the parietal-rhinal cortex. These data suggested that the disappearance of DA in the frontal cortex may be critical for the development of locomotor hyperactivity. In other words, the dopaminergic neurons projecting to the frontal cortex may exert an inhibitory control on locomotor behavior. However, these results do not completely exclude participation of other mesocortical or mesolimbic dopaminergic neurons. It is particularly interesting to note that this locomotor hyperactivity can be reversed by an acute injection of apomorphine or a chronic treatment with low doses of amphetamine (20). Since chronic amphetamine treatment has been used to reduce the hyperactive behavior observed in children with "minimal brain dysfunction," animals deprived of cortical and limbic dopaminergic innervation or with lesion in the tegmental ventral area may represent a useful physiopathological experimental model.

Effect of Stress on the Activity of the Mesocortical Dopaminergic System

In earlier studies we reported that a stress of long duration (180 min) induced by electric foot shocks increases the utilization of NE in various structures of the brain but does not influence DA utilization in the striatum (41). Therefore, animals previously treated with α-methylparatyrosine to block catecholamine synthesis were subjected to electric foot shock stress for 20 min, and DA levels were determined in various dopaminergic areas (43). As expected, the 20-min stress did not modify the activity of the nigrostriatal dopaminergic system (Fig. 3). The utilization of DA was accelerated in the nucleus accumbens but not in the tuberculum olfactorium (Fig. 3), indicating that dopaminergic neurons projecting to the two limbic structures do not behave similarly. The most striking effect was obtained in the frontal cerebral cortex where a 60% decrease in DA levels was observed in animals subjected

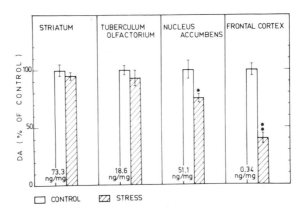

FIG. 3. Effect of 20 min of electric foot shock stress on the utilization of DA instructures innervated by the nigrostriatal, mesolimbic, or mesocortical dopaminergic system. DA levels were estimated 30 min after the injection of α-methyl-p-tyrosine (200 mg/kg) in tissues of control and stressed rats. The electric foot shock stress was applied 10 min after the injection of the catecholamine synthesis inhibitor. Numbers in bars represent absolute mean values of DA per mg of protein. Data expressed in percent of respective control values are the mean ± SEM of results obtained with groups of 6 rats. *p < 0.02; **p < 0.001 when compared with the respective controls. From Thierry et al. (43).

to electric foot shocks (Fig. 3). The intense activation of DA utilization seen in the frontal cortex during this stress situation suggests that the meso-corticofrontal dopaminergic system is involved in the cerebral circuitry of emotionality.

Self-Stimulation Behavior

Animals implanted with electrodes in certain sites of the brain learn to repeatedly press a lever which delivers central stimuli through these electrodes. Anatomical and pharmacological studies have revealed that the catecholamine-containing systems play an important role in this self-stimulation behavior [see for review German and Bowden (13)]. Some findings indicate that the mesocortical dopaminergic systems may also be implicated. Electrodes located in areas rich in dopaminergic cell bodies, i.e., the substantia nigra and the ventral tegmental area, support intracranial self-stimulation (13). Moreover, self-stimulation can be evoked from certain cortical areas. Routtenberg and Sloan (27) observed self-stimulation in rats with electrodes implanted in the medial frontal cortex or in the sulcal cortex on the dorsal lip of the rhinal sulcus. Self-stimulation sites were also found in the entorhinal and cingulate cortices but not in other neocortical areas (34). Neurons located in the sulcal and frontal cortex of the rat or in the orbitofrontal cortex of the monkey are activated during self-stimulation induced from different reward sites (26). Anesthetization of the sulcal pre-frontal cortex attenuates the self-stimulation evoked from the lateral hypothalamus and the pontine tegmentum (26). Moreover, unilateral electrolytic lesions of the cortex dorsal to the rhinal sulcus in rats markedly reduced the self-stimulation evoked from the substantia nigra (10). However, neurons in the prefrontal cortex which are activated during self-stimulation appear to be "closely related to but not essential for reward" (26). It is striking to observe that the sites from which self-stimulation behavior can be evoked in the cerebral cortex closely overlap those to which project the mesocortical dopaminergic system. On this basis changes in DA utilization in the rat frontal cortex were examined during self-stimulation from the tegmental ventral area. A 10-min session of self-stimulation induced a 34% decrease of DA levels and a 69% increase of dihydroxyphenylacetic acid (DOPAC), the main DA metabolite, in the frontal cortex revealing a significant activation of the mesocorticofrontal dopaminergic system (32). In these animals the utilization of DA in the nucleus accumbens was not significantly affected (32). Therefore, it can be concluded that the mesocortical dopaminergic system may modulate self-stimulation reward.

CONCLUSION

The dopaminergic innervation of the cerebral cortex is now well established. This innervation is circumscribed to defined areas. There is a striking convergence of data obtained with different experimental approaches. This includes the histofluorescence observations, the biochemical analysis of the distribution of DA, ^{3}H-DA uptake activity, and DA-sensitive adenylate cyclase, and finally the electrophysiological studies. The dopaminergic cell bodies projecting to the cerebral cortex are localized in the A10–A9 complex of dopaminergic cells, but the exact location of the neurons innervating individual cortical areas must still be determined. However, we already know that the frontal cortex is innervated by dopaminergic cells located mainly in the A10 group. An important problem has still to be elucidated: do the axons of the mesencephalic dopaminergic cells bifurcate to different cortical or limbic areas? Data already indicate that the activity of the mesocorticofrontal dopaminergic neurons of some mesolimbic dopaminergic neurons (nucleus accumbens, tuberculum olfactorium) and of the nigrostriatal dopaminergic neurons react differently to acute or chronic neuroleptic treatments, to electric foot shock stress, and finally during self-stimulation behavior. Moreover, after discrete lesions of the tegmental ventral area in rats, the correlation between the induced locomotor hyperactivity and the decrease in DA levels is better in the frontal cortex than in the nucleus accumbens. This suggests that the dopaminergic terminals in the frontal cortex and in the nucleus accumbens originate from distinct cell bodies. Such analysis should be extended to other cortical and limbic areas innervated by dopaminergic neurons. Since the mesocortical dopaminergic pathways represent links in integrated systems, the neurons involved in their regulation and those influenced by them should be identified to further clarify their functions.

ACKNOWLEDGMENTS

This research has been supported by grants from the INSERM, the CNRS, and the Société des Usines Chimiques Rhône Poulenc.

REFERENCES

1. Aghajanian, G. K., and Bunney, B. S. (1977): Pharmacological characterization of dopamine "autoreceptors" by microiontophoretic single cell recording studies. *Adv. Biochem. Psychopharmacol.*, 16:433–438.
2. Anden, N. E. (1972): Dopamine turnover in the corpus striatum and the limbic system after treatment with neuroleptic and antiacetylcholine drugs. *J. Pharm. Pharmacol.*, 24:905–906.
3. Beckstead, R. (1976): Convergent thalamic and mesencephalic projections to the anterior medial cortex in the rat. *J. Comp. Neurol.*, 166:403–416.
4. Berger, B., Tassin, J. P., Blanc G., Moyne, M. A., and Thierry, A. M. (1974): Histochemical confirmation for dopaminergic innervation of the rat cerebral cortex after destruction of the noradrenergic ascending pathways. *Brain Res.*, 81:332–337.
5. Berger, B., Thierry, A. M., Tassin, J. P., and Moyne, M. A. (1976): Dopaminergic innervation of the rat prefrontal cortex: A fluorescence histochemical study. *Brain Res.*, 106:133–145.
6. Bockaert, J., Premont, J., Glowinski, J., Tassin, J. P., and Thierry, A. M. (1977): Topographical distribution and characteristics of dopamine and β-adrenergic sensi-

tive adenylate cyclases in the rat frontal cerebral cortex striatum and substantia nigra. *Adv. Biochem. Psychopharmacol.,* 16:29–37.

7. Bockaert, J., Tassin, J. P., Thierry, A. M., Glowinski, J., and Premont, J. (1977): Characteristics of dopamine and β-adrenergic sensitive adenylate cyclases in the frontal cerebral cortex of the rat. Comparative effects of neuroleptics on frontal and striatal dopamine sensitive adenylate cyclases. *Brain Res.,* 122:71–86.

8. Bunney, B. S., and Aghajanian, G. K. (1976): Dopamine and norepinephrine innervated cells in the rat prefrontal cortex: Pharmacological differentiation using microiontophoretic techniques. *Life Sci.,* 19:1783–1792.

9. Carter, D. A., and Fibiger, H. C. (1977): Ascending projections of presumed dopamine containing neurons in the ventral tegmentum of the rat as demonstrated by horseradish peroxidase. *Neuroscience,* 2:569–576.

10. Clavier, R. M., and Corcoran, M. E. (1976): Attenuation of self stimulation from substantia nigra but not dorsal tegmental noradrenergic bundle by lesions of sulcal prefrontal cortex. *Brain Res.,* 113:59–69.

11. Crow, T. J., Deakin, J. F., and Longden, A. (1977): The nucleus accumbens: Possible site of antipsychotic action of neuroleptic drugs? *Psychol. Med.,* 7:213–221.

12. Fuxe, K., Hökfelt, T., Johansson, O., Jonsson, G., Lidbrink, P., and Ljüugdahl, A. (1974): The origin of the dopamine nerve terminals in limbic and frontal cortex. Evidence for mesocortico dopamine neurons. *Brain Res.,* 82:349–355.

13. German, D. C., and Bowden, D. A. (1974): Catecholamine systems as the neural substrate for intracortical self stimulation: A hypothesis. *Brain Res.,* 73:381–419.

14. Hökfelt, T., Ljungdahl, A., Fuxe, K., and Johansson, O. (1974): Dopamine nerve terminals in the rat limbic cortex: Aspects of the dopamine hypothesis of schizophrenia. *Science,* 184:177–179.

15. Julou, L., Scatton, B., and Glowinski, J. (1977): Acute and chronic treatment with neuroleptics: Similarities and differences in their action on nigrostriatal mesolimbic and mesocortical dopaminergic neurons. *Adv. Biochem. Psychopharmacol.,* 16:617–624.

16. Krettek, J. E., and Price, J. L. (1974): A direct input from the amygdala to the thalamus and the cerebral cortex. *Brain Res.,* 67:169–174.

17. Le Moal, M., Cardo, B., and Stinus, L. (1969): Influence of ventral mesencephalic lesions on various spontaneous and conditional behaviors in the rat. *Physiol. Behav.,* 4:567–574.

18. Le Moal, M., Galey, D., and Cardo, B. (1975): Behavioural effects of local injection of 6-hydroxydopamine in the medial ventral tegmentum in the rat. Possible role of the mesolimbic dopaminergic system. *Brain Res.,* 88:190–194.

19. Le Moal, M., Stinus, L., and Galey, D. (1976): Radiofrequency lesion of the ventral mesencephalic tegmentum: Neurological and behavioral considerations. *Exp. Neurol.,* 50:521–535.

20. Le Moal, M., Stinus, L., Simon, H., Tassin, J. P., Thierry, A. M., Blanc, G., Glowinski, J., and Cardo, B. (1977): Behavioral effects of a lesion in the ventral mesencephalic tegmentum. Evidence for involvement of A_{10} dopaminergic neurones. *Adv. Biochem. Psychopharmacol.,* 16:237–245.

21. Leonard, C. M. (1969): The prefrontal cortex of the rat. I. Cortical projection of the mediodorsal nucleus. II. Efferent corrections. *Brain Res.,* 12:321–343.

22. Lindvall, O., and Björklund, A. (1974): The organization of the ascending catecholamine neuron systems in the rat brain as revealed by the glyoxylic acid fluorescence method. *Acta Physiol. Scand. [Suppl.],* 412:1–48.

23. Lindvall, O., Björklund, A. K., and Divac, I. (1977): Organization of mesencephalic dopamine neurons projecting to neocortex and septum. *Adv. Biochem. Psychopharmacol.,* 16:39–46.

24. Lindvall, O., Björklund, A., Moore, R. Y., and Stenevi, U. (1974): Mesencephalic dopamine neurons projecting to neocortex. *Brain Res.,* 81:325–331.

25. Llamas, A., and Reinoso-Suarez, F. (1969): Projections of the substantia nigra and ventral tegmental mesencephalic area. In: *Third Symposium on Parkinson's Disease,* edited by F. J. Gillingham and I. M. L. Donaldson, pp. 82–87. Churchill-Livingstone, Ltd., Edinburgh and London.

26. Rolls, E. T., and Cooper, S. J. (1973): Activation of neurons in the prefrontal cortex by brain stimulation reward in the rat. *Brain Res.,* 60:351–368.
27. Routtenberg, A., and Sloan, M. (1972): Self stimulation in the frontal cortex of rattus norvegius. *Behav. Biol.,* 7:567–572.
28. Scatton, B., Boireau, A., Garret, C., Glowinski, J., and Julou, L. (1977): Action of the palmitic ester of pipotiazine on dopamine metabolism in the nigrostriatal meso-limbic and meso-cortical systems. *Naunyn Schmiedeberg's Arch. Pharmacol.,* 296: 169–175.
29. Scatton, B., Glowinski, J., and Julou, L. (1976): Dopamine metabolism in the mesolimbic and mesocortical dopaminergic systems after simple or repeated ad-ministration of neuroleptics. *Brain Res.,* 109:184–189.
30. Scatton, B., Thierry, A. M., Glowinski, J., and Julou, L. (1975): Effects of thiopro-perazine and apomorphine on dopamine synthesis in the mesocortical dopaminergic systems. *Brain Res.,* 88:389–393.
31. Simon, H., Le Moal, M., Galey, D., and Cardo, B. (1976): Silver impregnation of dopaminergic systems after radiofrequency and 6-OHDA lesions of the rat ventral tegmentum. *Brain Res.,* 115:215–231.
32. Simon, H., Stinus, L., Tassin, J. P., Blanc, G., Thierry, A. M., and Le Moal, M. (1977): Are the mesocorticolimbic dopaminergic neurons necessary for brain stimulation reward? XXVIIth International Congress of Physiological Sciences, Paris.
33. Squires, R. F. (1974): Effects of noradrenaline pump blockers on its uptake by synaptosomes from several brain regions, additional evidence for dopamine termi-nals in the frontal cortex. *J. Pharm. Pharmacol.,* 26:364–366.
34. Stein, L., and Roy, O. S. (1959): Self regulation of brain stimulating current in-tensity in the rat. *Science,* 130:570–572.
35. Tassin, J. P., Blanc, G., Stinus, L., Berger, B., Glowinski, J., and Thierry, A. M. (1976): Transport of dopamine in discrete areas of the striatum and of cerebral cortex in the rat. *Adv. Exp. Med. Biol.,* 69:337–345.
36. Tassin, J. P., Stinus, L., Simon, H., Blanc, G., Thierry, A. M., Le Moal, M., Cardo, B., and Glowinski, J. (1978): Relationship between the locomotor hyper-activity induced by A_{10} lesions and the destruction of the fronto cortical dopamin-ergic innervation in the rat. *Brain Res.,* 141:267–281.
37. Tassin, J. P., Stinus, L., Simon, H., Blanc, G., Thierry, A. M., Le Moal, M., Cardo, B., and Glowinski, J. (1977): Distribution of dopaminergic terminals in rat cerebral cortex: Role of dopaminergic mesocortical system in ventral tegmental area syndrome. *Adv. Biochem. Psychopharmacol.,* 16:21–28.
38. Tassin, J. P., Thierry, A. M., Blanc, G., and Glowinski, J. (1974): Evidence for a specific uptake of dopamine by dopaminergic terminals of the rat cerebral cortex. *Naunyn Schmiedeberg's Arch. Pharmacol.,* 282:239–244.
39. Tassin, J. P., Velley, L., Stinus, L., Blanc, G., Glowinski, J., and Thierry, A. M. (1975): Development of cortical and nigroneostriatal dopaminergic systems after destruction of central noradrenergic neurons in foetal and neonatal rats. *Brain Res.,* 83:93–106.
40. Thierry, A. M., Blanc, G., Sobel, A., Stinus, L., and Glowinski, J. (1973): Dopamin-ergic terminals in the rat cortex. *Science,* 182:499–501.
41. Thierry, A. M., Javoy, F., Glowinski, J., and Kety, S. S. (1968): Effect of stress on the metabolism of norepinephrine, dopamine and serotonin in the central nervous system. I. Modifications of norepinephrine turnover. *J. Pharmacol. Exp. Ther.,* 163: 163–171.
42. Thierry, A. M., Stinus, L., Blanc, G., and Glowinski, J. (1973): Some evidence for the existence of dopaminergic neurons in the rat cortex. *Brain Res.,* 50:230–234.
43. Thierry, A. M., Tassin, J. P., Blanc, G., and Glowinski, J. (1976): Selective ac-tivation of the mesocortical DA system motor stress. *Nature,* 263:242–244.
44. Trabucci, M., Govoni, S., Tonon, G., and Spano, P. (1976): Localization of dopa-mine receptors in the rat cerebral cortex. *J. Pharm. Pharmacol.,* 28:244–264.
45. Von Hungen, K., and Roberts, S. (1973): Adenylate cyclase receptors for adren-ergic neurotransmitters in rat cerebral cortex. *Eur. J. Biochem.,* 36:391–401.

Advances in Biochemical Psychopharmacology, Vol. 19,
edited by P. J. Roberts et al.
Raven Press, New York © 1978.

Transmitters for the Afferent and Efferent Systems of the Neostriatum and their Possible Interactions

Jin-Soo Kim

Neurobiologische Abteilung, Max-Planck Institute, 6 Frankfurt, Germany

Nineteen years ago Carlsson (15) discovered that the striatum (caudate nucleus plus putamen) contains a high concentration of dopamine. Since then dopamine has been considered to be not only a precursor of norepinephrine but also an independent transmitter in its own right in the striatum. There is now a growing body of evidence implicating dopamine as an inhibitory transmitter from cells arising in the pars compacta of substantia nigra and projecting to the striatum (2,3,7,8,16,21,23,27,29,32,60,61). The evidence can be summarized as follows: First, the dopamine content is higher in the striatum than in any other brain region. Second, when the fluorescence microscope is used, the histochemical localization of dopamine according to the Falck-Hillarp method is not within the cell bodies of striatal neurons but is within the nigrostriatal nerve terminals. The fractionation studies indicate that the striatal dopamine is mainly found in the synaptosomal fraction. Third, the destruction of the nigra or interruption of the nigrostriatal pathway results in a fall of dopamine concentration in the ipsilateral striatum. Fourth, dopamine is released from the striatum upon stimulation of the substantia nigra. Fifth, synaptic excitation in the striatum is inhibited by microiontophoretic application of dopamine or by electrical stimulation of the substantia nigra.

On the other hand, another important transmitter in the striatum is acetylcholine, which has an excitatory character (11,52,71). The source of the high striatal cholinergic activity is unknown. Several authors reported no change in cholinergic activity after lesions of several anatomically known afferent structures by using histochemical (48) and biochemical methods (49). These findings suggest that striatal cholinergic activity may be localized in interneurons of the striatum. However, our recent experiments indicate that some part of striatal acetylcholine originates from the centromedian-parafascicular complex of the thalamus.

Thus normal striatum needs a balance between excitatory cholinergic and inhibitory dopaminergic neurons (5,14,28). An imbalance of these antagonistic transmitters in the striatum results in extrapyramidal syndromes, especially Parkinson's disease. The constant loss of dopamine-producing

---

Present address: Department of Neurology, University of Ulm, 7959 Schwendi, Germany.

nerve cells of the substantia nigra and consequently a strong reduction of dopamine content in the striatum is the basis of Parkinson's disease. The rationale of classic anticholinergic drugs or L-DOPA treatment of Parkinson symptoms is the reduction of the cholinergic activity or the replacement of the dopamine deficiency in the striatum (77).

During the last few years, the evidence has accumulated which indicates that GABA is an inhibitory transmitter in the strionigral neuronal system (25,34,39,62,78). Furthermore, we have found recently the existence of a high glutamic acid-containing corticostriatal connection (41).

In the present chapter, therefore, we shall focus on the afferent and efferent transmitter pathways of the striatum and their possible interactions.

AFFERENT AND EFFERENT TRANSMITTER PATHWAYS OF THE STRIATUM

Striatal Afferent Systems

The striatum receives afferent connections mainly from the cortex, thalamus, and substantia nigra.

Nigrostriatal Connection

The evidence that a dopamine-containing neuron system projects from the substantia nigra and terminates in the striatum has been well documented by histochemical (2,3,16,29), biochemical (23,27,32,60,61), and electrophysiological studies (31,53). We have therefore tried to confirm these findings in the baboon, using dopamine and DOPA decarboxylase as indicators. We made unilateral hemitransections at the subthalamic level. One to two weeks postoperatively, there was a dramatic reduction of dopamine and DOPA decarboxylase in the caudate nucleus and the putamen ipsilateral to the

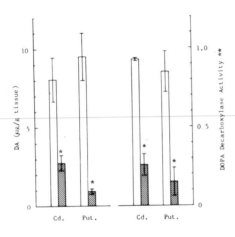

FIG. 1. Effect after 1–2 weeks of hemitransection at the subthalamic level on the dopamine and DOPA decarboxylase levels in the caudate nucleus and putamen of baboon. Open column, control side; hatched column, lesioned side. Each bar indicates mean ± SEM for 6 baboons. *p < 0.001; ** moles DOPA decarboxylated/kg/hr.

lesions (Fig. 1). These results are in fairly good agreement with earlier reports, and it can be safely said that the nigrostriatal pathway of the baboon is also dopaminergic as other mammalian brain.

Corticostriatal Connection

The existence of direct corticostriatal connections has been well established with the aid of various neuroanatomical methods in different species (17,18,35,36). Furthermore, intracellular and extracellular single-cell recordings have demonstrated that stimulation of the cerebral cortex evoked excitation in the caudate neurons (9,13,45,47). Although little is known about the biochemical nature of this pathway, a recent work by Spencer (69) showed that the excitatory response to cortical stimulation could be almost totally suppressed by iontophoretic application of glutamic acid diethylester, which suggests that either glutamic acid or aspartic acid is the excitatory transmitter in the corticostriatal pathway. Therefore, our investigation has focused on the amino acid neurotransmitters in the striatum of the rat after unilateral ablation of the frontal cortex. Figure 2 shows the extent of the frontal cortex lesion. One month after destruction of the left frontal cortex, the glutamic acid level was significantly decreased (-28%; $p < 0.001$) in the side ipsilateral to the lesion, whereas other amino acids remain unchanged (41) (Fig. 3).

In contrast to the glutamic acid data, we found practically no effect of lesions on striatal dopamine, norepinephrine, serotonin, and cholinergic systems (43). The decrease of only glutamic acid in the striatum after the frontal cortex lesion indicates that the frontal cortex is a source of glutamic acid in the striatum. To determine whether the effect of the frontal cortex

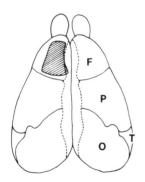

FIG. 2. Schematic drawing of dorsal and lateral views of rat brain. Hatching indicates area of frontal cortex removed by suction. F, frontal; P, parietal; O, occipital; T, temporal.

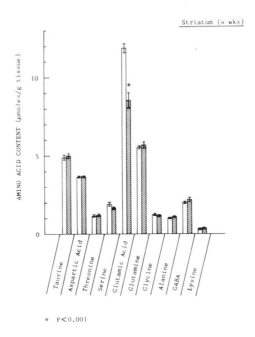

FIG. 3. Effect of left frontal cortex lesion on various amino acid levels in rat striatum. Open column, control side; hatched column, lesioned side. Each bar indicates mean ±SEM for 7 rats. * p < 0.001.

lesion on glutamic acid in the striatum is specific or not, we have chosen the hippocampus for comparison with the striatal data because of its high content of glutamic acid and its position adjacent to the frontal cortex lesion. However, Fig. 4 shows that no significant alterations in the amino acid levels were found in the hippocampus.

From these results together with the previous anatomical and electrophysiological findings, we proposed that the corticostriatal pathways are excitatory in nature and their transmitter is glutamic acid. Recent work from Divac et al. (22) and McGeer et al. (50), who reported that a similar cortex lesion caused reduction of glutamic acid uptake in the striatum, further supports our hypothesis.

Thalamostriatal Connection

The third afferent pathway to the striatum is the thalamostriatal pathway. The afferent input to the striatum was also investigated by neuroanatomical and electrophysiological methods. Recently the monosynaptic and excitatory nature of the centromedian-parafascicular complex input to the caudate nucleus was demonstrated by using intracellular recording technique (46). However, as far as we are aware, little evidence is available on what substance the transmitter is. To pursue this question, the selective unilateral coagulations of the centromedian-parafascicular complex were designed to determine the activities of choline acetyltransferase in caudate nucleus and

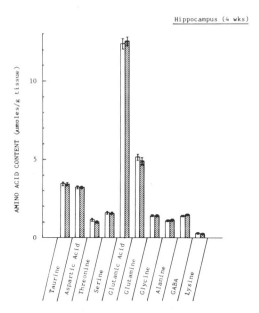

FIG. 4. Effect of left frontal cortex lesion on various amino acid levels in rat hippocampus. Open column, control side; hatched column, lesioned side. Each bar indicates mean ± SEM for 7 rats.

putamen of the cat. These experiments were based on the idea that the enzyme which is necessary for synthesis of the transmitter substance should be located in the nerve terminals and that the loss of enzyme activity may be considered to be an important sign of terminal degeneration. Indeed, the choline acetyltransferase activity is significantly decreased in the head and body of the caudate nucleus and the putamen (Fig. 5).

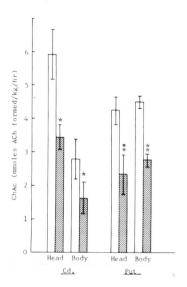

FIG. 5. Effect after 1 week of left centromedian-parafascicular complex lesion on choline acetyltransferase activity in the head and body of the caudate nucleus and putamen of cat. Open column, control side; hatched column, lesioned side Each bar indicates mean ± SEM for 7 cats. * $p < 0.05$; ** $p < 0.01$.

From this result, we can now conclude that the cholinergic input to the striatum is derived partly but not exclusively from the centromedian-parafascicular complex of thalamus. Some preliminary results have already been reported (29,74). Recently, Simke and Saelens (68) published similar results by using rats.

Striatal Efferent Systems

Strionigral and Striopallidal Connections

In 1971 γ-aminobutyric acid (GABA) was proposed as the inhibitory transmitter for strionigral pathway for the first time in our own biochemical and electrophysiological investigations. When the strionigral fibers of the rat and monkey were interrupted, the endogeneous content of GABA (39) and the activity of glutamic acid decarboxylase (GAD) (34) were significantly decreased in the substantia nigra. Furthermore, Okada and Hassler (56) reported that the stimulation of slices of the rat substantia nigra *in vitro* resulted in the release of GABA but not leucine. Electrophysiological studies by Precht and Yoshida (62) demonstrated that the neurons of the substantia nigra of the cat exhibit a distinct inhibitory postsynaptic potential during stimulation of the caudate nucleus. The blockade of caudate-evoked inhibition by picrotoxin suggests that GABA in the substantia nigra may be involved in chemical transmission. This view is further supported by Feltz (24) who demonstrated that the microiontophoretic application of GABA clearly depressed the firing rate of nigral cells.

Although the caudate nucleus sends axons to the pallidum as well as the substantia nigra, more recent electrophysiological work of Obata and Yoshida (55) indicated that the caudatopallidal fibers are GABAergic as are the caudatonigral fibers. However, McGeer et al. (51) and Hattori et al. (30) have reported results indicating that the primary sources of GABA in the substantia nigra is the pallidum. On the other hand, there are histochemical reports which suggest that the strionigral and striopallidal pathways are cholinergic (58,59).

Therefore, our investigation attempts to identify more clearly the transmitter substance for the strionigral and striopallidal pathways of the cat after unilateral ablation of the caudate nucleus. For this purpose, we have determined the GABA content and the activity of the enzyme which is involved in synthesis and degradation of GABA and acetylcholine in the substantia nigra and the pallidum of the cat after unilateral ablation of the caudate nucleus. Unilateral ablation in the caudate nucleus was performed by suction through the frontal cortex. Figure 6 shows that the caudate nucleus alone was removed by suction, leaving surrounding structures intact. Almost the entire nucleus was extracted. The results are summarized in Fig. 7. In both the substantia nigra and the pallidum, a strong reduction of GABA

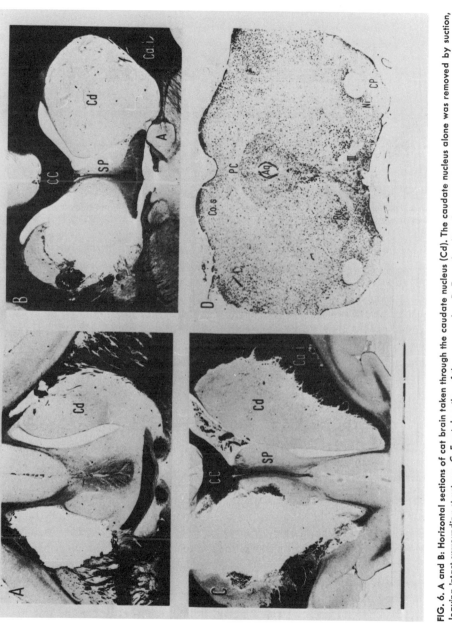

FIG. 6. A and B: Horizontal sections of cat brain taken through the caudate nucleus (Cd). The caudate nucleus alone was removed by suction, leaving intact surrounding structures. C: Frontal section of the same region. D: Frontal section demonstrating the areas of the substantia nigra (Ni) removed by metal puncher. A, B, and C are stained with Heidenheim-Woelcke and D with cresyl violet.

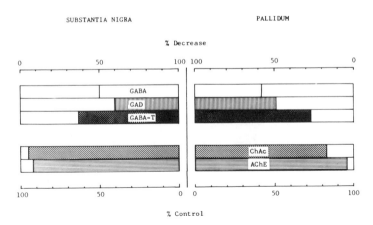

FIG. 7. Effect after 7 days of unilateral destruction of the caudate nucleus by suction on GABA, glutamic acid decarboxylase (GAD), GABA-transaminase (GABA-T), choline acetyltransferase (ChAc), and acetylcholinesterase (AChE) in the substantia nigra and pallidum of cat.

content is accompanied by a parallel loss of GAD (44). On the other hand, there is only a slight but significant decrease in GABA-transaminase, and practically no change in the cholinergic enzymes (44).

These results are in good agreement with our previous report (34,39). They may be extended, however, to show that the caudatopallidal pathway of the cat is GABAergic like the caudatonigral pathway. Both neuronal pools may be involved in an inhibition of the neurons of substantia nigra and pallidum. In addition, as far as our enzyme study indicates, the contribution of cholinergic fibers to the strionigral and striopallidal pathways is at most minimal.

TRANSMITTER INTERACTIONS IN THE EXTRAPYRAMIDAL SYSTEM

Dopaminergic-Cholinergic Interaction (6-Hydroxydopamine Study)

Evidence for the existence of a balance between cholinergic and dopaminergic neurons in the striatum has been reported mainly in pharmacological studies. Thus, cholinergic drugs like oxotremorine and physostigmine activate dopaminergic neurons and thus enhance the turnover of dopamine (1,20,54,67). On the other hand, anticholinergic drugs like atropine and scopolamine decrease the turnover of striatal dopamine (6,12,57). Furthermore, dopamine agonists (apomorphine and L-DOPA) have been shown to decrease the release of striatal acetylcholine, whereas dopamine antagonists (chlorpromazine and butyrophenon) antagonize this effect (19,33,66, 70,72). This view justifies usage of classic anticholinergic drugs for Parkinson's disease. A similar antagonistic relation has been found in harmaline experiments (42).

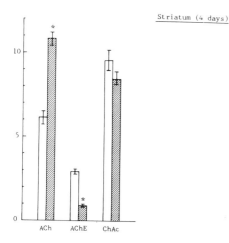

Striatum (4 days)

FIG. 8. Effect of 6-OHDA 4 days after intra-ventricular injection (200 μg/dose) on acetyl-choline, acetylcholinesterase, and choline acetyl-transferase in rat striatum. Open column, control; hatched column, 6-OHDA. Each bar indicates mean ± SEM for 12 rats. ACh, μg/g; AChE, moles acetylthiocholine degradated/kg/hr; ChAc mmoles acetylcholine formed/kg/hr. *p < 0.001.

Although the existence of dopaminergic-cholinergic interaction in the striatum is often mentioned (5,14,28), very few works have dealt with the effect of 6-hydroxydopamine (6-OHDA) on the cholinergic system in the striatum. Four days after a single intraventricular injection of 6-OHDA (200 μg/dose), there was a marked increase in the acetylcholine (ACh) (+ 70%) and a dramatic reduction of acetylcholinesterase (AChE) (− 77%), even though the choline acetyltransferase (ChAc) was hardly changed in the striatum (37) (Fig. 8). Therefore, the increased amount of ACh may reflect the depressed AChE found in the striatum. In time-interval studies after a single intraventricular injection of 6-OH-DA, a significant increase in ACh content was depicted at 2 days, rapidly reaching its maximum level at 4 days, thereafter gradually decreasing to an almost normal

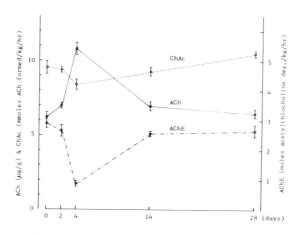

FIG. 9. Time course study of acetylcholine, acetylcholinesterase, and choline acetyltransferase in rat striatum after intraventricular injection of 6-OHDA (200 μg/dose). Each bar indicates mean ± SEM for 10 rats.

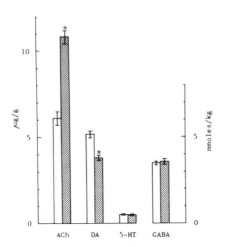

FIG. 10. Effect of 6-OHDA 4 days after intraventricular injection (200 μg/dose) on acetylcholine, dopamine, 5-hydroxytryptamine, and GABA levels in rat striatum. Open column, control; hatched column, 6-OHDA. Each bar indicates mean ± SEM for 12 rats. *p < 0.001.

level during the 28-day period (Fig. 9). As might be expected, the AChE is quite the reverse figure for ACh, and a slight decrease in ChAc was noted, although this effect should not be considered significant. There were no alterations of AChE or ChAc in the frontal cortex, hippocampus, or substantia nigra after the 6-OHDA.

Previous 6-OHDA studies have been primarily concerned with the influence of the drug on the catecholamine system. Therefore, the striatal dopamine was measured 4 days after 6-OHDA. As can be seen in Fig. 10, there is a highly significant decrease in dopamine content (-26%, $p < 0.001$) in the striatum with 6-OHDA. This result is in close agreement with the results of Bloom et al. (10) and Uretsky and Iversen (73), in rat whole brain dopamine levels after administration of 6-OHDA.

There were no significant changes in the level of serotonin and GABA in treated striatum when compared with the control (Fig. 10).

In conclusion, the present results indicate that a single intraventricular injection of 6-OHDA produces a toxic effect not only on the dopaminergic system but also on cholinergic neurons in the striatum. The marked increase in the ACh level in the striatum after 6-OHDA can be interpreted to be the result of a severely depressed AChE in the striatum. Although present results can not exclude the possibility that the blocking of the AChE is an independent action of 6-OHDA, it seems very probable that the drop in dopamine and the increase in ACh in the striatum are coordinated. The interaction between dopaminergic and cholinergic neurons in the striatum may be also present after 6-OHDA treatment.

Interaction of GABA and Dopamine Neurons

Little is known about functional correlations of the strionigral GABAergic system and the nigrostriatal dopaminergic reverberating neuron circuit. The systemic application of γ-hydroxybutyric acid (GHBA) or its precusor γ-butyrolactone, which are normal constituents of mammalian brain (64) and may be metabolites of GABA (63), causes a striking increase mainly in striatal dopamine levels without concomitant changes in the levels of serotonin and norepinephrine (26,65). Since GHBA does not have a direct effect on the enzymes synthesizing or metabolizing dopamine, it has been postulated that this compound acts to block impulse flow in the nigrostriatal pathway, thereby leading to a marked reduction in dopamine release in the striatum (75,76). Furthermore, Andén and Stock (4) reported that direct application of GHBA or GABA in the substantia nigra, but not in the striatum, causes an increase in the dopamine content of the rat striatum. It was suggested that the increased dopamine content of the striatum after direct nigral injection of GHBA or GABA may be due to an inhibition of the nerve impulse flow in the nigrostriatal dopamine neurons in the same way as seen after axotomy, and that this inhibitory action of GABA may be exerted directly on the dopamine neurons in the substantia nigra.

In this connection it is of interest that the well-known antipsychotic drug haloperidol significantly decreased GABA content in the striatum and the substantia nigra (Fig. 11) without change of either glutamic acid decarboxylase or GABA-transaminase activity (40). This may indicate that the decrease in GABA content is not due either to inhibition of synthesizing enzyme or to stimulation of catabolizing enzyme of GABA. Haloperidol alone produced a 35% depletion of dopamine content in the striatum (Fig. 12). However, administration of aminooxyacetic acid (AOAA), which inhibits GABA-transaminase, prior to haloperidol prevented reduction of dopamine, as can be seen in Fig. 12 (38). In contrast to dopamine content, there was no change in norepinephrine and serotonin levels (Fig. 12). There are many reports of increased turnover of dopamine following haloperidol

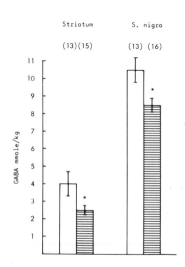

FIG. 11. Effect of haloperidol on GABA levels in rat striatum and substantia nigra. Open column, control; hatched column, haloperidol (10 mg/kg, i.p., 1 hr) Each bar indicates mean ± SEM. *p < 0.001; ( ) number of experiments.

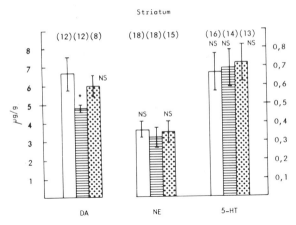

FIG. 12. Effect of haloperidol or aminooxyacetic acid plus haloperidol on dopamine, norepinephrine, and serotonin levels in rat striatum. Open column, control; hatched column, haloperidol (10 mg/kg, i.p., 1 hr); dotted column, AOAA + haloperidol (50 mg/kg, i.p., 2 hr, plus 10 mg/kg, i.p., 1 hr). Each bar indicates mean ± SEM. * p < 0.001; ( ) number of experiments.

treatment due to the blockade of the dopamine receptors. Therefore, we were interested in whether pretreatment with AOAA affects elevation of the striatal homovanillic acid (HVA) after haloperidol. Indeed, Fig. 13 shows that haloperidol alone increases the striatal HVA by more than 100% and AOAA pretreatment blocks the HVA-elevating property of haloperidol (38).

The mechanism of action of haloperidol on the extrapyramidal system may be explained as follows. Haloperidol decreases GABA content in strionigral neurons. The decreased GABA level in the strionigral neurons directly influences the dopaminergic neurons in the substantia nigra, which may result in decreased inhibition of dopaminergic nigrostriatal neurons and thereby

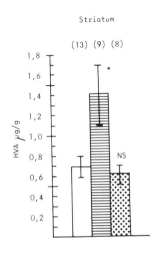

FIG. 13. Effect of haloperidol or aminooxyacetic acid plus haloperidol on homovanillic acid level in rat striatum. Open column, control; hatched column, haloperidol (10 mg/kg, i.p., 1 hr); dotted column, AOAA + haloperidol (50 mg/kg, i.p., 1 hr, plus 10 mg/kg, i.p., 1 hr). Each bar indicates mean ± SEM. * p < 0.001; ( ) number of experiments.

activate the turnover shown by the increase of HVA in the striatum. On the other hand, depletion of dopamine by haloperidol or a stimulatory effect of haloperidol on the turnover of dopamine was blocked by pretreatment of AOAA.

SUMMARY

The surgical denervation techniques have been widely employed as a tool to identify the neuronal origin of various neurotransmitters in the basal ganglia.

Besides the well known nigrostriatal dopaminergic pathway, there is a high glutamic acid-containing corticostriatal connection and the cholinergic thalamostriatal projection. On the other hand, it is strongly suggested that GABA is the transmitter for the strionigral and striopallidal efferent systems. Furthermore, no evidence was found to support strionigral or striopallidal cholinergic pathways.

From the 6-OHDA experiments, it is proposed that the 6-OHDA not only has a selective toxic effect on dopaminergic neurons, but also affects the cholinergic neurons in the striatum, and may provide further evidence for dopaminergic-cholinergic interaction in the striatum.

Finally, GABA may modulate dopamine metabolism in the striatum.

ACKNOWLEDGMENTS

The author is indebted to Prof. R. Hassler and Dr. A. Wagner, who participated in some of the experiments. The skillful technical assistance of Miss R. Koeberle is gratefully acknowledged.

REFERENCES

1. Andén, N. E., and Bédard, P. (1971): Influences of cholinergic mechanisms on the function and turnover of brain dopamine. *J. Pharm. Pharmacol.*, 23:460–462.
2. Andén, N. E., Carlsson, A., Dahlström, A., Fuxe, K., Hillarp, N. A., and Larsson, K. (1964): Demonstrating and mapping out of nigroneostriatal dopamine neurons. *Life Sci.*, 3:523–530.
3. Andén, N. E., Dahlström, A., Fuxe, K., and Larsson, K. (1965): Further evidences for the presence of nigro-striatal dopamine neurons in the rat. *Am. J. Anat.*, 116:329–333.
4. Andén, N. E., and Stock, G. (1973): Inhibitory effect of gamma-hydroxybutyric acid on the dopamine cells in the substantia nigra. *Naunyn-Schmiedeberg's Arch. Exp. Pathol. Pharmacol.*, 279:89–92.
5. Barbeau, A. (1962): The pathogenesis of Parkinson's disease. A new hypothesis. *Can. Med. Assoc. J.*, 87:802–807.
6. Bartholini, G., and Pletscher, A. (1971): Atropine-induced changes of cerebral dopamine turnover. *Experientia*, 27:1302–1303.
7. Bédard, P., Larochelle, L., Parent, A., and Poirier, L. (1969): The nigrostriatal

pathway: A correlative study based on neuroanatomical and neurochemical criteria in the cat. *Exp. Neurol.,* 25:365–377.

8. Bertler, A., Falck, B., Gottfries, C. G., Ljundgren, L., and Rosengren, E. (1964): Some observations on adrenergic connections between mesencephalon and cerebral hemispheres. *Acta Pharmacol. (Kbh.),* 21:283–289.

9. Blake, D. J., Zarzecki, P., and Somjen, G. G. (1976): Electrophysiological study of cortico-caudate projections in cats. *J. Neurobiol.,* 7:143–156.

10. Bloom, F. E., Algeri, S., Groppetti, A., Revuelta, A., and Costa, E. (1969): Lesions of central norepinephrine terminals with 6-hydroxydopamine: Biochemistry and fine structure. *Science,* 166:1284–1286.

11. Bloom, F. E., Costa, E., and Salmoiraghi, G. C. (1965): Anesthesia and the responsiveness of individual neurons of the caudate nucleus of the cat to acetylcholine, norepinephrine and dopamine administered by microelectrophoresis. *J. Pharmacol.,* 150:244–252.

12. Bowers, M. M. Jun., and Roth, R. H. (1972): Interaction of atropine-like drugs with dopamine-containing neurons in rat brain. *Br. J. Pharmacol.,* 44:301–306.

13. Buchwald, N. A., Price, D. D., Vernon, L., and Hull, C. D. (1973): Caudate intracellular response to thalamic and cortical inputs. *Exp. Neurol.,* 38:311–323.

14. Calne, D. B. (1970): *Parkinsonism: Physiology, Pharmacology and Treatment.* Edward Arnold Ltd., London.

15. Carlsson, A. (1959): The occurrence, distribution and physiological role of catecholamines in the nervous system. *Pharmacol. Rev.,* 11:490–493.

16. Carlsson, A., Falck, B., and Hillarp, A. (1962): Cellular localization of monoamines by a fluorescence method. *Acta Physiol. Scand. [Suppl. 196],* 56:1–26.

17. Carman, J. B., Cowan, W. M., and Powell, T. P. S. (1963): The organization of the cortico-striate connections in the rabbit. *Brain,* 88:525–562.

18. Carman, J. B., Cowan, W. M., Powell, T. P. S., and Webster, K. E. (1965): A bilateral cortico-striate projection. *J. Neurol. Neurosurg. Psychiatry,* 28:71–77.

19. Consolo, S., Ladinsky, H., and Garattini, S. (1974): Effect of several dopaminergic drugs and trihexyphenidyl on cholinergic parameters in the rat striatum. *J. Pharm. Pharmacol.,* 26:275–277.

20. Corrodi, H., Fuxe, K., Hammer, W., Sjöqvist, F., and Ungerstedt, U. (1967): Oxotremorine and central catecholamine neurons. *Life Sci.,* 6:2557–2566.

21. Dahlström, A., and Fuxe, K. (1964): Evidence for the existence of monoamine containing neurons in the central nervous system. I. Demonstration of monoamines in the cell bodies of brain stem neurons. *Acta Physiol. Scand. [Suppl. 232],* 62:1–55.

22. Divac, I., Fonnum, F., and Storm-Mathisen, J. (1977): High affinity uptake of glutamate in terminals of corticostriatal axons. *Nature,* 266:377–378.

23. Faull, R. L. M., and Laverty, R. (1969): Changes in dopamine levels in the corpus striatum following lesions in the substantia nigra. *Exp. Neurol.,* 23:332–340.

24. Feltz, P. (1971): γ-Aminobutyric acid and a caudato-nigral inhibition. *Can. J. Physiol. Pharmacol.,* 49:1113–1115.

25. Fonnum, F., Grofová, I., Rinvik, E., Storm-Mathisen, J., and Walberg, F. (1974): Origin and distribution of glutamate decarboxylase in substantia nigra of the cat. *Brain Res.,* 71:77–92.

26. Gessa, G. L., Vargiu, L., Crabai, F., Boero, G. C., Caboni, F., and Camba, R. (1966): Selective increase of brain dopamine induced by gamma-hydroxybutyrate. *Life Sci.,* 5:1921–1930.

27. Gumulka, W., Ramirez del Angel, A., Samanin, R., and Valzelli, L. (1970): Lesion of the substantia nigra: Biochemical and behavioral effects in rats. *Eur. J. Pharmacol.,* 10:79–82.

28. Hassler, R. (1972): Physiopathology of rigidity. In: *Fourth Symposium on Parkinson's Disease,* edited by J. Siegfried, pp. 20–45. Hans Huber Publ., Bern, Stuttgart, Vienna.

29. Hassler, R. (1975): A cholinergic centro-thalamic input to the strio-nigral and strio-pallidal systems. 10th International Congress on Anatomy, Tokyo, Abstr. 136.

30. Hattori, T., McGeer, P. L., Fibiger, H. C., and McGeer, E. G. (1973): On the source of GABA-containing terminals in the substantia nigra. Electron microscopic autoradiographic and biochemical studies. *Brain Res.,* 54:103–114.

31. Herz, A., and Zieglgänsberger, W. (1966): Synaptic excitation in the corpus striatum inhibited by microelectrophoretically administered dopamine. *Experientia*, 22:839–940.
32. Hornykiewicz, O. (1966): Dopamine (3-hydroxytyramine) and brain function. *Pharmacol. Rev.*, 18:925–964.
33. Javoy, F., Agid, Y., Bouvet, D., and Glowinski, J. (1974): Changes in neostriatal DA metabolism after carbachol or atropine microinjections into the substantia nigra. *Brain Res.*, 68:253–260.
34. Kataoka, K., Bak, I. J., Hassler, R., Kim, J. S., and Wagner, A. (1974): L-glutamate decarboxylase and choline acetyltransferase activity in the substantia nigra and the striatum after surgical interruption of the strio-nigral fibres of the baboon. *Exp. Brain Res.*, 19:217–227.
35. Kemp, J. M., and Powell, T. P. S. (1970): The cortico-striate projection in the monkey. *Brain*, 93:525–546.
36. Kemp, J. M., and Powell, T. P. S. (1971): The site of termination of afferent fibres in the caudate nucleus. *Philos. Trans. R. Soc. Lond. [Biol.]*, 262:413–427.
37. Kim, J. S. (1973): Effects of 6-hydroxydopamine on acetylcholine and GABA metabolism in rat striatum. *Brain Res.*, 55:472–475.
38. Kim, J. S. (1975): The influence of γ-aminobutyric acid upon the dopamine metabolism in rat. 6th International Congress on Pharmacology, Helsinki, Abstr. 401.
39. Kim, J. S., Bak, I. J., Hassler, R., and Okada, Y. (1971): Role of γ-Aminobutyric acid (GABA) in the extrapyramidal motor system. 2. Some evidence for the existence of a type of GABA-rich strio-nigral neurons. *Exp. Brain Res.*, 14:95–104.
40. Kim, J. S., and Hassler, R. (1975): Effects of acute haloperidol on the gamma-aminobutyric acid system in rat striatum and substantia nigra. *Brain Res.*, 88:150–153.
41. Kim, J. S., Hassler, R., Haug, P., and Paik, K. S. (1977): Effect of frontal cortex ablation on striatal glutamic acid level in rat. *Brain Res.*, 132:370–374.
42. Kim, J. S., Hassler, R., Kurokawa, M., and Bak, I. J. (1970): Abnormal movements and rigidity induced by harmaline in relation to striatal acetylcholine, serotonin, and dopamine. *Exp. Neurol.*, 29:189–200.
43. Kim, J. S., Hassler, R., Paik, K. S., and Schröder, N. (1977): Evidence for a high glutamic acid containing cortico-striatal pathway in rat brain. 6th International Meeting of the International Society of Neurochemists, Copenhagen, Abstr. 225.
44. Kim, J. S., Wagner, A., and Hassler, R. (1974): Effect of caudate lesion on GABA, and the activities of GAD, GABA-T, ChAc and AChE in the substantia nigra and the pallidum of the cat. *J. Pharmacol. (Paris) [Suppl. 2]*, 5:51.
45. Kitai, S. T., Kocsis, J. D., Preston, R. J., and Sugimori, M. (1976): Monosynaptic inputs to caudate neurons identified by intracellular injection of horseradish peroxidase. *Brain Res.*, 109:601–606.
46. Kocsis, J. D., Sugimori, M., and Kitai, S. T. (1977): Convergence of excitatory synaptic inputs to caudate spiny neurons. *Brain Res.*, 124:403–413.
47. Liles, S. L. (1974): Single-unit responses of caudate neurones to stimulation of frontal cortex, substantia nigra and entopeduncular nucleus in cats. *J. Neurophysiol.*, 37:254–265.
48. Lynch, G. S., Lucas, P. A., and Deadwyler, S. A. (1972): The demonstration of acetylcholinesterase containing neurons within the caudate nucleus of the rat. *Brain Res.*, 45:617–621.
49. McGeer, P. L., McGeer, E. G., Fibiger, H. C., and Wickson, V. (1971): Neostriatal choline acetylase and cholinesterase following selective brain lesions. *Brain Res.*, 35:308–314.
50. McGeer, P. L., McGeer, E. G., Scherer, U., and Singh, K. (1977): A glutamatergic corticostriatal path? *Brain Res.*, 128:369–373.
51. McGeer, P. L., McGeer, E. G., Wada, J. A., and Jung, E. (1971): Effect of globus pallidus lesions and Parkinson's disease on brain glutamic acid decarboxylase. *Brain Res.*, 32:425–431.
52. McLennan, H., and York, D. H. (1966): Cholinergic mechanisms in the caudate nucleus. *J. Physiol.*, 187:163–175.

53. McLennan, H., and York, D. H. (1967): The action of dopamine on neurons of the caudate nucleus. *J. Physiol. (Lond.)*, 189:393–402.
54. Nose, T., and Takemoto, H. (1974): Effect of oxotremorine on homovanillic acid concentration in the striatum in the rat. *Eur. J. Pharmacol.*, 25:51–55.
55. Obata, K., and Yoshida, M. (1973): Caudate-evoked inhibition and action of GABA and other substances on cat pallidal neurons. *Brain Res.*, 64:455–459.
56. Okada, Y., and Hassler, R. (1973): Uptake and release of GABA in slices of substantia nigra of rat. *Brain Res.*, 49:214–217.
57. O'Keeffe, R., Sharman, D. F., and Vogt, M. (1970): Effect of drugs used in psychoses on cerebral dopamine metabolism. *Br. J. Pharmacol.*, 38:287–304.
58. Olivier, A., Parent, A., Semard, H., and Poirier, L. J. (1970): Cholinesterasic, striatopallidal and striatonigral afferents in the cat and the monkey. *Brain Res.*, 18:273–282.
59. Poirier, L. J., Parent, A., Marchand, R., and Butcher, L. L. (1977): Morphological characteristics of the acetylcholinesterase containing neurons in the CNS of DFP-treated monkeys. Part 1. Extrapyramidal and related structures. *J. Neurol. Sci.*, 31:181–198.
60. Poirier, L. J., Sing, P., Sourkes, T. R., and Boucher, R. (1967): Effect of amine precursors on the concentration of striatal dopamine and serotonin in cats with and without unilateral brain stem lesion. *Brain Res.*, 6:654–666.
61. Poirier, L. J., and Sourkes, T. R. (1965): Influence of the substantia nigra on the catecholamine content of the striatum. *Brain*, 88:181–192.
62. Precht, W., and Yoshida, M. (1971): Blockade of caudate-evoked inhibition of neurons in the substantia nigra by picrotoxin. *Brain Res.*, 32:229–233.
63. Roth, R. H., and Giarman, N. J. (1969): Conversion in vivo of γ-aminobutyric to γ-hydroxybutyric acid in the rat. *Biochem. Pharmacol.*, 18:247–250.
64. Roth, R. H., and Giarman, N. J. (1970): Natural occurrence of gamma-hydroxybutyrate in mammalian brain. *Biochem. Pharmacol.*, 19:1087–1093.
65. Roth, R. H., and Suhr, Y. (1970): Mechanism of the hydroxybutyrate-induced increase in brain dopamine and its relationship to "sleep." *Biochem. Pharmacol.*, 19:3001–3012.
66. Sethy, V. H., and Van Woert, M. H. (1974): Regulation of striatal acetylcholine concentration by dopamine receptors. *Nature*, 251:529–530.
67. Sharman, D. F. (1966): Changes in the metabolism of 3,4-dihydroxyphenylethylamine (dopamine) in the striatum of the mouse induced by drugs. *Br. J. Pharmacol.*, 28:153–163.
68. Simke, J. P., and Saelens, J. K. (1977): Evidence for a cholinergic fiber tract connecting the thalamus with the head of the striatum of the rat. *Brain Res.*, 126:487–495.
69. Spencer, H. J. (1976): Antagonism of cortical excitation of striatal neurons by glutamic acid diethyl ester: Evidence for glutamic acid as an excitatory transmitter in the rat striatum. *Brain Res.*, 102:91–101.
70. Stadler, H., Lloyd, K. G., Gadea-Ciria, M., and Bartholini, G. (1973): Enhanced striatal acetylcholine release by chlorpromazine and its reversal by apomorphine. *Brain Res.*, 55:476–480.
71. Steg, G. (1969): Striatal cell activity during systemic administration of monoaminergic and cholinergic drugs. In: *Third Symposium on Parkinson's Disease*, edited by F. J. Gillingham and I. M. L. Donaldson, pp. 26–29. Livingstone, Edinburgh.
72. Trabucchi, M., Cheney, D., Racagni, G., and Costa, E. (1974): Involvement of brain cholinergic mechanisms in the action of chlorpromazine. *Nature*, 249:664–666.
73. Uretsky, N. J., and Iversen, L. L. (1970): Effects of 6-hydroxydopamine on catecholamines in the rat brain. *J. Neurochem.*, 17:269–278.
74. Wagner, A., Hassler, R., and Kim, J. S. (1975): Striatal cholinergic enzyme activities following discrete centro-median nucleus lesion in cat thalamus. 5th International Meeting of the International Society of Neurochemists, Barcelona, Abstr. 59.
75. Walters, J. R., and Roth, R. H. (1972): Effect of γ-hydroxybutyrate on dopamine and dopamine metabolites in the rat striatum. *Biochem. Pharmacol.*, 21:2111–2121.
76. Walters, J. R., Roth, R. H., and Aghajanian, G. K. (1973): Dopaminergic neurons:

Similar biochemical and histochemical effects of γ-hydroxybutyrate and acute lesions of the nigro-neostriatal pathway. *J. Pharmacol. Exp. Ther.,* 186:630–639.

77. Yahr, M. D., Duvoisin, R. C., Schear, M. J., Barrett, R. E., and Hoehn, M. M. (1969): Treatment of Parkinsonism with Levodopa. *Arch. Neurol.,* 21:343–354.

78. Yoshida, M., and Precht, W. (1971): Monosynaptic inhibition of neurons of the substantia nigra by caudato- nigral fibers. *Brain Res.,* 32:225–228.

Advances in Biochemical Psychopharmacology, Vol. 19,
edited by P. J. Roberts et al.
Raven Press, New York © 1978.

Studies on the Interactions Between the Substantia Nigra and the Neostriatum

G. W. Arbuthnott

M.R.C. Brain Metabolism Unit, University Department of Pharmacology, Edinburgh, EH8 9JZ Scotland

The clear description of the anatomy of the striatal dopamine-containing input from the substantia nigra (SN) (33,44) allowed a great deal of work, integrated around a specific biochemical pathway, to be linked with a visible anatomical substrate. The vision of these bright green neurons shining out of a largely dark brain also emphasizes our ignorance of the relationship of these visible neurons to the vast majority of invisible neurons which form the rest of the brain.

Under which conditions are the dopamine (DA) neurons active?

Which anatomical pathways are responsible for their activation?

What are the consequences of the activation for the animal?

What consequences follow the removal of the dopamine-containing cells?

Through which pathways in the brain are these consequences mediated?

Other authors in this volume will be dealing with the earlier questions to some extent, but this chapter deals with the final question. We wanted to find out whether the pathway from the neostriatum to the SN contributed to the control of the DA pathway itself, or if we had to think of the striatonigral fibers as an output carrying the consequences of changes in DA activation to the motor system of the animal.

The striatonigral pathway has a long and venerable history, and in one mammal or another it has been described using nearly every known anatomical technique (17,19,23,24,27,38,41,43,47). In spite of this we decided first to map the pathway in rats using the radioleucine tracing technique (13). This approach had the advantage over lesion studies that since the leucine is taken up exclusively into neuronal cell bodies it can be used to delineate the efferent pathways from structures which, like the striatum, have a multitude of fibers of passage. The large volume of previous work did not provide details of the complete course of the pathway in rats, and since it was in rats that our knowledge of the anatomy of the nigrostriatal system was based we thought the exercise worthwhile. In our early experiments we concentrated on the output from the head of the caudate nucleus (21,49), but we now have evidence for the topographical distribution of the fibers from the whole of the striatum to the substantia nigra.

TOPOGRAPHICAL DISTRIBUTION OF STRIATAL EFFERENTS

In these experiments we made three different types of injections of L(4–5,^{3}H)-leucine into the region of the striatum. Each injection carried approximately 12 μCi of leucine into a localized part of the striatal complex. The animals survived the operation by 3 to 4 days and were then perfused transcardially with 4% paraformaldehyde. The brains were postfixed in Bouin's fixative, and then prepared for paraffin sectioning. Sections were cut at 6 μm, mounted on slides, rehydrated, and coated with Kodak AR 10 stripping film. After exposure for 30 days at $-20°$C the film was developed and the sections stained through the emulsion with hematoxylin and eosin. The autoradiographs were studied under both light- and dark-field illumination by two independent observers. Figures 1 through 3 summarize their findings.

Dorsal Injections

The four animals in this group had injection sites well localized in the dorsal part of the head of the striatum. Figure 1 illustrates the distribution of

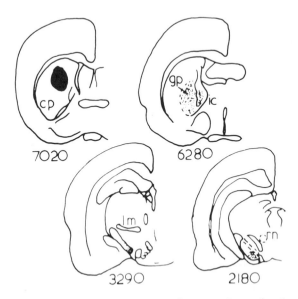

FIG. 1. Striatonigral pathway from the dorsal of striatum. Diagrams of coronal sections of rat brain re-drawn from the atlas of Konig and Klippel (31). Numbers below each diagram indicate the anterior plane from which the drawing was made. Black area indicates the injection site, and dotted areas the distribution of silver grains marking the striatonigral pathway. ac, anterior commissure; cc, crus cerebri; cp, striatum; gp, globus pallidus; hi, hippocampus; ic, internal capsule; ip, interpeduncular nucleus; lm, medial lemniscus; rn, red nucleus; sn, substantia nigra.

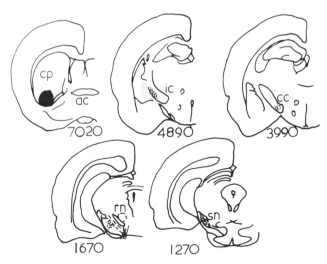

FIG. 2. Striatonigral pathway from the ventral striatum. Diagrams show the different entry points and the difference in distribution of radioactivity of the injections in the ventral area of striatum indicated. Abbreviations as in Fig. 1.

radioactivity as seen in the sections from these brains. Labeled fibers arising from the dorsal striatum entered the internal capsule ventrally and soon gathered into a compact bundle occupying the medioventral portion of the internal capsule. Densely labeled fibers appeared to leave the capsule and

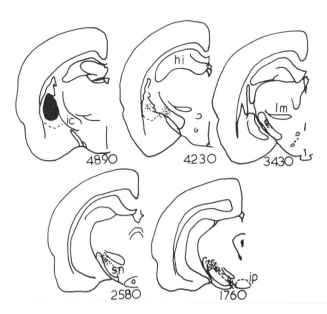

FIG. 3. Striatonigral pathway from the posterior striatum. The more lateral route and termination of the fibers arising from the posterior area of striatum are illustrated. Abbreviations as in Fig. 1.

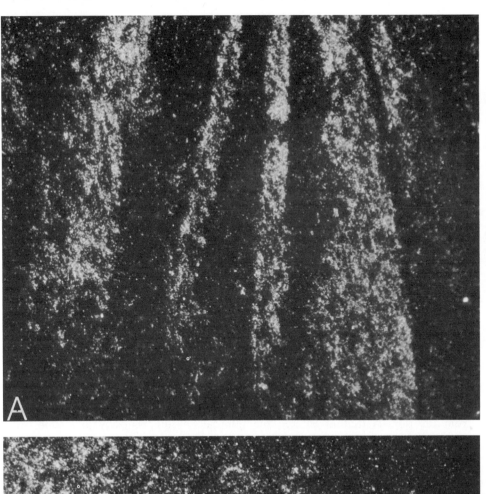

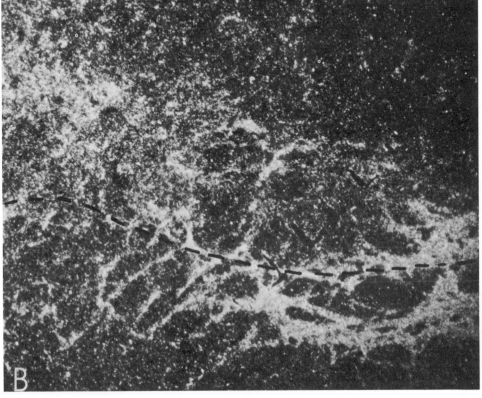

innervate the entire medial portion of the globus pallidus. As the labeled fibers enter the ventral part of the crus cerebri, they are distributed within the system of vertically oriented fascicles called the comb system of Edinger (35) (Fig. 4), from which they leave the crus to enter the anterior and medial portions of the SN. In accordance with earlier studies (24,26,27) of the termination of these fibers, it seems that there are few silver grains over the dorsal, zona compacta, region of SN.

Ventral Injections

In this group too a consistent localization of the injection was possible, and the anterior placement chosen allowed only minimal involvement of the globus pallidus. Figure 2 illustrates the grain distribution in these animals. It was not possible to distinguish labeled fibers of passage from fibers terminating in the globus pallidus in this material since the pathway seems to collect in the internal capsule on the far side of the ventral globus pallidus. The course of the fibers from ventral striatum in the internal capsule was only slightly more lateral than that from the dorsal sites. The area of termination in substantia nigra was, however, markedly different. In the anterior region the label was distributed clearly lateral to the area covered by the fibers from the dorsal site. At planes of section behind the exit of the third cranial nerve the entire zona reticulata was labeled. Although there was a detectable spread to the region of the larger cells in the zona compacta in these cases, this is still clearly a minor part of the terminal area.

Tail of the Striatum

Injections aimed at the tail region of the striatum were less successful. In only 2 of 7 animals did we achieve a clear localization of the injection site over the nucleus. Figure 3 is constructed from the results of the most successful injections, and the distribution was confirmed in some degree by all the animals in which accumulation of label was evident in the cells of the striatum. The entry of the fibers into the internal capsule is similar in these sections to that seen after the ventral injections, but the pathway occupies a more lateral part of the internal capsule as it descends. The innervation area in this case is the pars lateralis of the SN along with the most lateral portions of the pars reticulata. A spur of radioactivity extends along the zona compacta from the lateral SN in all the sections.

These results are in good agreement with the results of local injections of horseradish peroxidase into the SN. Although other projections are revealed

←

FIG. 4. Photomicrographs under dark-field illumination of the distribution of radioactivity (A) in the comb system of Edinger within the crus cerebri, and (B) in the SN. The dotted line marks the edge of cerebral peduncle. The calibration marks are 100 μm.

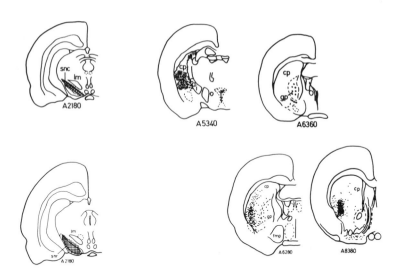

FIG. 5. The drawings on the left indicate the site of an injection of horseradish peroxidase (HRP). To the right are drawings of sections through the striatum at different anteroposterior planes. In these diagrams each dot represents a single cell which was labeled with antidromically accumulated HRP from the injection site. Most of the cells are more posterior in the striatum after the dorsal injection. fmp, medial forebrain bundle; snc, substantia nigra zona compacta; snr, substantia nigra zona reticulata.

by this technique, it is clear from Fig. 5 that the tail of the striatum contains labeled cells after injections in the dorsal substantia nigra which would have involved the lateral area seen in Fig. 3. On the other hand, the peroxidase which had been transported retrogradely from the injection site in the ventral substantia nigra was found mainly in the head of the striatum.

These anatomical results indicated two conclusions. Firstly, the topographical distribution of the striatonigral pathway in the rat was similar to that described in the cat and monkey (43,47); secondly, it was possible to lesion this pathway with a small lesion which would not damage the nigrostriatal DA neurons directly. The close similarity between the topographical arrangement of the DA system to the striatum and the striatal input to the same area was striking and suggested that parts of the striatum are linked to particular areas of nigra by connections in both directions. This arrangement would perhaps be an advantage if the striatonigral fibers carried information about the effectiveness of a DA input back to its source in SN.

The idea that the turnover of dopamine was under the control of the postsynaptic cells (11) had for a long time suggested that this striatonigral pathway might be the means whereby the DA blockade by neuroleptic drugs causes an increase in the turnover of dopamine (30). We therefore set out to test the effect of this reciprocal innervation on the control of dopamine turnover.

The lesions which we made in the striatonigral pathway were small enough not to reduce the dopamine content in the ipsilateral striatum by any significant amount and were largely confined to the crus cerebri. They caused

TABLE 1. Concentration of GABA and activity of GAD in SN

	Control SN	Intact side	Lesioned side
GABA	327.4 ± 168.9 (9)	321.7 ± 144.5 (6)	201.7 ± 125.3 (6)
GAD	61.2 ± 25.5 (6)	54.2 ± 9.0 (5)	41.4 ± 8.4 (5)

GABA in $\mu g/g$ ± SD (N) and GAD activity in nmoles/hr/mg protein ± SD (N) in normal rats (control SN) and in the SN on the two sides of unilaterally lesioned animals. The drop in both measures on the side of the lesion is significant $p < 0.005$ (paired t test).

a significant lowering of gamma-aminobutyric acid (GABA) concentration and lowered the glutamic acid decarboxylase (GAD) activity of the SN (Table 1). Nevertheless, they caused no change in the turnover of dopamine as measured by the concentration of the metabolites homovanillic acid (HVA) and dihydroxyphenylacetic acid (DOPAC) in the striatum. Alterations of the dopamine receptor activity with haloperidol or with apomorphine caused the same change in metabolite concentration on both the control side and the side of the lesion.

Perhaps the lesions were too small to change the effectiveness of the pathway (20). Against that interpretation is the report by Bedard and Larochelle (6) in which large knife cuts which removed the whole crus—as well as an unknown amount of other tissue—failed to block the effect of haloperidol on DA turnover.

Perhaps the GABA system compensated for the damage in the week which followed the lesions. That must remain a possibility until we know more about the response of GABA systems to injury, but the synthetic activity as judged by GAD was still grossly abnormal at the time of the experiment.

Perhaps the pathway concerned in the turnover is a lateral one which contains substance P and which escaped the lesion entirely. This may be a possibility if the major part of the substance P in striatum is posterior (28). Experiments to test this are in hand.

Perhaps the important pathway for feedback is the globus pallidus to SN pathway which was shown by Hattori et al. (26) to terminate predominantly on the dendrites of DA cells. That too seems unlikely since the path followed by these neurons is similar to that of the striatonigral fibers and so they too should have been lesioned in our experiments.

Perhaps after all there are enough alternative explanations of the feedback hypothesis to suggest that the striatonigral pathway subserves some other function. Undoubtedly, this is the most exciting interpretation of the results and it has recently received some direct support from the results of destruction of the cells in the striatum with kainic acid (12). If we accept this explanation, two questions follow:

1. What is the function or functions which the striatonigral pathway may subserve?
2. How is the "feedback" mediated?

Let us consider the second question first. The idea itself originates with pharmacological investigations (11), and so the neuronal mechanism for the feedback is not specified by those experiments. Indeed, there is evidence that there are other means of control which would account for the effects of neuroleptics on DA turnover without a neuronal feedback loop. The increase of the firing rate of individual cells in the SN after intravenous neuroleptics and its decrease after dopamine agonists at first seemed to support the idea that the drugs acted on the cells through a neuronal feedback loop (9). More recent experiments from the same workers (1) have on the contrary showed that the cells in the SN are sensitive to the iontophoretic application of neuroleptics and DA agonist drugs. It is possible that this local action of the drugs on cells in SN is reflected in the turnover changes. A similar result was obtained after local injection of drugs into the region of SN (25). That is, the drugs act on receptors which are on the postsynaptic cells in the striatum and also on the DA cells themselves. In confirmation of these studies we have recently obtained electrophysiological evidence that intravenous amphetamine has a direct effect on the cells of SN. In rats with successful striatonigral lesions (assessed histologically and behaviorally—see later), we have recorded from cells in the dorsal SN. An intravenous injection of amphetamine slows the firing rate of these cells just as it does in intact animals. Figure 6 illustrates one such cell response in an animal with the lesion site illustrated.

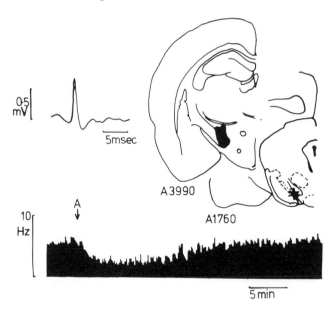

FIG. 6. Response of a cell in SN to amphetamine. The single-unit action potential (*top left*) was recorded at the point marked * in the diagram of the rat brain (*top right*). The firing rate of the cell is shown at the bottom of the figure. An injection of 1 mg/kg amphetamine at A caused a clear reduction in firing rate in spite of the lesion in the striatonigral pathway whose position is marked in the drawings of the brain. The lesion was made 17 days before the acute experiment in which the cell was recorded.

Our results are not in disagreement with those of Bunney and Aghajanian (8) since they base their suggestion that the effect of amphetamine on cells in the substantia nigra is mediated by a feedback loop on the acute effects of lesions. Like us they find that if the animal is allowed to recover from the acute effects of the lesion, then the influence of amphetamine on DA cell firing is intact.

Pharmacological experiments have also suggested that there may indeed be a class of "autoreceptors" which are more sensitive to the actions of low doses of apomorphine than the "postsynaptic" receptors in the striatum and which may mediate the effects on turnover which is observed (10). An interesting possibility for a mechanism whereby this action may be mediated is raised by the experiments on slices of the substantia nigra. The slices are able to release DA and increase their output of DA in response to an increase in the concentration of extracellular K^+ ions (22). A similar release of DA after excitation of the DA cells *in vivo* is suggested by the experiments of Korf et al. (32) and of Nieoullon et al. (36). This release may occur from dendrites in the SN (7) and may explain the effects of injury to the SN which causes an increase in the DA turnover (2) and also an increased firing rate in the cells of the region (45).

Such an esoteric explanation may not be necessary for the effects in the striatum, however, since it has been known for some time that the neuroleptics cause a typical increase in the turnover of DA in striatal slices *in vitro* (18). Clearly there are also mechanisms which will lead to an increase on the output of transmitter when the postsynaptic receptors are blocked which do not depend solely on an increase in the activity of the cell bodies. Whether these slices, like those of Misgeld (34), have an intact cholinergic mechanism or not is unknown, but it is tempting to ascribe at least a portion of the control of transmitter output in these cases to a presynaptic cholinergic action. Such a mechanism will also explain the ability of anticholinergics to reduce the effects of neuroleptics on DA turnover (3), as well as the effects of neuroleptics on acetylcholine output in the striatum (39).

The two explanations of the effects of neuroleptics on DA turnover, the one in the striatum and the other in the SN, are in no way mutually exclusive. Indeed, there is a growing body of evidence that the two ends of the nigrostriatal system are not so tightly linked as one might have thought. Eccleston and Nicolaou in the Brain Metabolism Unit have even demonstrated that the turnover of DA can be changed in opposite directions by the addition of an acute dose of haloperidol and also after apomorphine (Table 2). The results of Westerink and Korf (48) are in the same direction in that they show a different time course of the effect of neuroleptic in the two areas as well as a difference in the potency at the two sites, whereas Nieoullon et al. (36) show that SN and striatum do not release DA in the same manner.

Is there any evidence which would make the striatonigral pathway a good candidate for the feedback pathway? There has been a recent revival of

TABLE 2. HVA in striatum and SN

	Striatum	Substantia Nigra
Normal rats	1.4 ± 0.3 (34)	1.93 ± 0.5 (14)
Haloperidol	4.6 ± 1.3 (28)[a]	1.54 ± 0.4 (13)[b]
Apomorphine	0.9 ± 0.1 (24)[a]	2.53 ± 0.6 (19)[c]

HVA concentration in $\mu g/g$ ± SD (N) in normal striatum and SN and also 30 min after haloperidol 1 mg/kg and 10 min after apomorphine 1 mg/kg.
[a] $p < 0.001$ compared to control values in normal animals.
[b] $p < 0.05$.
[c] $p < 0.01$.

interest in the idea that GABA may control the turnover of DA. The experiments are in two groups because they use different measures of the effect of GABA. The behavioral experiments (16,29) suggest that the effect of increasing GABA with ethanolamine-O-sulfate (EOS) is similar to the effect of amphetamine and potentiates the effect of DA agonist drugs. This evidence can all be reinterpreted as an effect on the output system which carries the changes in DA cell activity on the way to the motor systems of the animal. Experiments on local injection of the GABA agonist muscimol (42) are interpreted this way.

The work by Dray et al. (15), on the other hand, suggests an increase in the turnover of DA as a result of EOS application which is not easily interpreted in these terms. The interpretation is even more confused by the reports of earlier workers who suggest exactly the opposite effect of GABA on DA turnover (4). Perhaps it is at the moment necessary to limit the discussion in that we simply admit the results of intracerebral injection on the SN to be anomalous.

We should now consider the first question, which concerned the likelihood of the striatonigral pathway having some other function. Even at the beginning of the 6-hydroxydopamine (6-OHDA) story it was clear that the DA system was not the only system destroyed by electrolytic lesions of the lateral hypothalamus. In contrast to the animals with 6-OHDA lesions, electrolytic lesions in the DA axons rarely—in our hands never—show supersensitivity (5). One obvious explanation of the anomaly was that the electrolytic lesions included another system whose function was to allow the output from the striatum to influence the motor system of the animal. The striatal efferents travel in the crus along with the DA fibers for most of their path, and even in the region of maximum separation are close enough to have been incorporated in many of the earlier lesion studies.

Is it possible that the striatonigral pathway is the output pathway? In favor of this suggestion, it is clear from behavioral testing that the animals turn in response to amphetamine and to apomorphine in the same way that animals do after electrolytic lesions in SN, (5). Animals with lesions histologically localized in the appropriate area of the crus cerebri and with clear reductions of GABA or GAD levels in SN turned between 150 and 200 times toward the side of the lesion after a dose of 2 mg/kg apomorphine intraperitoneally. The few animals in which a medial extension of the lesion caused a reduction in the DA concentration in the striatum also turned in the same way. That is, adding some damage to the DA system did not influence the turning due to the lesion.

Ungerstedt and Marshall (46) using similar arguments explored the hypothalamus for sites in which a lesion would block apomorphine-induced turning in unilaterally lesioned animals and block apomorphine-induced eating in animals with bilateral 6-OHDA lesions. In a recent publication (46) they show a diagram of the area most often affected by their lesions. It is the medial portion of the crus cerebri and coincides exactly with the position of the fibers from most of the head of the caudate on the way to the SN.

Until recently it seemed that one plausible explanation for the behavioral findings had nothing whatever to do with the striatonigral pathway. It was possible that the circling resulted from damage to the cortical efferents which also travel in the crus and which have a traditional role in the implementation of motor commands. The experiments of Dr. Crossman and his colleagues which were reported in Paris this year (14) render this explanation considerably less compelling. They were able to show that extensive decortication which certainly removed the sensorimotor cortex and a considerable area of association cortex as well, nevertheless had no demonstrable effect on the turning induced by drugs in animals with 6-OHDA lesions. Thus, although small lesions in the area of the descending projection of the striatum do cause a reversal of turning due to apomorphine, extensive damage to the major source of the other fibers which will have been damaged by the lesion does not have any similar effect.

The experiments with decorticate animals do call in question the simplest output for the striatum suggested (49). The likeliest output from the zona reticulata of the SN was via the thalamus to the cortical circuits. The other output from the SN to the reticular system (37,40) may now seem to be the best candidate for the output pathway through which changes in the nigrostriatal DA system have their dramatic effects on behavior.

ACKNOWLEDGMENTS

The experiments reported here were done in collaboration with I. F. Tulloch, A. K. Wright, M. Garcia-Munoz, and N. M. Nicolaou. I am grateful to Drs. Eccleston and Nicolaou for permission to publish Table 2, which contains their unpublished results.

REFERENCES

1. Aghajanian, G. K., and Bunney, B. S. (1977): Dopamine 'autoreceptors': Pharmacological characterization by microiontophoretic single cell recording studies. *Naunyn-Schmiedeberg's Arch. Pharmacol.*, 297:1–7.

2. Agid, Y., Javoy, F., and Glowinski, J. (1973): Hyperactivity of remaining dopaminergic neurones after partial destruction of the nigro-striatal dopaminergic system in the rat. *Nature [New Biol.]*, 245:150–152.
3. Anden, N.-E., and Bedard, P. (1971): Influences of cholinergic mechanisms on the function and turnover of brain dopamine. *J. Pharm. Pharmacol.*, 23:460–462.
4. Anden, N.-E., and Stock, G. (1973): Inhibitory effect of gamma-hydroxybutyric acid and gamma-aminobutyric acid on the dopamine cells in the substantia nigra. *Naunyn-Schmiedeberg's Arch. Pharmacol.*, 279:89–92.
5. Arbuthnott, G. W., and Crow, T. J. (1971): Relation of conversive turning to unilateral release of dopamine from the nigro striatal pathway in rats. *Exp. Neurol.*, 30:484–491.
6. Bedard, P., and Larochelle, L. (1973): Effect of section of the striatonigral fibres on dopamine turnover in the forebrain of the rat. *Exp. Neurol.*, 41:314–322.
7. Björklund, A., and Lindvall, O. (1975): Dopamine in dendrites of substantia nigra neurons: Suggestions for a role in dendritic terminals. *Brain Res.*, 83:531–537.
8. Bunney, B. S., and Aghajanian, G. K. (1976): d-Amphetamine-induced inhibition of central dopaminergic neurons: Mediation by a striato-nigral feedback pathway. *Science*, 192:391–393.
9. Bunney, B. S., Walters, J. R., Roth, R. H., and Aghajanian, G. K. (1973): Dopaminergic neurons: Effect of antipsychotic drugs and amphetamine on single cell activity. *J. Pharmacol. Exp. Ther.*, 195:560–571.
10. Carlsson, A. (1975): Receptor-mediated control of dopamine metabolism. In: *Pre- and Postsynaptic Receptors*, edited by E. Usdin and W. E. Bunney, Jr., pp. 49–66. Marcel Dekker, New York.
11. Carlsson, A., and Lindquist, M. (1963): Effect of chlorpromazine or haloperidol on formation of 3-methoxytyramine and normetanephrine in mouse brain. *Acta Pharmacol. Toxicol.*, 20:140–144.
12. Chiara, G. Di, Porceddes, M. L., Fratta, W., and Gessa, G. L. (1977): Postsynaptic receptors are not essential for DA feedback regulation. *Nature*, 267:270–272.
13. Cowan, W. M., Gottlieb, D. I., Hendrickson, A. E., Price, J. L., and Woolsey, T. A. (1972): The autoradiographic demonstration of axonal connections in the central nervous system. *Brain Res.*, 37:21–51.
14. Crossman, A. R., Sambrook, M. A., and Slater, P. (1977): Neurological basis of asymmetric movement after 6-hydroxydopamine lesions. Proceedings of the Paris Meeting of the International Union of Physiological Sciences, abst. No. 445.
15. Dray, A., Fowler, J. L., Oakley, N. R., and Simmons, M. E. (1977): Regulation of nigro-striatal DA neurotransmission in the rat. *Neuropharmacology*, 16:511–518.
16. Dray, A., Oakley, N. R., and Simmonds, M. A. (1975): Rotational behaviour following inhibition of GABA metabolism unilaterally in the rat substantia nigra. *J. Pharm. Pharmacol.*, 27:627–629.
17. Edinger, L. (1911): *Vorlesungen uber den Bau der nervozen Zentralorgane, Vol. 1*, Ed. 8. Vogel, Leipzig.
18. Farnebo, L.-O., and Hamberger, B. (1971): Drug-induced changes in the release of ^{3}H monoamines from field stimulated rat brain slices. *Acta Physiol. Scand. [Suppl.]*, 371:35–44.
19. Fonnum, F., Grofova, I., Rinvik, E., Storm-Mathisen, J., and Walberg, F. (1974): Origin and distribution of glutamate decarboxylase in substantia nigra of the cat. *Brain Res.*, 71:77–92.
20. Gale, K., and Hong, S. (1977): Interaction of dopamine (DA), GABA and SP in striatonigral neural regulation. *Fed. Proc.*, 36:394.
21. Garcia-Munoz, M., Nicolaou, N. M., Tulloch, I. F., Wright, A. K., and Arbuthnott, G. W. (1977): Striato-nigral fibres—feedback loop or output pathway? *Nature*, 265:363–365.
22. Geffen, L. B., Jessel, T. M., Cuello, A. C., and Iversen, L. L. (1976): Release of dopamine from dendrites in rat substantia nigra. *Nature*, 260:258–260.
23. Grofova, I. (1975): The identification of striatal and pallidal neurons projecting to substantia nigra. An experimental study by means of retrograde axonal transport of horseradish peroxidase. *Brain Res.*, 91:286–291.

24. Grofova, I., and Rinvik, E. (1970): An experimental electron microscopical study on the striatonigral projection in the cat. *Exp. Brain Res.,* 11:249–262.
25. Groves, P. M., Wilson, C. J., Young, S. J., and Rebec, G. V. (1975): Self-inhibition by dopaminergic neurons. *Science,* 190:522–529.
26. Hattori, T., Fibiger, H. C., and McGeer, P. L. (1975): Demonstration of a pallidonigral projection innervating dopaminergic neurons. *J. Comp. Neurol.,* 162:487–504.
27. Hattori, T., McGeer, D. L., Fibiger, H. C., and McGeer, E. G. (1973): On the source of GABA-containing terminals in the substantia nigra. Electron microscopic, autoradiographic, and biochemical studies. *Brain Res.,* 54:103–114.
28. Hong, J. S., Yang, H.-Y. T., Racagni, G., and Costa, E. (1977): Projections of substance P containing neurons from neostriatum to substantia nigra: *Brain Res.,* 122:541–544.
29. Iversen, S. D. (1977): Striatal function and stereotyped behaviour. In: *Psychobiology of the Striatum,* edited by A. R. Cools, A. H. M. Lohman, and J. H. L. van den Berken, pp. 99–118. North Holland Publishing Co., Amsterdam.
30. Kim, J. S., Bak, I. J., Hassler, R., and Okada, Y. (1979): Role of γ-aminobutyric acid (GABA) in the extrapyramidal motor system. 2. Some evidence for the existence of a type of GABA-rich strio-nigral neurons. *Exp. Brain Res.,* 14:95–104.
31. Konig, J. F. R., and Klippel, R. A. (1963): *The Rat Brain.* Williams & Wilkins Co., Baltimore.
32. Korf, J., Zielman, M., and Westerink, B. H. C. (1976): Dopamine release in substantia nigra. *Nature,* 260:257–258.
33. Lindvall, O., and Björklund, A. (1974): The organisation of the ascending catecholamine neuron systems in the rat brain: As revealed by the glyoxylic acid fluorescence method. *Acta Physiol. Scand. [Suppl.],* 412:1–48.
34. Misgeld, U. (1977): Locally evoked field potentials and unitary activity in striatal slices of the rat. Proceedings of the Paris Meeting of the International Union of Physiological Sciences, abst. No. 1528.
35. Nauta, W. J. H., and Mehler, W. R. (1966): Projections of the lentiform nucleus in the monkey. *Brain Res.,* 1:3–42.
36. Nieoullon, A., Cheramy, A., and Glowinski, J. (1977): Release of dopamine in vivo from cat substantia nigra. *Nature,* 266:375–377.
37. Nieuwenhuys, R. (1977): Aspects of the morphology of the striatum. In: *Psychobiology of the Striatum,* edited by A. R. Cools, A. H. M. Lohman, and J. H. L. van den Bercken, pp. 1–20. North Holland Publishing Co., Amsterdam.
38. Niimi, K., Ikeda, T., Kawamura, S., and Inoshita, H. (1970): Efferent projections of the head of the caudate nucleus in the cat. *Brain Res.,* 21:327–343.
39. Racagni, G., Cheney, D. L., Trabucchi, M., and Costa, E. (1976): In vivo actions of clozapine and haloperidol on the turnover rate of acetylcholine in rat striatum. *J. Pharmacol. Exp. Ther.,* 196:323–332.
40. Rinvik, E., Grofova, I., and Ottersen, O. P. (1976): Demonstration of nigrotectal and nigroreticular projections in the cat by axonal transport of proteins. *Brain Res.,* 112:388–394.
41. Rosegay, H. (1944): An experimental investigation of the connections between the corpus striatum and the substantia nigra in the cat. *J. Comp. Neurol.,* 80:292–310.
42. Scheel-Kruger, J., Arnt, J., and Magelund, G. (1977): Behavioural stimulation induced by muscimol and other GABA agonists injected into the substantia nigra. *Neurosci. Lett.,* 4:351–356.
43. Szabo, J. (1962): Topical distribution of the striatal efferents in the monkey. *Exp. Neurol.,* 5:21–36.
44. Ungerstedt, U. (1971): Stereotaxic mapping of the monoamine pathways in the rat brain. *Acta. Physiol. Scand. [Suppl.],* 367:1–48.
45. Ungerstedt, U., Ljungberg, T., Ranje, Ch., Schultz, W., and Tulloch, I. (1977): Neuronal transmission and animal behaviour—a search for correlations in the central dopamine pathways. Proceedings of the Paris Meeting of the International Union of Physiological Sciences, abst. 11.36.
46. Ungerstedt, U., and Marshall, J. F. (1975): Nerve degeneration in functional studies: Experiments illustrating the problem of lesion specificity and compensatory

supersensitivity. In: *Chemical Tools in Catecholamine Research, Vol. 1,* edited by G. Jonsson, T. Malmfors, and C. Sachs, pp. 311–318. North-Holland Publishing Co., Amsterdam.

47. Voneida, T. J. (1960): An experimental study of the course and destination of fibres arising in the head of the caudate nucleus in the cat and monkey. *J. Comp. Neurol.,* 115:75–87.

48. Westerink, B. H. C., and Korf, J. (1976): Comparison of effects of drugs on dopamine metabolism in the substantia nigra and the corpus striatum of the rat brain. *Eur. J. Pharmacol.,* 40:131–136.

49. Wright, A. K., Arbuthnott, G. W., Tulloch, I. F., Garcia-Munoz, M., and Nicolaou, N. M. (1977): Are the striatonigral fibres the feedback pathway? In: *Psychobiology of the Striatum,* edited by A. R. Cools, A. H. M. Lohman, and J. H. L. van den Bercken, pp. 31–50. North-Holland Publishing Co., Amsterdam.

Advances in Biochemical Psychopharmacology,
edited by P. J. Roberts et al.
Raven Press, New York © 1978.

Brain Dopamine Metabolism and Behavioral Problems of Farm Animals

D. F. Sharman

*Agricultural Research Council, Institute of Animal Physiology,
Babraham, Cambridge CB2 4AT England*

Man has bred strains of animals for providing food that are behaviorally better suited to the restrictive environments of his farming practices than the original wild stock. However, problems of behavior can still arise particularly when a different method of animal husbandry is introduced. Some of these problems involve an external behavioral manifestation that leads to an economic disadvantage and are sometimes referred to as vices. The common vices in farm animals usually involve oral activity and include tail biting in pigs, wool biting in sheep, crib biting in horses, and some forms of "licking sickness or disease" in cows. Russell (21) observed that investigators of diseases of livestock in Europe agreed that the symptoms which are collectively termed "licking disease" are due to different causes in different areas. The symptoms can be associated with osteomalacia and with phosphorus deficiency but have also been attributed to copper deficiency and to a deficiency or imbalance of dietary sodium, potassium, or chloride. The behavioral disorder is sometimes called pica, since licking or chewing activity leads to the ingestion of substances other than foodstuffs with deleterious consequences. Abnormal licking or chewing activity in farm animals has also been ascribed to "boredom," and it is being recognized that such anomalous behavior can be the response of the animal to an inadequate environment (15). Thus there appear to be a group of abnormal oral activities in farm animals that can be regarded as stereotyped behavior patterns insofar as they are aberrant and repetitive, which show many similarities although they are apparently caused by different dietary or environmental deficiencies. They may, in fact, represent a common behavioral response that occurs when the sensory input is reduced by lack of environmental stimuli or is modified by disease or dietary deficiency processes. Stereotyped behavior patterns in addition to those involving oral activity are well known in both farm and zoo animals (17,19,20), but this discussion will be confined to those stereotypies that involve the mouth and lips. Meyer-Holzapfel (20) described how a simple repetitive behavior pattern can be either developed into a more complex activity or attenuated to a more simple activity. For example, pacing up and down along the edge of the area in which an animal is confined can develop into more complex figure-of-eight patterns or can be reduced to head weaving. Thus, the abnormal behavior patterns described in farm animals as vices may be noticed only when additions to the initial repetitive response to an environmental inadequacy have reached a stage that interferes with the output from the system under which the animals are kept or are sufficiently bizarre to warrant attention.

There is pharmacological evidence that dopaminergic neurons in the brain might be involved in abnormal oral behavior in farm animals. In the 1870s Feser (6–14) described the effects of the then newly discovered drug apomorphine in several domesticated species of animals and birds. He observed that the behavioral symptoms that occurred after the administration of apomorphine were similar to those of "licking sickness" in cattle or wool biting in sheep and concluded that the same part of the brain was affected in these conditions as that affected by apomorphine. Since apomorphine is thought to act by stimulating dopamine receptors in the brain, the conclusion of Feser suggests that dopaminergic neurons in the brain might be involved in the production of such abnormal oral behavior. In the pig, apomorphine causes an intense snout rubbing activity which closely resembles the normal rooting activity of this animal. In most cases snout rubbing is accompanied by chewing movements and salivation. Snout rubbing directed toward the flank of other animals can be seen in young piglets and is sometimes intense enough to be described as a vice. A description of snout rubbing as a vice in weaned pigs was given by Allison (3). Although tail biting is probably the most common oral vice in pigs, it is possible that this is the result of an additional behavioral component that increases the complexity of the initial behavioral response to a restrictive environment. The initial response may be not noticed because it can closely resemble normal rooting behavior.

In my experiments on the use of neuroleptics in pigs, I have often observed intense snout rubbing as an unwelcome side effect. The observations of Ahtee and Buncombe (2) and Ahtee (1) that metoclopramide produced catalepsy and also increased the striatal homovanillic acid content in mice led me to try this drug in the pig. The intravenous administration of a dose in the region of 3 mg/kg of metoclopramide was followed by a period lasting 1 to 15 min during which the pig was quiet, showed "cataleptic" postures, and could be handled easily. This was followed by the onset of stereotyped behavior resembling that following apomorphine, snout rubbing being the major component. Metoclopramide, however, will antagonize the behavioral effects of apomorphine in the pig, but a larger dose of metoclopramide does not antagonize the snout rubbing seen after metoclopramide. When metoclopramide was given intraperitoneally in a dose of 6.5 mg/kg there was an increase in the concentration of homovanillic acid and dihydroxyphenylacetic acid, metabolites of dopamine, in the brain, although this dose by this route of administration did not produce stereotyped snout rubbing.

The increase in the concentrations of the acidic metabolites of dopamine in the brain is thought to be a result of an increase in the activity of the dopaminergic neurons. Over the past few years Dr. Fry and myself (*in preparation*) have obtained evidence that suggests that this effect need not be the result of the blockade of postsynaptic dopamine receptors on cells in the striatum that subserve the behavioral characteristics depressed by neuroleptic drugs. If the increased release of dopamine is due to an action of these drugs at another site, then it might be expected that with certain drugs in some species, the blockade of the receptors involved with behavior might be absent or the receptors might be less sensitive to the action of the drugs than those involved in the activation of the dopaminergic neurons. In this case, one might see a behavioral response similar to that seen after drugs which are thought to act by stimulating dopamine receptors in the brain. The pig appears to be such a species, and metoclopramide (as well as other neuroleptics) is such a drug in the pig.

Unfortunately, it is difficult to obtain a sufficient number of pigs to allow a detailed examination of this aspect of abnormal oral behavior in this species. However, I have looked for another species showing a similar response to metoclopramide in which the neurochemical changes in response to such drugs can be investigated and which might help to define the regions of the brain involved in the onset of abnormal oral behavior.

The guinea pig was domesticated as a source of food by the South American Indians before the Spaniards arrived, and it shows many similarities with our own farm animals. Coulon (5) has demonstrated that young guinea pigs can develop abnormal chewing activity if separated from their mother at birth. They will also show cross-sucking, a behavioral vice that can occur in farm animals.

Recently, we have studied the responses of guinea pigs to neuroleptic drugs and to metoclopramide. The experiments with the latter drug have produced results that are comparable with those seen in the pig. Metoclopramide in a dose of 50 mg/kg (s.c.) produced little behavioral effect and did not cause catalepsy. However, this dose antagonized the behavioral effects of apomorphine (1 mg/kg s.c.). In doses of 75 mg/kg s.c. and above, metoclopramide regularly induced an intense nose rubbing activity often accompanied by gnawing and by rapid ballismic movements particularly of the forelimbs. Twisting of the head has also been observed, and in some cases convulsions have developed.

The response to metoclopramide in the guinea pig, as in the pig, resembles the response to apomorphine, but differences are more apparent in the rodent. The response to apomorphine consists mainly of stereotyped gnawing activity, but nose rubbing can occur, whereas nose rubbing appears to be the major component of the response to metoclopramide with gnawing as a secondary component. The abnormal oral activity following metoclopramide can be antagonized by oxiperomide but not by haloperidol. The experiments of Costall and Naylor (4) showed that the behavioral responses in guinea pigs to an intrastriatal injection of dopamine were also inhibited by oxiperomide but not by haloperidol. It would thus seem that the abnormal oral behavior following metoclopramide is due to the release of dopamine within the striatum, and analysis of regions of the guinea pig striatum has demonstrated an increase in the concentration of homovanillic acid following the administration of metoclopramide in a dose that causes abnormal oral behavior.

The evidence obtained from experiments with apomorphine and metoclopramide in the pig and the guinea pig suggests that dopamine receptors in the brain can be involved in the production of abnormal oral behavior, but there seems to be more than one type or group of receptors involved since in the guinea pig relatively low doses of metoclopramide or haloperidol will block the response to apomorphine, but the behavioral response to metoclopramide was not blocked by haloperidol.

In the pig we have found no drug that will antagonize the snout rubbing induced by metoclopramide. Studies on snout rubbing in pigs induced by environmental manipulation have been carried out (Fry, Sharman, and Stephens, *in preparation*). Intense snout rubbing was induced by not allowing early weaned piglets to suck. The concentrations of the acidic metabolites of dopamine, homovanillic acid, and 3,4-dihydroxyphenylacetic acid were estimated in parts of the brain known to have a dopaminergic innervation. These results were compared with similar measurements made in early weaned piglets that were allowed to suck when fed at a rubber teat until satisfied and in which snout rubbing occurred much less frequently. The only differences observed were small but significant decreases in the concentration of homovanillic acid in the nucleus accumbens and the putamen in those piglets that were not allowed to suck. There was no evidence of an overall increased release of dopamine, but it is possible that a very small part of a brain area receiving a dopaminergic input is involved and its contribution was missed.

We are then left with at least two further points to consider. Firstly, does repetitive, stereotyped behavior cause the release of dopamine in the brain, and does the animal carry out a repeated behavior pattern in order to replace release of dopamine that has been decreased because of a reduced sensory input? Possibly an increased release of dopamine from one set of terminals could result in the diffusion of the transmitter to receptor sites usually responding to release from other adjacent terminals. An alternative suggestion is that the dopaminergic neurons which innervate cells concerned with the repeated behavior also innervate cells concerned with other functions. The involvement of dopaminergic neuron systems in reward mechanisms (16) could lend support to this hypothesis. Kiley (18) has discussed the possibility that stereotypies might be considered as a cutoff mechanism to divert attention from an unacceptable environment. Secondly, the dopaminergic neuronal system which innervates those cells that respond to apomorphine might act as modulator of the behavior pattern that is repeated, and the reduction in the concentration of homovanillic acid might reflect a reduced dopamine release in an attempt to correct the stereotyped abnormal behavior.

In conclusion, it seems that dopamine receptors in the brain can be involved in the generation of stereotyped, abnormal oral behavior in animals. When similar anomalous behavior occurs as a result of disease, dietary deficiency, or environmental inadequacy, the role of the dopaminergic neuronal systems in the brain is yet to be defined.

REFERENCES

1. Ahtee, L. (1975): The effect of drugs on metoclopramide-induced catalepsy and increase in striatal homovanillic acid content. *Br. J. Pharmacol.*, 53:460P.
2. Ahtee, L., and Buncombe, G. (1974): Metoclopramide induces catalepsy and increases striatal homovanillic acid content in mice. *Acta Pharmacol. Toxicol.*, 35: 429–432.
3. Allison, C. J. (1976): Snout rubbing as a vice in weaned pigs. *Vet. Rec.*, 98:254–255.
4. Costall, B., and Naylor, R. J. (1975): Neuroleptic antagonism of dyskinetic phenomena. *Eur. J. Pharmacol.*, 33:301–312.
5. Coulon, J. (1971): Influence de l'isolement social sur le comportement du Cobaye. *Behaviour*, 38:93–120.
6. Feser, Prof. (1873): Die in neuester Zeit in Anwendung gekommenen Arzneimittel. *Z. praktische Veterinairwissenschaft*, 273–278.
7. Feser, Prof. (1873): Die in neuester Zeit in Anwendung gekommenen Arzneimittel. *Z. praktische Veterinairwissenschaft*, 302–306.
8. Feser, Prof. (1874): Die in neuester Zeit in Anwendung gekommenen Arzneimittel. *Z. praktische Veterinairwissenschaft*, 84–89.
9. Feser, Prof. (1874): Die in neuester Zeit in Anwendung gekommenen Arzneimittel. *Z. praktische Veterinairwissenschaft*, 147–157.
10. Feser, Prof. (1874): Die in neuester Zeit in Anwendung gekommenen Arzneimittel. *Z. praktische Veterinairwissenschaft*, 310–317.
11. Feser, Prof. (1874): Die in neuester Zeit in Anwendung gekommenen Arzneimittel. *Z. praktische Veterinairwissenschaft*, 335–343.
12. Feser, Prof. (1874): Die in neuester Zeit in Anwendung gekommenen Arzneimittel. *Z. praktische Veterinairwissenschaft*, 371–377.
13. Feser, Prof. (1875): Die in neuester Zeit in Anwendung gekommenen Arzneimittel. *Z. praktische Veterinairwissenschaft*, 64–71.
14. Feser, Prof. (1975): Apomorphinum hydrochloratum, ein Heilmittel gegen die sog. Lecksucht der Rinder, Schafe und Schweine. *Z. praktische Veterinairwissenschaft*, 111–113.
15. Fraser, A. F. (1974): *Farm Animal Behaviour.* Bailliere Tindall, London.
16. German, D. C., and Bowden, D. M. (1974): Catecholamine systems as the neural substrate for intracranial self-stimulation: A hypothesis. *Brain Res.*, 73:381–419.
17. Hediger, H. (1950): *Wild Animals in Captivity.* Butterworth and Co., London, and Academic Press, New York. Republished (1964): Dover Publications, New York, and Constable and Co. Ltd., London.
18. Kiley, M. (1974): Behavioural problems of some captive and domestic ungulates. International Symposium on the Behaviour of Ungulates and its Relation to Management, Calgary, Alberta, Canada, 2–5 November, 1971. International Union for Conservation of Nature and Natural Resources, Morges, Switzerland.
19. Kiley-Worthington, M. (1977): *Behavioural Problems of Farm Animals.* Oriel Press, London.

20. Meyer-Holzapfel, M. (1968): *Abnormal Behaviour in Zoo Animals,* edited by M. W. Fox. W. B. Saunders Co., Philadelphia.
21. Russell, F. C. (1944): Minerals in pasture deficiencies and excesses in relation to animal health. Imperial Bureau of Animal Nutrition Technical Communication No. 15, Rowett Institute, Bucksburn, Aberdeen, Scotland.

Advances in Biochemical Psychopharmacology, Vol. 19,
edited by P. J. Roberts et al.
Raven Press, New York © 1978.

Effect of Centrally Acting Drugs on Regional Dopamine Metabolism

B. H. C. Westerink

Laboratory for Pharmaceutical and Analytical Chemistry, Department of Clinical Chemistry, Groningen University, Groningen, The Netherlands

Neuropharmacological, biochemical, and behavioral studies have proven that different centrally acting drugs—such as neuroleptics, analgesics, central stimulants, cholinomimetics, anticholinergics, γ-hydroxybutyric acid, monoamine depleting drugs including reserpine and oxypertine, ergot drugs and LSD, anesthetics, ethanol and (in combination with neuroleptics) aminooxyacetic acid, *p*-chlorophenylalanine, and benzodiazepines—interact with dopaminergic neurotransmission via different mechanisms. The fact that most centrally acting drugs interfere with dopamine (DA) utilization and synthesis in the brain is surprising if one considers that the number of dopaminergic neurons in the rat brain was estimated to be 3,500 (2), which equals 0.0003% of the central neurons. The apparent sensitivity of the dopaminergic system to drug treatment could be responsible for the wide variety of clinical disorders, such as schizophrenia, motoric behavior, parkinsonism, anorexia nervosa, sleep and sedation, and tardive dyskinesia, in which DA is believed to play an important role. That such complex behavioral phenomena can be understood by analyzing some thousands of neurons is amazing for statistical reasons and warrants a (more) critical evaluation of the experimental data.

AIMS AND SCOPE

Changes in DA formation or utilization cause, within minutes, pronounced changes in the levels of the two main metabolites, 3,4-dihydroxyphenylacetic acid (DOPAC) and homovanillic acid (HVA), whereas the formation of 3-methoxytyramine (3-MT) is of interest after inhibition of monoamine oxidase (MAO). Measurement of the levels of these metabolites therefore can be used as a sensitive method to detect changes in the turnover of DA. A recently developed sensitive concurrent assay of DA, DOPAC, HVA, and 3-MT (33) allowed us to investigate the influence of various drugs on DA metabolism in different rat brain areas (28–32). In this chapter we will discuss our observations on three DA-containing neuronal structures which differ fundamentally in morphology: the nerve terminal-rich areas localized in the forebrain, the retina, and the cell bodies/dendrites localized in the mesencephalon (in this study referred to as the substantia nigra).

Firstly, our findings in the nerve terminal areas of striatum, nucleus accumbens, and tuberculum olfactorium will be described. The significance of the distinction between the pattern of regional DA metabolism with different types of neuroleptics will be discussed. Secondly, the formation of HVA in the retina and the striatum after various drug treatments will be compared. The aim of this study was to investigate whether the mechanism of drug action is dependent on or independent of the connections of dopaminergic neurons with other neuronal systems. Thirdly, our data obtained from studies on DA metabolism in the substantia nigra will be discussed in view of a possible dopaminergic neurotransmission in this brain region.

NERVE TERMINAL AREAS

Various authors have suggested that the extrapyramidal and antipsychotic actions of neuroleptics might be due to a blockade of dopaminergic neurotransmission in the striatum and mesolimbic-mesocortical system, respectively (3,12,26,27,35). Neuroleptics devoid of extrapyramidal side effects (the atypical neuroleptics), e.g., clozapine, sulpiride, and thioridazine, increased HVA or DOPAC levels in limbic structures somewhat more than in the striatum of rodents (3,7,12). By treating rats with neuroleptics in combination with probenecid, Bartholini (4) could demonstrate a stronger HVA accumulation in limbic structures after clozapine, sulpiride, or thioridazine than after more traditional neuroleptics, e.g., haloperidol and chlorpromazine. We studied the effects of different doses of 11 neuroleptics and 14 nonneuroleptics in the striatum and the limbic structures, nucleus accumbens, and tuberculum olfactorium (28). To index drugs according to their relative potency for increasing DA metabolites in striatal versus limbic brain structures, we calculated ratios of percentage DOPAC and HVA increase between striatum, nucleus accumbens, and tuberculum olfactorium. The drugs were further grouped as follows: neuroleptics, atypical neuroleptics (clozapine, sulpiride, and thioridazine), and a heterogeneous group termed nonneuroleptics. Of the six possible ratios of DOPAC and HVA levels in the three dopaminergic regions, two are shown graphically in Figs. 1 and 2. The data confirm reports of regional differences between the action of atypical neuroleptics and of the classic neuroleptics, as the atypical neuroleptics showed a relatively stronger DOPAC and HVA increase in the two limbic regions (3,4,7,12). The differentiation was clear when DOPAC levels in the striatum were compared with those in the tuberculum olfactorium (Fig. 2). No differences were seen between the two groups of neuroleptics when the two limbic structures were compared. It appeared, however, that the heterogeneous group of nonneuroleptic drugs showed ratios which were similar to those of the atypical neuroleptics. We therefore conclude that although there

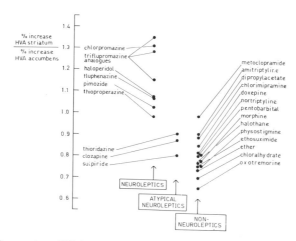

FIG. 1. Ratios of percentage HVA increase between striatum and nucleus accumbens for neuroleptics, atypical neuroleptics, and nonneuroleptics. In some cases the average ratios were derived from different dosages or times of application of the drug (28–30).

is a clear distinction between the pattern of regional DA metabolism with clozapine, sulpiride, and thioridazine on the one hand and the classic neuroleptics on the other, such an action is not specific and therefore not necessarily related to the antipsychotic actions of these neuroleptics. DA metabolism in mesolimbic regions, in contrast to striatal tissue, seems to respond more to atypical neuroleptics and nonneuroleptics than to classic neuroleptics.

The question arises whether percentage changes in DOPAC and HVA can be considered to reflect changes in DA turnover. Some of the drugs

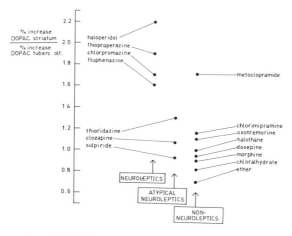

FIG. 2. Ratios of percentage DOPAC increase between striatum and tuberculum olfactorium for neuroleptics, atypical neuroleptics, and nonneuroleptics (28,30).

studied were used in relatively high doses, such as morphine (20 mg kg⁻¹)
and sulpiride (50 mg kg⁻¹). Interference with the active transport mechanism
of DOPAC and HVA out of the brain can seriously complicate the interpretation of drug-induced changes in metabolite levels. Some drugs such as
amphetamine and γ-hydroxybutyric acid (GHBA) are known to induce
changes in DA release which are not well reflected in the levels of DOPAC
and HVA (13,24). Kehr et al. (20) reported, however, that the effects of
amphetamine and GHBA on 3-MT levels during MAO inhibition showed
a good correlation with the presumed changes in DA release. DOPAC and
HVA are probably formed on different sites, and the "simplification" of DA
metabolism caused by MAO inhibition obviously masks the complex interaction between DOPAC and HVA formation. The finding that 3-MT is not
able to leave the brain during MAO inhibition (*unpublished results*) excludes
interference with efflux mechanisms during drug treatment. We therefore
investigated the effects of various drugs on the 3-MT accumulation during
MAO inhibition in different brain regions. Figure 3 shows that the observed
pattern of 3-MT levels after haloperidol, sulpiride, or morphine treatment
are identical with the regional patterns of the acid metabolites earlier described (Figs. 1 and 2). Next the question arises if a neuroleptic-induced
percentage change in the levels of DA metabolites in a given brain structure
can be considered as an index of DA-receptor blockade. In this connection it
is of interest to note that amphetamine induced pronounced differences in
3-MT levels in the striatum and limbic structures (Fig. 4). Amphetamine is
believed to act presynaptically as an indirect dopaminergic agonist by releasing DA of a hypothesized functional DA-pool (9,11). Figure 4 provides

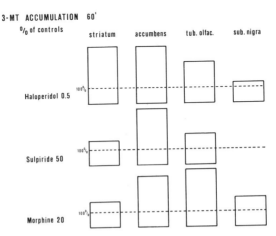

FIG. 3. Effects (% of controls) of haloperidol, sulpiride, and morphine HCl (mg/kg⁻¹) on 3-MT formation in
striatum, nucleus accumbens, tuberculum olfactorium, and substantia nigra after pargyline (75 mg kg⁻¹)
treatment. Pargyline and the drug under investigation were administered 60 min before sacrifice (microwave fixation). N ≥ 5.

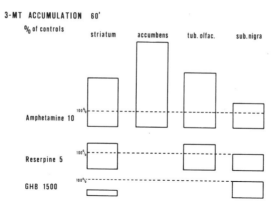

FIG. 4. Effects (% of controls) of (+)-amphetamine sulfate, reserpine, and GBH on 3-MT formation in striatum, nucleus accumbens, tuberculum olfactorium, and substantia nigra after pargyline treatment. See also legend of Fig. 3.

some evidence that this pool is more responsive in the nucleus accumbens and tuberculum olfactorium than in the striatum. For one of the DA pools to show regional differences in responsiveness after treatment with different neuroleptics is unknown but not unlikely. It should be noted that the atypical neuroleptics are applied in relatively high doses, which increases the possibility of complex interactions with different DA pools. We therefore conclude that a percentage change of the levels of DA metabolites in a given brain structure cannot be considered directly as an index of DA-receptor blockade. In this regard it is of interest to note that the inhibition of the DA-sensitive adenylate cyclase by clozapine showed no regional preference in the forebrain structures (6).

Crow et al. (12) interpreted the stronger rise of HVA levels in the nucleus accumbens observed after thioridazine pretreatment as a result of a more effective blockade of DA receptors in this brain region. The suggestion that DA-receptor blockade in the nucleus accumbens—a limbic structure innervated by some hundred dopaminergic neurons—might be responsible for the clinical efficacy of neuroleptic drugs (12,27) may lead to an oversimplification of the biological mechanisms underlying antischizophrenic pharmacotherapy. The relation between schizophrenia and DA-receptor blockade is further complicated by the clinical and pharmacological properties of metoclopramide and propranolol. Metoclopramide is known to provide certain types of extrapyramidal effects in man, to induce catalepsy, and to increase DA turnover in rats, but is devoid of antipsychotic actions (22). It is interesting to note that metoclopramide is similar to the classic neuroleptics in displaying an exceptional pattern of regional DA metabolism (Figs. 1 and 2). In addition, we studied (28) the influence of a high dose of propranolol, recently found to have antipsychotic potency (34), on DA metabolism. We found, however, no statistically significant effect in any of the dopaminergic regions studied. The data on metoclopramide and propranolol suggest that the increased DA turnover observed in the striatum as well as in the limbic areas after neuroleptic treatment is more likely to be correlated with the extrapyramidal side effects of these drugs.

RETINA

The presence of dopaminergic processes in the retina (17) allows one to study the influence of drugs on DA metabolism in a neuronal environment which is relatively simple in comparison with the nigrostriatal and related structures. Table 1 shows that various neuroleptics increased HVA formation, whereas apomorphine decreased HVA levels in the retina. Similar changes of DA metabolism induced by various neuroleptics and apomorphine in the striatum as well as the retina strongly suggest that these drugs are able to act independently on the connections of dopaminergic neurons with other neuronal systems. These findings are of significance for the understanding of feedback mechanisms which are believed to be initiated after interaction of agonists or antagonists at DA receptors. A neuronal feedback model (8,10,15) which is often used to explain the increased DA turnover observed after DA-receptor blockade is not supported by our findings in the retina, as it is not likely that complex neuronal feedback loops are present in the retinal amacrine cell layer. The data obtained from the retina are in accordance with the "autoreceptor" model (20) which suggests that the amount of transmitter released per nerve impulse is regulated via a local mechanism involving presynaptic DA receptors localized on cell bodies, dendrites, and/or nerve terminals of dopaminergic neurons.

TABLE 1. *Effects of various types of drugs on HVA levels (±SEM, N) in retinal samples (total eyes) and striatum of the rat*

Drug	Dose (mg kg^{-1})	Killed after injection (min)	Retina (ng eye^{-1})	Striatum (μg g^{-1})
Saline	—	60	4.3 ± 0.2 (12)	0.45 ± 0.01 (20)
Apomorphine	5.0	45	2.7 ± 0.3 (10)[b]	0.17 ± 0.03 (5)[b]
Clozapine	15	120	5.2 ± 0.4 (9)[a]	1.24 ± 0.08 (7)[b]
Cis-flupenthixol	2.0	120	11.0 ± 0.7 (3)[b]	2.57 ± 0.18 (3)[b]
Trans-flupenthixol	2.0	120	4.4 ± 0.3 (3)	0.45 ± 0.03 (3)
Haloperidol	1.0	120	9.9 ± 0.5 (4)[b]	2.97 ± 0.27 (9)[b]
Morphine	20	120	4.9 ± 0.6 (8)	1.09 ± 0.04 (12)[b]
Oxotremorine	1.0	60	4.6 ± 0.3 (9)	0.90 ± 0.09 (6)[b]
Probenecid	200	120	8.8 ± 0.6 (4)[b]	1.03 ± 0.07 (12)[b]
Probenecid controls	200	75	8.0 ± 0.6 (7)	1.25 ± 0.05 (7)
Probenecid + morphine	200 + 20	75	6.7 ± 0.6 (5)	2.40 ± 0.18 (5)
Probenecid + oxotremorine	200 + 1.0	75	7.7 ± 0.6 (6)	1.92 ± 0.08 (6)

Data from ref. 32.
Different from control: [b] $p < 0.001$; [a] $p < 0.02$.

Morphine and oxotremorine did not induce a rise in HVA levels in the retinal samples as was seen in the striatum (Table 1). If morphine and oxotremorine affect DA metabolism by indirect mechanisms dependent on the neuronal organization of the striatum and the substantia nigra, it is conceivable that such a response is absent from retinal tissue.

SUBSTANTIA NIGRA

Recent histological studies revealed the presence of DA in the dendrites of dopaminergic cells in the substantia nigra (5,18). The possible existence of dendrodendritic dopaminergic transmission in the substantia nigra is of significance for a better understanding of feedback mechanisms and of the coordination between dopaminergic neurons. Evidence for dopaminergic neurotransmission in the substantia nigra was provided by recent studies which indicated that DA can be released from dendrites and/or cell bodies in the rat substantia nigra by antidromic stimulation *in vivo* (21) or K^+ stimulation *in vitro* (14). In addition, a DA-sensitive adenylate cyclase has been demonstrated in homogenates of the substantia nigra (23).

Detailed information about the impulse activity of dopaminergic neurons during various drug treatments has been obtained by extracellular recording of dopaminergic neurons in the zona compacta of the rat substantia nigra (1). For the various drugs examined a good correlation was found between the effects of these drugs on the firing of dopaminergic neurons and their ability to increase or decrease the levels of DOPAC in the striatum (25). We investigated whether this correlation between impulse flow activity and DA metabolism also exists in the substantia nigra (31). The influence of various treatments on DA metabolism in the substantia nigra and striatum in comparison with the reported changes in nigral cell activities (1,25) is summarized in Table 2. In the case of amphetamine and GHBA, rats were pretreated with a MAO inhibitor (19) (Fig. 4). Although the DOPAC and HVA rise in both structures after chloralhydrate treatment can be explained by an increased impulse flow of dopaminergic neurons, it remains unexplained that haloperidol—also known to increase the activity of dopaminergic cells—causes a negligible DOPAC and HVA increase in the substantia nigra compared with a pronounced and long-lasting increase in the striatum. The presence of functional DA release in the substantia nigra was also questioned by the absence of decreased 3-MT formation after GHBA treatment, which is in strong contrast with the 3-MT decrease observed in the striatum. Evidence for DA release by amphetamine in the substantia nigra could only be obtained using a high dose of this drug (10 mg kg^{-1}). In contrast with the findings on haloperidol, amphetamine, and GHBA, it was found that apomorphine decreased DA metabolism in both striatum and substantia nigra, which gives some support for the existence of a DA receptor in the substantia nigra. The relation between impulse flow activity and decreased DA turnover

TABLE 2. Comparison of changes in nigra cell activities (1,8,25) with concomitant changes in DA metabolite levels in the striatum and the substantia nigra after various treatments

Treatment	Influence on nigral cell activity	DA metabolite investigated	Effect on DA metabolism in nigra (% of controls)	Effect on DA metabolism in striatum (% of controls)
(+)-Amphetamine sulfate, 5 mg/kg^{-1}, 60 min[c]	Decrease	3-MT	110	257
Apomorphine, 5 mg/kg^{-1}, 45 min	Decrease	HVA	65[b]	35[b]
Chloralhydrate, 400 mg/kg^{-1}, 60 min	Increase	HVA	184[b]	204[b]
GHBA, 1,500 mg/kg^{-1}, 60 min[c]	Decrease	3-MT	102	31[b]
Morphine HCl, 20 mg/kg^{-1}, 120 min	Unknown	HVA	235[b]	265[b]
Haloperidol, 1 mg/kg^{-1}, 120 min	Increase	HVA	110	500[b]
Oxotremorine, 1 mg/kg^{-1}, 60 min	Unknown	HVA	235[b]	205[b]
Electrical stimulation median forebrain bundle (21)	Increase	DOPAC	150[a]	185[a]
Partial lesion DA fibers, "diencephalic lesions"	Increase (16)	HVA	88	460–1200[b]

Different from control: [a] p < 0.01; [b] p < 0.001.
[c] After pargyline treatment (75 mg/kg^{-1}, 60 min).

observed after apomorphine treatment is, however, complicated by the fact that apomorphine was also able to exert its effect on striatal DA turnover when the impulse flow in dopaminergic neurons was prevented by axotomy of the nigrostriatal tract (20).

Two drugs whose effects on the nigral cell activity are not well documented were investigated: morphine and oxotremorine. Both drugs induced a rapid and similar percentage increase in DOPAC and HVA levels in the substantia nigra as well as the striatum. These findings suggest that the interaction of these drugs with DA turnover does not differ in the two structures studied.

The observed effects of electrical stimulation, apomorphine, or chloralhydrate treatment on DA metabolism contrast with the results of haloperidol, amphetamine, and GHBA experiments with respect to the question of possible functional DA release in the substantia nigra. In this context an experiment should be discussed in which discrete lesions were made in the diencephalon (Fig. 5). If small electrolytic or mechanical lesions were placed lateral, dorsal, or ventral to the nigrostriatal pathway, a dramatic and long-lasting increase in the levels of DOPAC and HVA levels occurred at the operated side (occasionally animals were seen which displayed a rise over 1,200% of the metabolite levels when compared with the intact side). As chronic experiments revealed that such lesions removed about 50% of the dopaminergic innervation of the striatum, we conclude that the observed increased DA metabolism resulted from partial destruction of the nigrostriatal dopaminergic bundle. This dramatic and acute increase in striatal DOPAC and HVA levels illustrates that dopaminergic neurons do not act

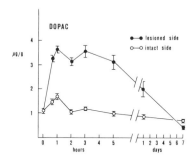

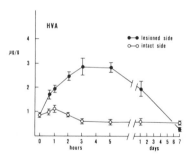

FIG. 5. Time-response curves of changes in bilateral DOPAC and HVA levels (μg/g $\pm$ SEM, $N \geq 5$) in the striatum after partial unilateral lesions ("diencephalic lesions") of the nigrostriatal pathway.

in an uncoordinated fashion, and that rapidly acting compensatory mechanisms are able to modify the output of this system within minutes. About the mechanism underlying the observed rise in DA metabolism we can only speculate. Groves et al. (16) reported recently a pronounced increase in the firing rate of nigral cells 15 to 20 min after the placement of "anterior diencephalic lesions," of which the extent was comparable to those applied in our study. The similarity in time response between the firing of nigral cells described by these authors and the rise of DOPAC and HVA levels depicted in Fig. 5 is striking. It seems therefore likely that the observed rise in striatal DA metabolism is the result of an increased activity of the remaining intact neurons. In strong contrast with the striatum and limbic nerve terminal areas, the rise of DA metabolite levels did not occur in the substantia nigra.

If we summarize the effects of different drug treatments, electrical stimulation, and diencephalic lesions on DA metabolism in striatum and substantia nigra (Table 2), a complex picture appears. Our data point to differences as well as to similarities in the regulation of DA metabolism in the terminal areas and the substantia nigra, and therefore fail to provide consistent evidence for dopaminergic neurotransmission within the substantia nigra.

If DA is compartmentalized in the brain, it might be possible that the relative size of the DA pools differs between the substantia nigra and nerve terminal areas. Figure 4 shows the absence of reserpine-sensitive DA metabolism in the substantia nigra. If the "functional" DA pool present in the substantia nigra is easily exhausted, it is conceivable that this pool is not reflected in the metabolite levels during the described experiments. Some support for this hypothesis is given by the findings of relatively low DA levels in the substantia nigra.

REFERENCES

1. Aghajanian, G. K., and Bunney, B. S. (1973): Central dopaminergic neurons: Neurophysiological identification and responses to drugs. In: *Frontiers in Catecholamine Research,* edited by E. Usdin and S. Snyder, pp. 641–648. Pergamon Press, Oxford.
2. Andén, N.-E., Fuxe, K., Hamberger, B., and Hökfelt, T. (1966): A quantitative study on the nigro-neostriatal dopamine neuron system in the rat. *Acta Physiol. Scand.,* 67:306–312.
3. Andén, N.-E., and Stock, G. (1973): Effect of clozapine on the turnover of dopamine in the corpus striatum and the limbic system. *J. Pharm. Pharmacol.,* 25:346–348.
4. Bartholini, G. (1976): Differential effect of neuroleptic drugs on dopamine turnover in the extrapyramidal and limbic system. *J. Pharm. Pharmacol.,* 28:429–433.
5. Björklund, A., and Lindvall, O. (1975): Dopamine in dendrites of substantia nigra neurons: Suggestions for a role in dendritic terminals. *Brain Res.,* 83:531–537.
6. Bochaert, J., Tassin, J. P., Thierry, A. M., Glowinski, J., and Premont, J. (1977): Characterization of dopaminergic and β-adrenergic sensitive adenylate cyclases in the frontal cortex of the rat. *Brain. Res.,* 122:71–86.
7. Bowers, M. B., and Rozitis, A. (1974): Regional differences in homovanillic acid

concentrations after acute and chronic administration of antipsychotic drugs. *J. Pharm. Pharmacol.,* 26:743–745.

8. Bunney, B. S., and Aghajanian, G. K. (1976): d-Amphetamine-induced inhibition of central dopaminergic neurons: Mediation by a striato-nigral feedback pathway. *Science,* 192:391–393.

9. Carlsson, A., Fuxe, K., Hamberger, B., and Lindqvist, M. (1966): Biochemical and histochemical studies on the effects of imipramine-like drugs and (+)amphetamine on central and peripheral catecholamine neurones. *Acta Physiol. Scand.,* 67:481–497.

10. Carlsson, A., and Lindqvist, M. (1963): Effect of chlorpromazine or haloperidol on formation of 3-methoxytyramine and normetanephrine in mouse brain. *Acta Pharmacol. Toxicol.,* 20:140–144.

11. Carlsson, A., Lindqvist, M., Fuxe, K., and Hamberger, B. (1966): The effect of (+)amphetamine on various central and peripheral catecholamine-containing neurones. *J. Pharm. Pharmacol.,* 18:128–130.

12. Crow, T. J., Deakin, J. F. W., Johnstone, E. C., and Longden, A. (1976): Dopamine and schizophrenia. *Lancet,* 563–566.

13. Da Prada, M., and Keller, H. (1976): Baclofen and γ-hydroxybutyrate: Similar effects on cerebral dopamine neurones. *Life Sci.,* 19:1253–1264.

14. Geffen, L. B., Jessell, T. M., Cuello, A. C., and Iversen, L. L. (1976): Release of dopamine from dendrites in rat substantia nigra. *Nature,* 260:258–260.

15. Groves, P. M., Wilson, C. J., Young, S. J., and Rebec, G. V. (1975): Self-inhibition by dopaminergic neurons. *Science,* 190:522–529.

16. Groves, P. M., Young, S. J., and Wilson, C. J. (1976): Self-inhibition by dopaminergic neurones: Disruption by (±)-α-methyl-p-tyrosine pretreatment or anterior diencephalic lesions. *Neuropharmacology,* 15:755–762.

17. Häggendal, J., and Malmfors, T. (1965): Identification and cellular localization of the catecholamines in the retina and the choroid of the rabbit. *Acta Physiol. Scand.,* 64:58–66.

18. Hajdu, F., Hassler, R., and Bak, I. J. (1973): Electron microscopic study of the substantia nigra and the strio-nigral projection in the rat. *Z. Zellforsch.,* 146:207–221.

19. Kehr, W. (1976): 3-Methoxytyramine as an indicator of impulse-induced dopamine release in rat brain in vivo. *Naunyn-Schmiedeberg's Arch. Pharmacol.,* 293:209–215.

20. Kehr, W., Carlsson, A., Lindqvist, M., Magnusson, T., and Atack, C. (1972): Evidence for a receptor-mediated feedback control of striatal tyrosine hydroxylase activity. *J. Pharm. Pharmacol.,* 24:744–747.

21. Korf, J., Zieleman, M., and Westerink, B. H. C. (1976): Dopamine release in substantia nigra? *Nature,* 260:257–258.

22. Peringer, E., Jenner, P., Donaldson, I. M., and Marsden, C. D. (1976): Metoclopramide and dopamine receptor blockade. *Neuropharmacology,* 15:463–469.

23. Phillipson, O. T., and Horn, A. S. (1976): Substantia nigra of the rat contains a dopamine sensitive adenylate cyclase. *Nature,* 261:418–420.

24. Roffler-Tarlov, S., Sharman, D. F., and Tegerdine, P. (1971): 3,4-Dihydroxyphenylacetic acid and 4-hydroxy-3-methoxyphenylacetic acid in the mouse striatum: A reflection of intra- and extra-neuronal metabolism of dopamine? *Br. J. Pharmacol.,* 42:343–351.

25. Roth, R. H., Murrin, L. C., and Walters, J. (1976): Central dopaminergic neurons: Effects of alterations in impulse flow on the accumulation of dihydroxyphenylacetic acid. *Eur. J. Pharmacol.,* 36:163–171.

26. Scatton, B., Thierry, A. M., Glowinski, J., and Julou, L. (1975): Effects of thioproperazine and apomorphine on dopamine synthesis in the mesocortical dopaminergic systems. *Brain Res.,* 88:389–393.

27. Stevens, J. R. (1973): An anatomy of schizophrenia? *Arch. Gen. Psychiatry,* 29:177–189.

28. Westerink, B. H. C., Jejeune, B., Korf, J., and Van Praag, H. M. (1977): On the significance of regional dopamine metabolism in the rat brain for the classification of centrally acting drugs. *Eur. J. Pharmacol.,* 42:179–190.

29. Westerink, B. H. C., and Korf, J. (1975): Influence of drugs on striatal and limbic homovanillic acid concentrations in the rat brain. *Eur. J. Pharmacol.,* 33:31–40.
30. Westerink, B. H. C., and Korf, J. (1976): Regional rat brain levels of 3,4-dihydroxyphenylacetic acid and homovanillic acid: Concurrent fluorometric measurement and influence of drugs. *Eur. J. Pharmacol.,* 38:281–291.
31. Westerink, B. H. C., and Korf, J. (1976): Comparison of effects of drugs on dopamine metabolism in the substantia nigra and the corpus striatum of rat brain. *Eur. J. Pharmacol.,* 40:131–136.
32. Westerink, B. H. C., and Korf, J. (1976): Effects of drugs on the formation of homovanillic acid in the rat retina. *Eur. J. Pharmacol.,* 40:175–178.
33. Westerink, B. H. C., and Korf, J. (1977): Rapid concurrent fluorimetric assay of noradrenaline, dopamine, 3,4-dihydroxyphenylacetic acid, homovanillic acid and 3-methoxytyramine in milligram amounts of nervous tissue after isolation on Sephadex G 10. *J. Neurochem.,* 29:697–706.
34. Yorkston, N. J., Zaki, M. K. U., Malik, R. C., Morrison R. C., and Havard, C. W. H. (1974): Propranolol in the control of schizophrenic symptoms. *Br. Med. J.,* IV:633.
35. Zivkovic, B., Guidotti, A., Revuelta, A., and Costa, E. (1975): Effect of thioridazine, clozapine and other antipsychotics on the kinetic state of tyrosine hydroxylase and the turnover rate of dopamine in striatum and nucleus accumbens. *J. Pharmacol. Exp. Ther.,* 194:37–46.

Advances in Biochemical Psychopharmacology, Vol. 19,
edited by P. J. Roberts et al.
Raven Press, New York © 1978.

Adaptational Phenomena in Neuroleptic Treatment

I. Møller Nielsen, A. V. Christensen, and J. Hyttel

*Department of Pharmacology and Toxicology, H. Lundbeck & Co. A/S,
DK 2500 Copenhagen-Valby, Denmark*

Neuroleptics are generally accepted to cause receptor blockade in central dopaminergic neuron systems. The antipsychotic effect of these substances is thought to be related to their dopamine (DA) receptor blocking effect. However, receptor blockade is a dynamic phenomenon that causes counter-regulatory adaptation, which must be taken into account when considering the mode of action of these drugs. Thus it might well be that the antipsychotic effect is not based on receptor blockade in dopaminergic neurons, but rather on the adaptational consequence of this receptor blockade, which in essence is a facilitation of dopaminergic nerve transmission.

We have studied these phenomena in mice after a single dose of neuroleptic as well as after repeated dosages. As a model for dopamine receptor blockade, we have used antagonism against methylphenidate-induced compulsive gnawing in mice. Mice treated with a standard subcutaneous dose of 60 mg/kg methylphenidate will when placed on corrugated paper bite holes in the paper. This effect is antagonized by neuroleptics (6). Figure 1 (*upper curve*) indicates the time course of inhibition induced by the neuroleptic teflutixol for each time a new group of mice was tested. One hundred percent inhibition is present on the day of injection and the following day, after which inhibition disappears.

When given apomorphine (10 mg/kg s.c.) normal mice do not show compulsive gnawing. Groups of mice were given teflutixol and tested with apomorphine at varying intervals thereafter, each time a new group of mice was tested. On days 0 and 1, where the methylphenidate test had shown complete receptor blockade no gnawing was seen with apomorphine (Fig. 1, *lower curve*), but on days 3 to 6 an intensive gnaw compulsion was seen in 100% of animals tested. Since gnawing is not seen in normal mice, this is interpreted as supersensitivity to the DA agonist apomorphine. That an increased sensitivity of DA receptors is present is also indicated by the fact that 4 days following a single dose of teflutixol the dose-response curve of methylphenidate is shifted to the left. The supersensitive reaction to dopaminergic agonists may be antagonized only by DA receptor blocking agents, but higher doses are needed to achieve antagonism than in normosensitive animals.

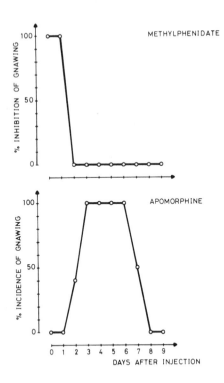

FIG. 1. Influence of a single dose of teflutixol on methylphenidate- and apomorphine-induced stereotypies. Ordinate indicates in case of methylphenidate (upper graph) percentage inhibition and in case of apomorphine (lower graph) percentage occurrence of gnawing. All treatments performed i.p. on day zero.

A supersensitivity phase has been shown to occur following the decline of receptor blockade with all neuroleptics tested. Even penfluridol, which does not induce detectable receptor blockade in mice and rats, induces supersensitivity after repeated administration, 5 × 5 mg/kg p.o. The degree of supersensitivity is dose dependent as may be seen from Fig. 2 (1).

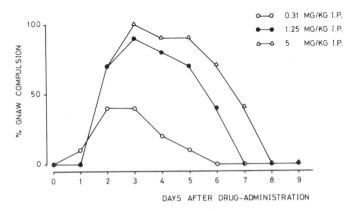

FIG. 2. Time course of teflutixol-induced potentiation of apomorphine. Teflutixol was given i.p. on day zero in doses of: O——O 0.31 mg/kg; ●——● 1.25 mg/kg; and △——△ 5 mg/kg. At various times after these treatments apomorphine 10 mg/kg s.c. was given and % animals gnawing estimated.

It is well established that blockade of DA receptors leads to an increased turnover of DA. The question of what might happen during the supersensitivity phase was studied in mice given a single injection of teflutixol (Fig. 3). During the period of receptor blockade on days 0, 1, and 2, the [^{14}C]DA formed from [^{14}C]tyrosine was significantly increased, but on days 3, 4, and 5 when supersensitivity was present the accumulation of [^{14}C]DA was significantly decreased, after which it returned to normal levels (3). When the concentrations of homovanillic acid (HVA) and dihydroxyphenyl-acetic acid (DOPAC) were studied after a single dose of teflutixol, a marked increase was found during the receptor blockade phase whereas it was decreased during the supersensitivity phase (Fig. 4) (4). Thus receptor blockade was followed by increased synthesis and release, whereas supersensitivity was followed by decreased synthesis and release. In the supersensitivity phase teflutixol is still capable of inducing an acute increase in DA synthesis rate which is not significantly different from that in untreated animals (5).

When a neuroleptic is given by repeated dosage, one would expect that

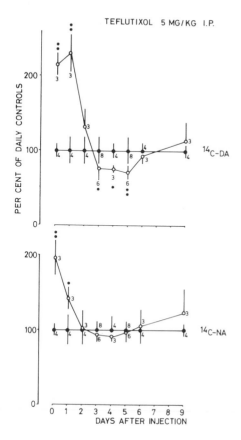

FIG. 3. Accumulation of ^{14}C-DA (upper) and ^{14}C-NA (lower) formed from ^{14}C-tyrosine in mouse brain at different times after an intraperitoneal injection of teflutixol (5 mg/kg, day 0). Each point is the mean ± S.D. (vertical bars). * p < 0.05; ** p < 0.01.

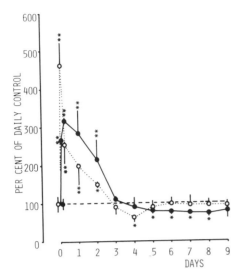

FIG. 4. Content of DOPAC (O·····O) and HVA (●———●) in mouse corpus striatum after treatment with teflutixol (5 mg/kg i.p. at day 0). Each point represents the mean ± S.D. (vertical bars) of 2–6 determinations. * $p < 0.01$; ** $p < 0.001$.

the receptor blockade induced by each medication would be capable of overcoming the effect of any induced supersensitivity. This, however, is not the case. Groups of mice were treated with an oral daily dose of 1.25 mg/kg teflutixol and tested with apomorphine 2 hr after the last dose at various times during treatment (Fig. 5). As expected, no compulsive gnawing occurred after the first doses, but as dosing continued an increasing tendency

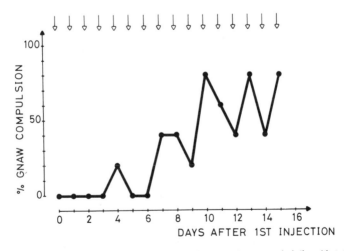

FIG. 5. Incidence of apomorphine-induced gnaw compulsion in mice treated daily with teflutixol 1.25 mg/kg p.o. (↓). Animals were tested with apomorphine 2 h after the preceding dose teflutixol.

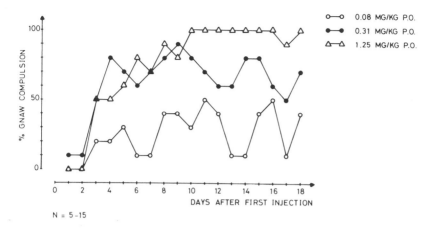

FIG. 6. Apomorphine potentiation after daily repeated doses of teflutixol. ○——○, 0.08 mg/kg p.o.; ●——●, 0.31 mg/kg p.o.; △——△ 1.25 mg/kg p.o.; N = 5–15 pairs per group.

to compulsive gnawing appeared. Since 2 hr after daily dosage should represent the peak time of receptor blockade, this finding is surprising.

When animals are tested 24 hr after the daily dosage, supersensitivity is even more marked. At this time it could be shown that the induction of supersensitivity was dose dependent (Fig. 6). A daily dose of 0.08 mg/kg p.o. produced only marginal supersensitivity, whereas 1.25 mg/kg induced supersensitivity in 100% of mice after 10 days of treatment, and 0.31 mg also produced marked supersensitivity. Even when, in an attempt to overcome supersensitivity, we administered increasing dosages of teflutixol, supersensitivity still occurred (Fig. 7).

It was furthermore investigated whether a dose of teflutixol (0.08 mg/kg p.o.) in itself too small to induce appreciable supersensitivity would be able

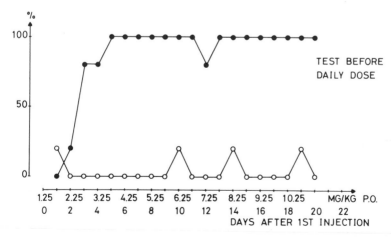

FIG. 7. Apomorphine potentiation ●——● and methylphenidate antagonism ○——○ in mice daily dosed with teflutixol in increasing dose. Tested before the daily dose. N = 5–10 pairs per group.

to maintain supersensitivity once induced by a higher dose (1.25 mg/kg p.o.) (Fig. 8). Under these circumstances the supersensitivity was sustained more than 30 days. The level of apomorphine gnawing was significantly higher than that obtained with 0.08 mg/kg alone.

In accordance with the increasing development of supersensitivity during treatment, the accumulation rate of DA was increased after the first doses of teflutixol (Fig. 9). However, after the fourth dose the increase in DA accumulation rate was no longer significant, and at the end of treatment it had returned to control level even at the time of peak effect, 2 hr after dosage. Accumulation rate below normal level was not seen under these circumstances.

These experiments indicate that the effect of neuroleptics on DA neuron systems is a dynamic process. First, receptor blockade is induced which is accompanied by an increase in DA turnover. When the receptor blockade has declined the receptor is not left in the same condition as it was before the induction of receptor blockade. It has increased its sensitivity to DA agonists which in turn results in a decreased DA turnover, in other words, decreased dopaminergic firing. When the neuroleptic is given by repeated administration, the daily dose of neuroleptic becomes less and less effective in overcoming the effect of increased agonist sensitivity, and this leads to a return in the synthesis rate of DA from the initially increased level to normal levels.

These phenomena must be taken into consideration when discussing the mode of action of neuroleptics. If these events also apply to the clinical effect of neuroleptics, then antipsychotic effect would not necessarily be related to blockade of DA receptors *per se* but to the resulting supersensitivity, i.e., facilitation of DA transmission. Receptor blockade is the immediate effect, but it is declining during repeated administration and thus does not correlate with the onset of antipsychotic effect. In this connection one should

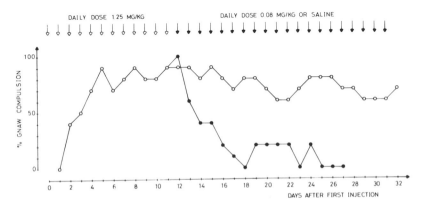

FIG. 8. Apomorphine gnawing after daily teflutixol treatment (1.25 mg/kg p.o.) for 12 days. Thereafter 0.08 mg/kg p.o. O——O or saline ●——● for the rest of the period. N = 10 pairs per group.

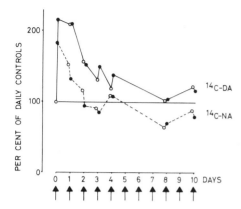

FIG. 9. Accumulation of ^{14}C-DA and ^{14}C-NA formed from ^{14}C-tyrosine in mouse brain two hours (●) and 22 hours (○) after a daily oral dose of teflutixol 1.25mg/kg (arrows). Each point is the mean of 3 determinations.

mention that both supersensitivity and antipsychotic effect take some time to develop, and that neither phenomenon is subject to tolerance development.

Another conclusion would be that supersensitivity could be the cause of tardive dyskinesia. This would seem an attractive hypothesis and more in keeping with current thinking. But whereas antipsychotic effect occurs in most patients after a few weeks' treatment, tardive dyskinesia develops in only a few patients and only after much longer time of treatment. Furthermore, tardive dyskinesia persists much longer than the functional supersensitivity would be expected to remain. It would appear that some kind of true denervation supersensitivity is involved in these cases. Another aspect which comes to mind is the alleged antidepressive effect of some neuroleptics. It may be possible that mood elevation may be related to supersensitivity development. One interesting observation in this respect is that of Corsini et al. (2) who treated depressed patients with a combination of chlorimipramine and haloperidol. Haloperidol was then discontinued while chlorimipramine treatment continued. Within 2 days they observed a dramatic remission of depressive symptoms which was ascribed to the development of supersensitivity after haloperidol withdrawal. Teflutixol, which is a much more potent inducer of supersensitivity than haloperidol, might be a better choice for further testing of this principle.

Whatever the clinical implication may be, such adaptational phenomena do undoubtedly occur when strong receptor blocking neuroleptics are given to humans and need to be considered when discussing the mode of action of neuroleptics.

REFERENCES

1. Christensen, A. V., Fjalland, B., and Møller Nielsen, I. (1976): On the supersensitivity of dopamine receptors, induced by neuroleptics. *Psychopharmacology,* 48:1–6.

2. Corsini, G. W., Masala, C., DelZompo, M., Piccardi, M. R., and Magoni, A. (1975): Potentiation of the antidepressant effect of chlorimipramine following haloperidol withdrawal. Sixth International Congress of Pharmacology, p. 453, abst. 1080.

3. Hyttel, J. (1975): Long-term effects of teflutixol on the synthesis and endogenous levels of mouse brain catecholamines. *J. Neurochem.*, 25:681–686.

4. Hyttel, J. (1977): Levels of HVA and DOPAC in mouse corpus striatum in the supersensitivity phase after neuroleptic treatment. *J. Neurochem.*, 28:227–228.

5. Hyttel, J., and Møller Nielsen, I. (1976): Changes in catecholamine concentration and synthesis rate in mouse brain during the "supersensitivity" phase after treatment with neuroleptic drugs. *J. Neurochem.*, 27:313–315.

6. Pedersen, V., and Christensen, A. V. (1972): Antagonism of methylphenidate-induced stereotyped gnawing in mice. *Acta Pharmacol. Toxicol.*, 31:488–496.

Advances in Biochemical Psychopharmacology, Vol. 19,
edited by P. J. Roberts et al.
Raven Press, New York © 1978.

Self-Inhibitory Dopamine Receptors: Their Role in the Biochemical and Behavioral Effects of Low Doses of Apomorphine

G. Di Chiara, G. U. Corsini, G. P. Mereu, *A. Tissari, and G. L. Gessa

Institute of Pharmacology, University of Cagliari, 09100 Cagliari, Italy

In mice, rats, and man, small doses of apomorphine cause sedation and sleep and other behavioral changes which have been considered to be mediated by the stimulation of a specific population of dopamine (DA) receptors, called by Carlsson (3) "autoreceptors," whose stimulation leads to decreased dopaminergic function.

Although the term "autoreceptor," by indicating an "autoregulatory" role, is essentially a functional one, it is currently used in an anatomical sense to imply the localization of these receptors on the dopaminergic neuron itself.

Therefore, autoreceptors include (Fig. 1): (a) the presynaptic DA receptors, located on dopaminergic nerve terminals, controlling the synthesis and release of the transmitter (6,15,19); (b) somatic and dendritic receptors,

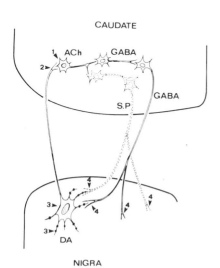

FIG. 1. Possible localization of DA receptors regulating DA synthesis and dopaminergic neuronal activity. 1, Postsynaptic DA receptors; 2, presynaptic DA receptors; 3, DA receptors located on the soma and on the dendrites of DA neurons; 4, nigral DA-sensitive adenylate cyclase; 2, 3, and 4 are included in the term "self-inhibitory DA-receptors."

* Permanent address: Department of Pharmacology, University of Helsinki, Helsinki, Finland.

whose stimulation results in decreased rate of firing of dopaminergic neuron (2).

Recently, the presence of a DA-sensitive adenylate cyclase has been demonstrated in the pars reticulata of the substantia nigra (22,30,35). This nigral DA receptor is located on axonal terminals of neurons originating in the striatum (16,36). It has been suggested (36) that the activation of this enzyme by DA released by dendrites of dopaminergic neurons results in enhanced release of an inhibitory transmitter (e.g., GABA) or, vice versa, in a reduction of the release of an excitatory one (e.g., substance P). If nigral adenylate cyclase is a third type of DA receptor controlling the activity of the DA neuron, then one should extend the term "autoreceptor," in its pure functional significance, to these newly discovered receptors. However, since the term "autoreceptor" is so heavily linked to the concept of a localization on the membrane of the DA neuron, which does not apply to nigral DA-sensitive cyclase, we propose to replace it with that of "self-inhibitory" DA receptors. This term specifies the kind of influence these receptors have on DA synthesis and on dopaminergic firing but leaves open the question of their localization.

BIOCHEMICAL AND ELECTROPHYSIOLOGICAL EVIDENCE FOR SELF-INHIBITORY DA RECEPTORS

Much of the evidence for the existence of self-inhibitory DA receptors has been gained from studies with apomorphine. *In vitro* apomorphine inhibits DA synthesis and release from striatal slices and synaptosomes (6,15,19). *In vivo* apomorphine decreases DA synthesis in doses far smaller than those necessary to cause stereotypy and motor hyperactivity, i.e., those needed to stimulate striatal and/or limbic postsynaptic DA receptors (14,38).

Apomorphine decreases DA synthesis in "silent" dopaminergic neurons, that is, after interruption of impulse flow (by axotomy or by systemic administration of gamma-butyrolactone) (23,39). Since in such conditions the effects of a neuronal feedback loop are eliminated and apomorphine inhibition of DA synthesis is prevented by neuroleptics, apomorphine response is considered to be mediated by the stimulation of receptors located on the presynaptic membrane.

Electrophysiological evidence for the action of apomorphine on DA autoreceptors in the substantia nigra has been provided by the studies of Bunney and Aghajanian who showed that apomorphine inhibits the firing rate of dopaminergic neurons not only after systemic administration but also when applied by microiontophoresis directly into DA neurons in the pars compacta of the substantia nigra. Moreover, intravenous or locally applied apomorphine inhibits the activity of dopaminergic neurons after surgical interruption of the striatonigral feedback neuronal loop. As for the inhibition of DA synthesis, also the inhibitory effect of apomorphine on DA firing is antagonized by neuroleptics (2).

KAINIC ACID-INDUCED DESTRUCTION OF POSTSYNAPTIC DA RECEPTORS

We have recently shown that the destruction of postsynaptic DA receptors by the intrastriatal injection of kainic acid fails to decrease the inhibitory effect of apomorphine on DA synthesis. Since these results might be considered a definite proof that postsynaptic DA receptors are not essential for apomorphine effect on DA synthesis and for dopaminergic feedback regulation, they will be discussed in some detail. The intrastriatal injection of kainic acid (2.5 μg), a rigid analogue of glutamic acid, produces a degeneration of striatal perikarya but leaves intact dopaminergic terminals (11,27). Consistently, kainic acid causes a decrease in the basal adenylate cyclase activity in striatal homogenates and completely abolishes the stimulant effect of DA on this enzyme (13,26,32) (Table 1).

The behavioral changes following kainic acid injection are the functional indication that striatal perikarya are initially stimulated and then destroyed by such treatment. For 3 to 4 hr after treatment, rats exhibit rolling and turning contralateral to the injected side.

However, by 24 hr rats display for many days homolateral torsion of the body and homolateral turning. The latter becomes more vigorous after the administration of 0.1 to 0.5 mg/kg of apomorphine. Haloperidol reverses the homolateral turning into a contralateral one. Ten days after the unilateral administration of kainic acid, when the caudate nucleus appears devoid of

TABLE 1. *Effect of intrastriatal administration of kainic acid on basal and DA-stimulated adenylate cyclase activity of striatal homogenates*

Dopamine concentration	Adenylate cyclase activity (pmoles cAMP/min/mg protein)	
	Control side	Lesioned side
Basal	210 ± 15	130 ± 12
1×10^{-6} M	285 ± 16^a	128 ± 13 ns
1×10^{-5} M	395 ± 20^a	132 ± 15 ns
1×10^{-4} M	420 ± 26^a	135 ± 10 ns

Rats were injected with 3 μg of kainic acid in the right and with saline in the left striatum and were sacrificed 10 days later. The caudate of each side was homogenized and assayed individually for adenylate cyclase activity. Each value is the mean $\pm$ SEM of 5 determinations run in triplicate.

ns, not significantly different from basal values.

[a] $p < 0.001$.

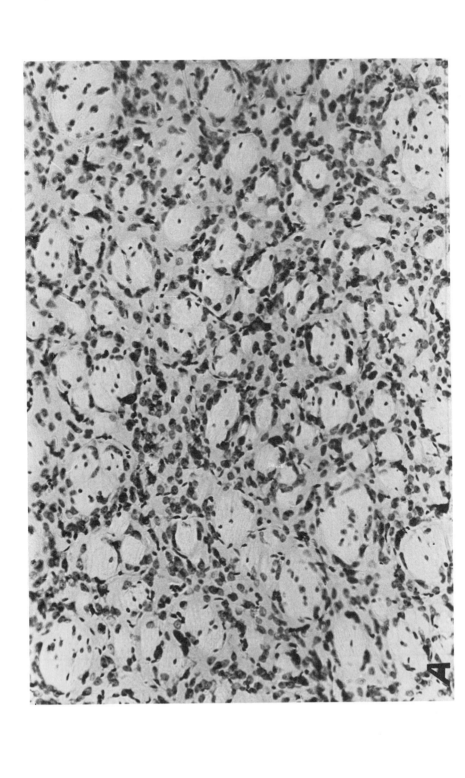

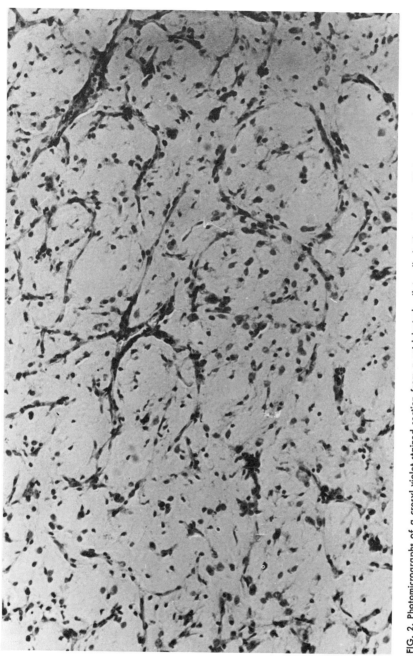

FIG. 2. Photomicrographs of a cresyl violet-stained section from a rat injected unilaterally in the striatum with kainic acid (3 μg) 10 days earlier. A: Control striatum; B: kainic acid-injected striatum. Magnification ×10.

neuronal perikarya (Fig. 2), DA concentrations are not altered but there is an increase of dihydroxyphenylacetic acid (DOPAC) level in the injected striatum (Fig. 3). Apomorphine administration (0.5 and 0.1 mg/kg s.c.) produces a more pronounced decrease in DOPAC content in the kainic injected side than in the control one. The effect of apomorphine is prevented by haloperidol in a competitive manner. Thus, the complete loss of post-synaptic DA receptors fails to prevent not only the action of apomorphine but also the stimulant action of haloperidol on DA metabolism. Indeed, haloperidol at the dose of 0.5 mg/kg causes a greater accumulation of DOPAC in the kainic-lesioned striatum than in the intact one. Moreover, a dose of 0.03 mg/kg of haloperidol, which is insufficient to enhance DOPAC level in the intact striatum, causes a significant increase in the kainic-injected side (Fig. 3) (12,13).

The changes in the level of the DA metabolite reflect an increase in DA synthesis. Consistently, haloperidol enhances and apomorphine decreases the formation of DOPA (after inhibition of the aromatic amino acid decarboxy-lase by NSD 1015), both in the intact and in the kainic-lesioned caudate (Fig. 4).

Therefore, these results constitute the first evidence that DA receptors located on the membrane of DA neurons control DA synthesis *in vivo*.

Although these results also indicate that postsynaptic DA receptors in the caudate nucleus are not essential for the action of apomorphine and haloperi-dol on DA synthesis, they are not against the existence of a neuronal strio-nigral loop controlling DA synthesis and firing of dopaminergic neurons. Indeed, the fact that kainic acid increases DOPAC levels and activates

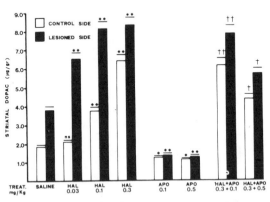

FIG. 3. Effects of haloperidol (HAL) and apomorphine (APO) on DOPAC concentrations in control and kainic-lesioned striatum. Rats were injected with 3 μg of kainic acid in the right striatum and with saline in the left one. After 10 days, rats were given haloperidol or apomorphine and were sacrificed 90 and 45 min, respectively, after drug administration. Each value is the mean ± SEM of the number of determi-nations indicated in parentheses. * $p < 0.01$; ** $p < 0.001$; ns, not significantly different in respect to the values of the homolateral striatum of rats administered with saline. † $p < 0.01$; †† not significantly different in respect to the values of the homolateral striatum of rats administered with haloperidol alone.

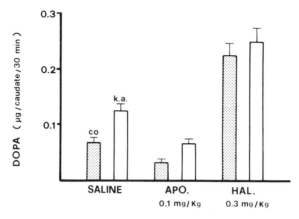

FIG. 4. Effects of haloperidol and apomorphine on DOPA accumulation in control striata and in striata lesioned 3 days before with kainic acid (3.0 μg). Rats were treated with NSD-1015 (100 mg/kg) 30 min before sacrifice. Haloperidol (i.p.) and apomorphine (s.c.) were administered 60 and 45 min before sacrifice. Each value is the mean ± SEM of at least 6 experiments.

tyrosine hydroxylase in the injected caudate indicates that kainic acid has eliminated an inhibitory neuronal input to the dopaminergic neurons. One possible candidate for such inhibitory input is the GABAergic strionigral pathway (24,28). In conclusion, our results indicate that the site of action of neuroleptics and apomorphine in modifying DA synthesis may also reside on the DA autoreceptors. In agreement with such a conclusion, Garcia-Munoz et al. (17) have recently reported that the electrolytic lesion of the GABA-containing striatonigral pathway does not affect the increase in DA turnover after administration of haloperidol. However, unlike the kainic-induced lesion, the electrolytic lesion does not seem to affect DA metabolism.

FUNCTIONAL CHANGES INDUCED BY SMALL DOSES OF APOMORPHINE IN RODENTS

The above evidence indicates that apomorphine acts as an agonist on self-inhibitory DA receptors. The question now arises as to whether some of the behavioral changes induced by low doses of apomorphine are indeed due to the stimulation of such receptors. To answer such a question implies clarification of the functional role of self-inhibitory receptors and of DA itself. Low doses of apomorphine, insufficient to elicit stereotypy and hyperactivity, produce a number of effects in rats and mice such as hypomotility, sedation, sleep, repeated yawnings, recurrent episodes of erection, and ejaculation.

Are any of these effects due to the stimulation of self-inhibitory DA receptors? Are they due to the stimulation of DA receptors at all?

We will now refer to our studies on the sedative and hypnotic effect of apomorphine in rats since they suggest that DA plays an important role on the sleep-wakefulness mechanism, a role which was considered to be exclusive for norepinephrine and serotonin (20).

SEDATION AND SLEEP IN RODENTS

Minute doses of apomorphine (10 to 50 μg/kg) decrease motor activity in mice and rats. This effect is especially evident when the animals are placed in a new environment, a condition in which the untreated animals show maximal increase in exploratory activity (14,38).

The inhibitory effect of apomorphine is dose and time related to a decrease in DOPAC levels (14) and in DOPA formation in DA-rich brain regions (38). This fact has suggested that the hypomotility is due to the inhibitory action of apomorphine via presynaptic DA receptors.

We have demonstrated (14) the dopaminomimetic nature of the inhibitory effect of apomorphine on exploratory behavior by showing that this effect can be blocked by neuroleptics at doses which, *per se,* do not influence motor activity or brain DOPAC. In fact, small doses of different neuroleptics, such as haloperidol, benzperidol, droperidol, and sulpiride, are able to prevent both the hypomotility and the fall in brain DOPAC produced by apomorphine (Table 2, Fig. 5). Interestingly, neuroleptics are not equally active in preventing the sedative effect of apomorphine and its effect on DA synthesis. Indeed, a maximal nonsedative dose of clozapine was found to be completely ineffective in preventing these apomorphine responses. On the con-

TABLE 2. Effects of various neuroleptics on the hypomotility and brain DOPAC decrease produced by apomorphine

Neuroleptic	Dose (mg/kg^{-1})	Motility (% of control)	DOPAC (μg/g^{-1})
Control	—	100 ± 11	0.185 ± 0.008
None	—	25 ± 3.2	0.095 ± 0.006
Benzperidol	0.050	85 ± 9.5	0.180 ± 0.010
Droperidol	0.050	80 ± 7.5	0.178 ± 0.009
Haloperidol	0.050	75 ± 8.5	0.175 ± 0.008
Pimozide	0.300	83 ± 9.3	0.182 ± 0.009
Sulpiride	10.0	87 ± 8.5	0.192 ± 0.010
Trifluperidol	0.050	27 ± 3.0	0.098 ± 0.007
Clozapine	0.50	23 ± 2.5	0.097 ± 0.006

All neuroleptics were administered intraperitoneally 20 min before apomorphine (0.1 mg/kg^{-1} s.c.); mice were placed in the motility cages (4 mice/cage) 10 min after apomorphine administration and motility counted for 20 min. At the end of the motility test, the animals were killed and DOPAC assayed fluorimetrically according to Di Chiara et al. (*in preparation*). Each value is the mean ± SEM of 4 determinations. All neuroleptics, except trifluperidol and clozapine, significantly (p < 0.01) modified motility and brain DOPAC with respect to apomorphine alone.

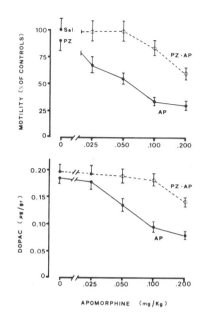

FIG. 5. Antagonism by pimozide of the hypo-motility and decrease of brain DOPAC produced by apomorphine in mice. Pimozide (0.3 mg/kg^{-1} intraperitoneally) was administered 20 min before apomorphine. Apomorphine was administered subcutaneously, and 10 min later the animals (4/cage) were placed in the motility meters (Motron, Sweden), and motility counted for 20 min. Mice were killed at the end of the motility test and DOPAC assayed fluorometrically according to Di Chiara et al. (*unpublished*). The effect of pimozide on apomorphine hypomotility was calculated as % of the motility obtained after pimozide alone. The results are the mean ± SEM of 4 experiments. Open circles indicate a significant difference ($p < 0.01$) with respect to apomorphine alone. Solid circles, apomorphine; open circles, pimozide and apomorphine.

trary, sulpiride seems to be the most selective in blocking self-inhibitory DA receptors.

This compound does not produce catalepsy or other extrapyramidal changes for doses up to 100 mg/kg, whereas a dose of 1 to 10 mg/kg prevents the inhibitory effect of apomorphine on DA synthesis and on motor activity in both mice and rats. Obviously, the important question arises as to whether the ability to block preferentially the self-inhibitory DA receptors may contribute to some therapeutic as well as side effects of antipsychotic agents. Small doses of sulpiride enhance motor activity in rats accustomed to the motility cage, suggesting that under such conditions DA neurons are tonically inhibited by DA.

In order to clarify whether the decreased motor activity reflects a true sedative effect, we studied the effect of low doses of apomorphine on the EEG pattern of freely moving rats (29).

Due to the rapid inactivation of apomorphine, we studied its effect on the EEG only during the first hour following an acute administration of the drug.

A dose of apomorphine of 1 mg/kg produced stereotyped behavior. Moreover, in agreement with previous results (21), it caused a marked reduction of total sleep. In fact, the percentage of total sleep, over the 60 min recording time, fell from 15.9% in saline-treated rats to 4.2% after apomorphine. The residual amount of sleep was due to a brief episode of SWS which usually occurred either a few minutes after treatment or at the end of recording period; i.e., presumably at the time apomorphine concentration in the CNS was idoneous to cause central depression.

In contrast to the above results, doses of apomorphine of 100 µg/kg or lower caused behavioral sedation and increased the amount of total sleep. This effect was already maximal with a dose of apomorphine as low as 25.0 µg/kg, which increased the amount of total sleep to 56% of the recording time. The enhancement of total sleep corresponded mainly to SWS (89% of total sleep). However, the small doses of apomorphine also increased the amount of REM sleep, usually with one or two episodes of REM sleep occurring toward the end of the recording period (Table 3).

Following the small doses of apomorphine, the behavior of the animal was coherent with the EEG activity. Moreover, as previously reported (1), small doses of apomorphine caused recurrent episodes of yawning and penile erection.

To clarify the dopaminomimetic nature of the hypnotic effect of low doses of apomorphine, we studied whether this effect might be prevented by different neuroleptics such as pimozide, benzperidol, and sulpiride (Table 4).

Neuroleptics, at the dose and time schedule used, did not influence the overt behavior of the animals and did not modify the amount of total sleep, SWS, and REM sleep of the animals. However, they prevented the hypnotic effect of apomorphine.

The finding that selective blockers of DA receptors prevented the hypnotic effect of apomorphine indicates that this effect is mediated by a stimulation of DA receptors.

The fact that the effect of small doses is the mirror image of that of high doses (i.e., arousal) suggests that the hypnotic effect is due to a decreased dopaminergic transmission, and therefore it is mediated by the stimulation of DA self-inhibitory receptors. However, it is possible that DA receptors responsible for sleep are a special kind of postsynaptic DA receptors located in DA terminal areas as the basal ganglia, limbic system, or the hypothalamus, different from DA receptors responsible for motor stimulation, stereotypy, and arousal for being more sensitive to the action of the transmitter.

A similar problem arises regarding the receptors responsible for the other

TABLE 3. Effects of different doses of apomorphine on sleep in the rat

Apomorphine µg/kg s.c.	No. of recordings	No. of animals	% of total recording time (1 hr) spent in:		
			Total sleep	SWS	REM sleep
Saline	10	8	15.94 ± 1.29	14.12 ± 1.21	1.82 ± 0.33
1000	4	4	4.22 ± 0.85^a	4.22 ± 0.85^a	—
100	8	7	62.86 ± 5.10^a	61.40 ± 4.42^a	1.46 ± 0.52
50	8	8	53.57 ± 4.80^a	50.06 ± 4.21^a	3.51 ± 0.48^a
25	8	7	54.36 ± 7.85^a	49.78 ± 5.12^a	4.58 ± 0.58^a
12.5	8	6	31.76 ± 4.82^b	29.30 ± 4.18^b	2.26 ± 0.34
6.2	8	7	18.25 ± 2.32	16.17 ± 2.08	2.08 ± 0.22

Each value is the mean ± SE obtained from the reported number of recordings.
^{a} p < 0.001.
^{b} p < 0.01, in respect to saline-treated animals.

TABLE 4. Antagonism by neuroleptics of the hypnotic effect of apomorphine (A), 25 µg/kg s.c.

Neuroleptic µg/kg i.p.		Time before A or saline min	Saline	No. of recordings	No. of animals	Total sleep as % of total recording time (1 hr)		
						A	No. of recordings	No. of animals
Saline		30	16.32 ± 1.58	8	6	58.50 ± 7.26[a]	8	7
Pimozide	50	120	18.12 ± 3.12	4	4	28.35 ± 3.86[b]	8	7
Benzperidol	50	30	17.54 ± 2.84	4	4	21.75 ± 4.35[b]	8	8
Sulpiride	100	30	20.85 ± 4.31	4	3	29.32 ± 4.32[b]	8	6

Each value is the mean ± SE obtained from the reported number of recordings.
[a] $p < 0.001$, in respect to saline treatment.
[b] $p < 0.001$, in respect to apomorphine alone.

effects induced by low doses of apomorphine, namely, yawning, erection, and ejaculation. Since these changes are also prevented by DA-receptor blockers, they are dopaminomimetic in nature; however, it is not clear if the DA receptors involved can be identified with self-inhibitory receptors.

BEHAVIORAL CHANGES INDUCED BY SMALL DOSES OF APOMORPHINE IN HUMANS

In man the emetic action of apomorphine prevents the possibility of using doses higher than 50 μg/kg. Presumably this is the reason why no effects attributable to postsynaptic DA receptor stimulation are observable, except in parkinsonian patients in which apomorphine has a known therapeutic efficacy (37). However, it is likely that in such condition postsynaptic DA receptors in the basal ganglia present a supersensitivity to the drug.

On the other hand, in humans it is possible to study some effects of apomorphine which cannot be observed in animals, such as the therapeutic

TABLE 5. Neurological and mental syndromes ameliorated by apomorphine

Parkinson's disease	Schwab 1951, Duby 1972
Huntington's chorea	Tolosa 1974, Corsini 1977
Tardive diskinesia	Marsden 1975, Tolosa 1974
Gilles De La Tourette syndrome	Feinberg 1975
Spasmodic torticollis	Granacher 1975
Acute dystonia	Gessa 1972, Corsini 1977
Schizophrenia	Bleuler 1911, Feldman 1945, Corsini 1976, Davis 1977
Mania	Feldman 1945, Corsini 1976

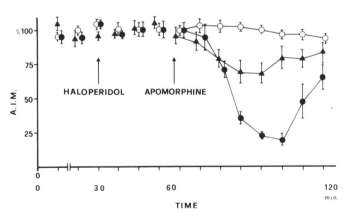

FIG. 6. Prevention of the apomorphine-induced improvement on abnormal involuntary movements (AIM) by haloperidol. Open circles: haloperidol 2 mg i.m. + saline i.m.; closed circles: saline + apomorphine* i.m.; closed triangles: haloperidol 2 mg + apomorphine* i.m. (* = highest nonemetic dose for each patient.)

effects in neurological and psychiatric conditions and different subjective effects (Table 5).

Some of the effects exerted by apomorphine in man may be considered to result from the stimulation of DA self-inhibitory receptors. Thus, nonemetic doses of apomorphine have been found to dramatically ameliorate the abnormal involuntary movements (AIM) in patients with Huntington's chorea (10), an effect which is prevented by haloperidol and sulpiride, indicating that it is mediated by stimulation of DA receptors (Fig. 6).

Such findings are in apparent contrast with the accepted view that increased dopaminergic activity is responsible for the neurological disturbances present in Huntington's chorea (5).

However, the antichoreic effect of apomorphine may well be explained with a preferential stimulation of self-inhibitory DA receptors resulting in inhibition of dopaminergic transmission. A similar mechanism may be involved in the dramatic improvement brought about by apomorphine on neuroleptic-induced tardive dyskinesia (4,34).

Consistent with a preferential action on self-inhibitory DA receptors, we found that low doses of apomorphine reduced the psychotic symptoms in some actively ill schizoaffective patients, rather than exacerbated their psy-

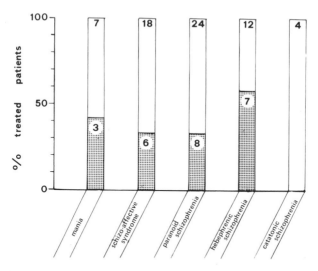

FIG. 7. Antipsychotic effect of acute apomorphine administration in various groups of patients. Apomorphine (1 mg i.m.) was administered in unmedicated patients of either sex ages 13–35. Two physicians independently evaluated the type of disease on the basis of the clinical picture and evolution of the syndrome. Antipsychotic effects of apomorphine were assessed by a quantal response (i.e., present or absent on the basis of a temporary reduction of the symptoms evaluated by means of a modified overall rating scale). Columns from left to right indicate: mania, schizoaffective syndrome, paranoid schizophrenia, hebephrenic schizophrenia, and catatonic schizophrenia. The figures at the top of the columns represent the number of cases. The shaded area indicates percent of patients beneficially influenced by the drug, and the figures at the top of the shaded area indicate the number of patients beneficially influenced by apomorphine.

chotic symptoms which would have been predicted from a DA-receptor supersensitivity hypothesis of schizophrenia. Apomorphine's effect was of short duration (20 to 50 min), after which the patients returned to their previous psychotic condition, but the amelioration included most features of the psychotic symptomatology (8). Similar results have been reported by Smith et al. (33) (Fig. 7).

SEDATION AND SLEEP INDUCED BY NONEMETIC DOSES OF APOMORPHINE IN HUMANS

Acute intramuscular injection of nonemetic doses of apomorphine (1 mg) was found to cause sedation and behavioral sleep in a high percentage of normal and schizophrenic subjects (9). As in animal studies, the sedative effect was prevented by haloperidol, pimozide, and, particularly, sulpiride, suggesting that the effect is due to the stimulation of DA receptors (Table 6).

However, as for the hypnotic effect in rats, the problem arises as to whether DA receptors responsible for sedation and sleep in humans are DA self-inhibitory receptors or a special kind of postsynaptic DA receptors sensitive to low concentrations of the transmitter.

Moreover, although the above results indicate that nonemetic doses of apomorphine facilitate falling asleep. the use of a single intramuscular administration of the drug does not clarify what may be the influence of apomorphine on sleep parameters. In fact, the short half-life of apomorphine does allow one to distinguish direct effects of the drug from rebound compensatory changes in sleep parameters.

To clarify this problem, we have recently studied the effect of intravenous infusion of apomorphine on human sleep (7). Apomorphine was given to 10 volunteers (4 men and 6 women) at a nonemetic dose, ranging according to the patient from 10 to 15 μg/min. The infusion began at 10 P.M., when the subjects would normally fall asleep, and lasted for 240 min. The results, summarized in Table 7, indicate that apomorphine infusion totally suppressed REM sleep and decreased by more than 90% the amount of delta

TABLE 6. *Prevention by neuroleptics of the sedative and hypnotic affect of apomorphine (A) in normal subjects.*

Pretreatment (30' before A)	mg(i.m.)	A mg(i.m.)	N	Subjects (%) showing sedation	sleep
Saline	—	1.0	12	8(66)	4(33)
Haloperidol	1.0	1.0	12	2(17)	0
Pimozide	1.0	1.0	12	1(8)	0
Sumpiride	10.0	1.0	12	2(17)	0

Drugs were given according to a latin square design at an interval of 5 days.
N = subjects treated.

TABLE 7. *Sleep patterns during apomorphine infusion (180 min) and placebo infusion*

Sleep parameter	Apomorphine	Placebo
Sleep latency (min)	20.8 ± 14.1	25.3 ± 8.5
Percent S1	10.3 ± 4.2[a]	6.5 ± 3.1
" S2	59.5 ± 17.5[b]	33.8 ± 10.6
" S3	13.4 ± 11.2	15.2 ± 7.1
" S4	5.1 ± 8.1[c]	29.8 ± 11.4
" SREM	0.0 ± 0.0[b]	9.7 ± 8.3
" W (interspersed)	11.7 ± 11.9	5.0 ± 5.2
Total sleep time	179.2 ± 14.1	174.7 ± 8.5

Stage percentages are referred to total sleep time.
Each value is the mean ± SE from 10 subjects.
[a],[b],[c] Significantly different at $p < 0.05$, < 0.01, < 0.001 level, respectively, calculated with the paired t-test.

sleep. Thus, the EEG pattern during apomorphine infusion is characterized almost exclusively by the presence of stages 1 and 2 sleep (Table 7).

The effect of apomorphine on sleep was prevented by haloperidol and sulpiride in doses which did not modify sleep parameters *per se*.

Although there is reason to assume that apomorphine-induced changes in sleep parameters are due to stimulation of DA receptors, it is unlikely that these receptors may be ascribed to the DA self-inhibitory receptors. In fact, the effects of apomorphine are opposite to those observed in humans with specific inhibitors of catecholamine synthesis (40) and with DA receptor blockers (31).

On the other hand, the suppressant effect of apomorphine on REM sleep resembles that obtained with amphetamine and with the intravenous infusion of L-DOPA (18).

In humans, unlike the effect observed in rodents, apomorphine does not produce insomnia. It is possible that the doses of apomorphine that can be used in humans are insufficient to affect DA receptors involved in arousal. However, species differences in sleep mechanisms are well known (20). The physiological implication of the above results might be that stimulation of some kind of DA receptors might be involved in the onset of light sleep, which in turn facilitates progression into the other sleep components. However, an abnormal persistence of DA stimulation such as that produced by apomorphine infusion would maintain NREM light sleep and prevent the development of a normal sleep. Interestingly, marked decreases in the amount of REM sleep and delta sleep have been noted in acute schizophrenics (25), a condition in which DA hyperstimulation has been suggested.

CONCLUSIONS

By evaluating the information presented above, one can draw the following conclusions including self-inhibitory DA receptors.

1. Apomorphine caused a series of biochemical, neurological, psychological, and behavioral changes that are prevented by specific blockers of DA receptors, suggesting that these responses are mediated through stimulation of such receptors.

2. Some changes such as the decreased motor activity in rodents, the therapeutic effect of the drug in Huntington's chorea and tardive dyskinesia, and perhaps the antipsychotic effect might be due to a decreased dopaminergic transmission and therefore might result from stimulation of self-inhibitory DA receptors.

Note Added in Proof

After this work was completed we found that destruction of postsynaptic dopamine receptors by intrastriatal kainic acid prevents the haloperidol-induced activation of striatal tyrosine-hydroxylase but not the stimulation of DA-synthesis estimated *in vivo* on the accumulation of 3,4-dihydroxyphenyl-alanine after inhibition of aromatic amino acid decarboxylase. This indicates the existence of two DA-receptor-mediated mechanisms regulating DA-synthesis *in vivo:* one depends on the presence of postsynaptic DA-receptors and capable of producing a stable activation of tyrosine-hydroxylase whereas the other is not associated to a persistent conformational change of tyrosine-hydroxylase and is possibly mediated by presynaptic DA-receptors. The results also indicate that the activation of striatal tyrosine-hydroxylase by neuroleptics is unrelated to blockade of presynaptic DA-receptors.

REFERENCES

1. Baraldi, M., and Benassi-Benelli, A. (1975): Apomorphine-induced penile erections in adult rats. *Riv. Farm. Ter.,* VI:147–149.
2. Bunney, B. S., and Aghajanian, G. K. (1975): In: *Pre- and Postsynaptic receptors,* edited by E. Usdin and W. E. Bunney, Jr., pp. 89, Marcel Dekker, New York.
3. Carlsson, A. (1975): In: *Pre- and Postsynaptic receptors,* edited by E. Usdin and W. E. Bunney, Jr., pp. 49–65. Marcel Dekker, New York.
4. Carroll, B. J., Curtis, G. C., and Kokmen, E. (1977): Paradoxical response to dopamine agonists in tardive dyskinesia. *Am. J. Psychiatry,* 134:785–789.
5. Chase, T. (1973): Biochemical and pharmacologic studies of monoamines in Huntington's chorea. *Adv. Neurol.,* 1:553.
6. Christiansen, J., and Squires, R. F. (1974): Antagonistic effects of apomorphine and haloperidol on rat striatal synaptosomal tyrosine hydroxylase. *J. Pharm. Pharmacol.,* 26:367–369.
7. Cianchetti, C., Masala, C., Corsini, G. U., Mangoni, A., and Gessa, G. L. (1978): *Life Sci. (in press).*
8. Corsini, G. U., Del Zompo, M., Manconi, S., Cianchetti, C., Mangoni, A., and Gessa, G. L. (1976): In: *Symposium on Non-Striatal Dopaminergic Neurons,* edited by G. L. Gessa and E. Costa, p. 645. Raven Press, New York.
9. Corsini, G. U., Del Zompo, M., Manconi, S., Onali, P. L., Mangoni, A., and Gessa, G. L. (1977): Evidence for dopamine receptors in human brain mediating sedation and sleep. *Life Sci.,* 20:1613–1618.

10. Corsini, G. U., Onali, P. L., Masala, C., Cianchetti, C., Mangoni, A., and Gessa, G. L. (1978): *Arch. Neurol. (in press)*.
11. Coyle, J. T., and Schwarcz, R. (1976): Lesion of striatal neurones with kainic acid provides a model for Huntington's chorea. *Nature*, 263:244–246.
12. Di Chiara, G., Porceddu, M. L., Fratta, W., and Gessa, G. L. (1977): Postsynaptic receptors are not essential for dopaminergic feedback regulation. *Nature*, 267:270.
13. Di Chiara, G., Porceddu, M. L., Spano, P. F., and Gessa, G. L. (1977): Haloperidol increases and apomorphine decreases striatal dopamine metabolism after destruction of striatal dopamine-sensitive adenylate cyclase by kainic acid. *Brain Res.*, 130:374–382.
14. Di Chiara, G., Porceddu, M. L., Vargiu, L., Argiolas, A., and Gessa, G. L. (1976): Evidence for dopamine receptors mediating sedation in the mouse brain. *Nature*, 264:564–567.
15. Farnebo, L. O., and Hamberger, B. (1971): Drug-induced changes in the release of ^{3}H-monoamines from field-stimulated rat brain slices. *Acta Physiol. Scand.* [*Suppl. 84*], 371:35–44.
16. Gale, K., Guidotti, A., and Costa, E. (1977): Dopamine-sensitive adenylate cyclase: Location in substantia nigra. *Science*, 195:503–505.
17. Garcia-Munoz, M., Nicolau, N. M., Tulloch, I. F., Wright, A. V., and Arbuthnott, G. W. (1977): Feedback loop or output pathway in striato-nigral fibres? *Nature*, 265:363–365.
18. Gillin, J. C., Post, R. M., Wyatt, R. J., Goodwin, F. K., Snyder, F., and Bunney, W. E., Jr. (1973): REM inhibitory effect of L-dopa infusion during human sleep. *EEG Clin. Neurophysiol.*, 35:181–186.
19. Iversen, L. L., Rogawski, M. A., and Miller, R. J. (1975): Comparison of the effects of neuroleptic drugs on pre- and postsynaptic dopaminergic mechanisms in the rat striatum. *Mol. Pharmacol.*, 12:251–262.
20. Jouvet, M. (1972): The role of monoamines and acetylcholine-containing neurons in the regulation of the sleep-waking cycle. *Ergebn. Physiol.*, 64:166–307.
21. Kafi, S., and Gaillard, J. M. (1976): Brain dopamine receptors and sleep in the rat: Effects of stimulation and blockade. *Eur. J. Pharmacol.*, 38:357–363.
22. Kebabian, J. W., Petzold, G. L., and Greengard, P. (1972): Dopamine-sensitive adenylate cyclase in caudate nucleus of rat brain, and its similarity to the "dopamine receptor." *Proc. Natl. Acad. Sci. U.S.A.*, 69:2145–2149.
23. Kehr, W., Carlsson, A., Lindqvist, M., Magnusson, T., and Atack, C. V. (1972): Evidence for a receptor-mediated feedback control of striatal tyrosine hydroxylase activity. *J. Pharm. Pharmacol.*, 24:744–746.
24. Kim, J. S., Bak, I. J., Hassler, R., and Okada, Y. (1971): Role of γ-aminobutyric acid (GABA) in the extrapyramidal motor system. *Exp. Brain Res.*, 14:95–104.
25. Kupfer, D. J., Wyatt, R. J., Scott, J., and Snyder, F. (1970): Sleep disturbance in acute schizophrenic patients. *Am. J. Psychiatry*, 126:1213–1223.
26. McGeer, E. G., Innanen, V. T., and McGeer, P. L. (1976): Evidence on the cellular localisation of adenyl cyclase in the neostriatum. *Brain Res.*, 118:356–358.
27. McGeer, E. G., and McGeer, P. L. (1976): Duplication of biochemical changes of Huntington's chorea by intrastriatal injections of glutamic and kainic acids. *Nature*, 263:517–519.
28. McGeer, P. L., McGeer, E. G., Wada, J. A., and Jung, E. (1971): Effects of globus pallidus lesions and Parkinson's disease on brain glutamic acid decarboxylase. *Brain Res.*, 32:425–431.
29. Mereu, G. P., Scarnati, E., Paglietti, E., Chessa, P., Di Chiara, G., and Gessa, G. L. (1978): *Neuropharmacology (in press)*.
30. Phillipson, O. T., and Horn, A. S. (1976): Substantia nigra of the rat contains a dopamine-sensitive adenylate cyclase. *Nature*, 261:418–420.
31. Sagalés, T., and Erill, S. (1975): Effects of central dopaminergic blockade with pimozide upon the EEG stages of sleep in man. *Psychopharmacology*, 41:53–56.
32. Schwarcz, R., and Coyle, J. T. (1977): Striatal lesions with kainic acid: Neurochemical characteristics. *Brain Res.*, 127:235–249.
33. Smith, R. C., Tamminga, C. A., and Davis, J. M. (1977): Effect of apomorphine on schizophrenic symptoms. *J. Neural Transm.*, 40:171–176.

34. Smith, R. C., Tamminga, C. A., Haraszti, J., Pandey, G. N., and Davis, J. M. (1977): Effect of dopamine agonists in tardive dyskinesia. *Am. J. Psychiatry*, 134:763–768.
35. Spano, P. F., Di Chiara, G., Tonon, G., and Trabucchi, M. (1976): A dopamine-stimulated adenylate cyclase in rat substantia nigra. *J. Neurochem.*, 27:1565–1568.
36. Spano, P. F., Trabucchi, M., and Di Chiara, G. (1977): Localization of nigral dopamine-sensitive adenylate cyclase on neurons originating from corpus striatum. *Science*, 196:1343–1345.
37. Strain, F., Micheler, E., and Benkert, O. (1972): *Pharmakopsychiatrie Neuro-Psychopharmakologie*, 5:198.
38. Strömbom, U. (1976): Catecholamine receptor agonists: Effects on motor activity and rate of tyrosine hydroxylation in mouse brain. *Naunyn-Schmiedeberg's Arch. Pharmacol.*, 262:167–176.
39. Walters, J. R., and Roth, (1974): Dopaminergic neurons: Drug-induced antagonism of the increase in tyrosine hydroxylase activity produced by cessation of impulse flow. *J. Pharmacol. Exp. Ther.*, 191:82–91.
40. Wyatt, R. J., Chase, T. N., Kupper, D. J., Scott, J., Snyder, F., Sjoerdsma, A., and Engel, K. (1971): Brain catecholamines and human sleep. *Nature*, 233:63–65.

Advances in Biochemical Psychopharmacology, Vol. 19,
edited by P. J. Roberts et al.
Raven Press, New York © 1978.

Neurochemistry of Parkinson's Disease: Relation Between Striatal and Limbic Dopamine

*Kathleen S. Price, *Irene J. Farley, and **Oleh Hornykiewicz

*Clarke Institute of Psychiatry, Toronto M5T 1R8, Canada; and **Institute of Biochemical Pharmacology, University of Vienna, A-1090 Vienna, Austria

The behavior of dopamine (DA) in the striatum and related brainstem nuclei (caudate nucleus, putamen, globus pallidus, substantia nigra) in patients with Parkinson's disease is well established (see ref. 13). For the purpose of this discussion two previously made observations are particularly relevant. First, as a rule, in the caudate nucleus of parkinsonian patients the decrease of DA is distinctly less severe than in the putamen (3). On the neuropathological level this distinct pattern of striatal DA deficiency can be related to the characteristic pattern of cell loss in the substantia nigra in Parkinson's disease. It is now well established that in Parkinson's disease, especially its idiopathic variety, there is in general a typical pattern of nigral cell loss, with rostral portions of the nucleus suffering less severe damage than caudal portions (3,12). This characteristic pattern of nigral cell loss seems to determine the pattern of DA decrease in the striatal nuclei; it has repeatedly been demonstrated that the rostral portions of the substantia nigra preferentially project to the caudate nucleus and the caudal portions to the putamen (20,21). Second, the decrease of DA in the striatum is causally related to the extrapyramidal deficits of Parkinson's disease. Specifically, the degree of DA decrease in the caudate nucleus has been demonstrated to be positively correlated with the degree of akinesia, one of the major motor deficits of the parkinsonian disorder (3).

Despite these well-established correlations, the following question has been suggesting itself for some time: Are there, besides the striatal DA deficiency, other neurochemical factors involved in the pathophysiology of the parkinsonian motor deficits, especially akinesia? Based on experimental evidence obtained in laboratory animals, recently structures of the limbic forebrain system have been implicated in motor behavior (see ref. 6). In this respect, the nucleus accumbens (septi) has received considerable attention. On a previous occasion we have discussed the possible involvement of limbic norepinephrine (whose levels were found to be subnormal in the parkinsonian brain) in the symptomatology of Parkinson's disease (8). Since several of the limbic forebrain structures are also rich in DA (see ref. 11), it seemed of interest to examine the behavior of limbic DA and its main metabolite homovanillic acid (HVA) in Parkinson's disease, comparing it with the behavior of DA and HVA in the striatal nuclei. Apart from a possible involvement in motor dysfunction, the possibility of changes of limbic DA metabolism seemed of some interest in relation to the well-known changes in mood and affect seen in patients with Parkinson's disease. In this respect, the limbic forebrain has often been proposed as a possible seat of changes underlying mood disorders and the schizophrenic disturbance (16).

The following discussion will be subdivided into three parts: (a) distribution of limbic DA and HVA in normal human brain; (b) behavior of limbic DA in Parkinson's disease; and (c) functional considerations resulting from the reported data.

MATERIALS AND METHODS

The following report is based on biochemical analyses of postmortem material which was obtained and handled as described elsewhere (8–10). Details on the Parkinsonian material (4 cases) have been presented in previous reports (8,9). DA was assayed either spectrofluorimetrically after separation on Dowex columns or by means of a radioenzymatic procedure (see ref. 10). In our hands values obtained by either of the methods were in good agreement. HVA was determined spectrofluorimetrically (see ref. 10).

RESULTS AND DISCUSSION

Limbic Dopamine and Homovanillic Acid in Normal Human Brain

Table 1 summarizes the data on the distribution of DA and HVA in the limbic forebrain structures of control subjects. These results are compared

TABLE 1. *Human brain dopamine and homovanillic acid in limbic forebrain regions—comparison with striatum*

Brain region	Dopamine	Homovanillic acid	Molar ratio HVA/DA
	(μg/g wet tissue)		
Nucleus accumbens	3.79 ± 0.82 (8)	4.38 ± 0.64 (8)	1.1
Bed nucleus of the stria terminalis	0.77 ± 0.08 (5)	1.86 (2)	2.2
Medial olfactory area	0.75 ± 0.15 (7)	3.57 ± 0.63 (6)	4.4
Lateral olfactory area	0.61 ± 0.10 (4)	4.43 ± 0.23 (5)	6.7
Lateral hypothalamus	0.51 ± 0.08 (4)	1.96 ± 0.28 (3)	3.6
Ventral septum	0.24 ± 0.03 (4)	1.46 (2)	6.1
Parolfactory gyrus	0.35 ± 0.09 (4)	0.98 (2)	2.6
Caudate nucleus	4.52 ± 0.63 (8)	6.08 ± 0.51 (8)	1.2
Putamen	5.37 ± 0.70 (8)	11.40 ± 1.63 (8)	2.0

The figures are means ± SEM; number of examined cases in parentheses.

with the DA and HVA concentrations measured in the nuclei of the striatum (caudate nucleus and putamen).

Dopamine

It can be seen from Table 1 that by far the highest level of limbic DA was detected in the subcortical region of the nucleus accumbens (3.79 μg/g). Other areas of the subcortical component of the limbic forebrain, i.e., bed nucleus of the stria terminalis, medial and lateral olfactory areas, hypothalamus and the septum, contained no more than $\frac{1}{5}$ to $\frac{1}{16}$ of the accumbens level. In the examined areas of the limbic lobe (as defined by Broca), only the parolfactory gyrus (area 25 of Brodmann) contained appreciable levels of DA, about $\frac{1}{10}$ of the accumbens level; all other limbic cortical areas had DA concentrations below the 0.1 μg/g mark. Thus, in the human brain the limbic DA seems to possess a comparatively narrow localization. This is in apparent contrast to the distribution of limbic DA in laboratory animals; thus, in the rat, levels of DA 35% to 100% of those measured in the accumbens and/or caudate nucleus have been reported for the olfactory tubercle, the area of the medial forebrain bundle, the anterior amygdaloid area, and the nucleus of the diagonal tract (5).

Homovanillic Acid

In general, the distribution pattern of limbic HVA followed the DA pattern. However, there were on the quantitative level some important differences. Thus, in the medial and lateral olfactory areas as well as the ventral septum, the concentration of HVA exceeded that of DA by a factor of approximately 4.5 to 7; this predominance of the DA metabolite is in contrast to the other DA-containing limbic regions (i.e., nucleus accumbens, bed nucleus of the stria terminalis, lateral hypothalamus, parolfactory gyrus), as well as the nuclei of the striatum, in which structures the ratio of HVA to DA ranged from 1.1 (for the nucleus accumbens) to 3.6 (for the lateral hypothalamus). The possible significance of this difference will be discussed in the section dealing with the behavior of limbic DA and HVA in Parkinson's disease (see below).

Possible Relation Between the Accumbens and Caudate Dopamine

An interesting detail of the human limbic DA study is the observation (see Table 1) that the DA and HVA concentrations measured in the human nucleus accumbens were quantitatively similar to those found in the caudate nucleus, being in both structures distinctly less than in the putamen. These similarities and differences, respectively, are also reflected in the respective molar ratios of HVA to DA which were, for the caudate nucleus and the accumbens 1.2 and 1.1, respectively; for the putamen, however, this ratio was 2.0. In this respect, it is also noteworthy that the HVA/DA ratios in the bed nucleus of the stria terminalis (2.2) and the parolfactory gyrus (2.6) were closer to the ratio calculated for the putamen than that of the caudate nucleus. Although the similarity between the caudate and accumbens DA may be accidental, there is reason to believe (see ref. 10) that it may reflect a possibly close anatomical relationship between these two subcortical gray masses. This possibility is further discussed in the following section.

Metabolic Changes of Limbic Dopamine in Parkinson's Disease

Dopamine and Homovanillic Acid

Of all limbic forebrain regions analyzed in this study, three areas showed a marked decrease of their DA levels in parkinsonian material. These regions were the parolfactory gyrus, the lateral hypothalamus, and the nucleus accumbens. The other two limbic areas examined in the parkinsonian brain, namely, the medial and lateral olfactory areas, had DA concentrations which were well within the control range. In contrast to DA, the concentrations of HVA were decreased in all analyzed limbic regions, including the medial and lateral olfactory areas. This is shown diagrammatically in Fig. 1. In order to explain this regionally different behavior of DA and HVA, it seems reasonable to assume that in those areas in which there was an approximately parallel decrease of both DA and HVA (similar to that seen in the caudate

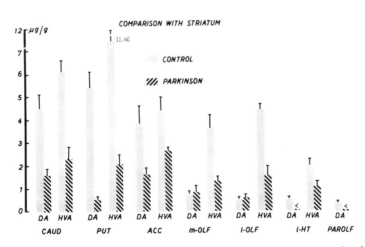

FIG. 1. Behavior of dopamine (DA) and homovanillic acid (HVA) in limbic forebrain regions in patients with Parkinson's disease. Number of parkinsonian cases examined: 4. Number of control cases: see Table 1. ACC, nucleus accumbens; CAUD, caudate nucleus; l-HT, lateral hypothalamus; l-OLF, lateral olfactory area; m-OLF, medial olfactory area; PAROLF, parolfactory gyrus; PUT, putamen.

nucleus and putamen), this change was due to a degeneration of DA terminals innervating the affected areas. In contradistinction, for those areas in which there was an obvious lack of parallelism between DA and HVA, that is to say, where only the HVA levels were decreased (medial and lateral olfactory areas), it may be assumed that (a) there was, in the material examined, no degeneration of the DA terminals innervating these areas (cf. unchanged DA levels); (b) the decrease of HVA in these areas may have been due to degeneration, as a consequence of Parkinson's disease, of DA fibers passing through these basal forebrain regions to reach those distally located structures (e.g., accumbens and parolfactory gyrus) whose DA innervation is greatly reduced in Parkinson's disease. This explanation is directly supported by an analogous behavior of the HVA contained in the nigrostriatal DA fibers passing through the internal capsule (which in man contain but traces of DA); in Parkinson's disease this internal capsule HVA is also greatly decreased, apparently as a consequence of the degeneration of the nigrostriatal DA tract passing through this area (14); (c) in addition, the fact that in normal human material (see preceding section) the molar ratio HVA/DA specifically in the regions of the medial and lateral olfactory areas (as well as the septum) considerably exceeded the ratio calculated for regions known to contain DA terminals (caudate nucleus, putamen, nucleus accumbens) suggests that a high proportion of the HVA in the former regions most probably is contained in DA fibers of passage.

Is There a Common Anatomical Substrate for the Limbic and Striatal Dopamine Changes in Parkinson's Disease?

Of special interest is the observation that from a quantitative point of view the decrease of DA in the parolfactory gyrus (less than 10% DA remaining) was similar in degree to the DA decrease seen in the putamen (9% DA remaining), similarly, the DA decrease in the nucleus accumbens (42% DA remaining) was of the same magnitude as that measured in the caudate nucleus (35% DA remaining). This observation raises the intriguing possibility that the dopaminergic innervation of the parolfactory gyrus may be anatomically related to that of the putamen, whereas the dopaminergic innervation of the nucleus accumbens may be related to that of the caudate nucleus. (The similarities between the accumbens and striatal DA have already been pointed out; see preceding section.) In other words, the dopaminergic fibers innervating the limbic parolfactory gyrus and the nucleus accumbens may stem from those portions of the substantia nigra which innervate the putamen and caudate nucleus, respectively. In respect to the nucleus accumbens this possibility is at variance with fluorescence-histochemical evidence obtained in the rat suggesting that the bulk of the accumbens DA may be contained in neurons originating in the area A10 of the midbrain tegmentum (see ref. 11). However, in the cat, lesions of the substantia nigra sparing the A10 area have been reported to cause a marked decrease of the DA level in the ipsilateral nucleus accumbens (18). Thus, the possibility can not be disregarded that in some (higher) species, at least part of the dopaminergic innervation of the nucleus accumbens may have an anatomical origin common with that of the caudate nucleus. Since morphologically the nucleus accumbens can be classified as being part of the striatal complex (1), the accumbens DA may represent, as it were, the striatal heritage of this limbic structure. In respect to the possible nigral origin of at least some of the dopaminergic innervation of the human parolfactory gyrus, the report may be relevant that in the rat, the substantia nigra, besides projecting to the striatum, also sends DA fibers to the limbic motor cortex, especially the anterior cingulate gyrus (4).

In this context, it is important to note that although widespread, the decrease of DA in Parkinson's disease did not affect all dopaminergically innervated forebrain regions. This is shown by the apparent lack of changes in such important DA-containing regions as the medial and lateral olfactory areas. In other words, in Parkinson's disease there probably is no systemic degeneration of (all) DA neurons in the brain; this indirectly supports the notion that those DA systems (striatal and limbic) that do degenerate may in fact have a common anatomical origin.

Possible Functional Consequences of the Disturbed Limbic Dopamine Metabolism in Parkinson's Disease

Motor Functions—Possible Role of Accumbens Dopamine in Parkinsonian Akinesia

There exists a large body of experimental evidence showing that manipulations of the accumbens DA (in the rat) produce marked effects on the animal's locomotor activity (see ref. 6). This point is particularly well illustrated by microinjection experiments showing that direct application of DA into the nucleus accumbens produced a marked locomotor hyperactivity of the animal (19). Also, it has recently been made quite likely that the nucleus accumbens represents the principal anatomical site for the locomotor hyperactivity elicited by amphetamine (15), which is generally assumed to be mediated through the brain's dopaminergic mechanisms. In view of these observations, the possibility suggests itself that the changes in limbic (especially accumbens) DA metabolism found in patients with Parkinson's disease may be related to some of the motor deficits typical of this disorder.

The limited material available for this study did not permit any meaningful correlations to be made between the degree of DA decrease in the nucleus accumbens and the motor deficits presented by the patients. As mentioned above, in a previous study a positive correlation was observed between the degree of DA loss in the caudate nucleus and the symptom of akinesia (3). Since in our present parkinsonian material we have demonstrated close parallelism between the caudate and accumbens DA loss, a relationship between loss of accumbens DA and severity of akinesia does indeed suggest itself. Hence, we should like to propose that parkinsonian akinesia should be viewed as being the result of a combined caudate-accumbens DA deficiency rather than being exclusively due to DA loss in the caudate nucleus. This hypothesis is in accord with the above quoted laboratory data implicating accumbens DA in locomotor acitivity. Accordingly, the term "striatal DA deficiency," when applied to the symptom of parkinsonian akinesia, should in our view be understood as including the disturbance of the dopaminergic mechanisms in the nucleus accumbens.

Psychic Functions

Apart from being involved in motor behavior, the limbic forebrain has traditionally been implicated in affective disorders as well as behavioral disturbances characteristic of the schizophrenic illness (16). Therefore, our finding of a disturbed DA metabolism in some of the limbic forebrain structures, especially the parolfactory gyrus and lateral hypothalamus, suggests that DA changes in these limbic regions may in fact be an important factor in the etiology of affective disturbances commonly observed in patients with Parkinson's disease. Recently, a functional hyperactivity of limbic DA mechanisms has been proposed as a possible factor in schizophrenia (see refs. 17 and 22). If pursued logically, the latter suggestion leads directly to the conclusion that because of the widespread loss of limbic DA the incidence of schizophrenia in patients with Parkinson's disease should be extremely low. However, this notion is not supported by a recent report describing the appearance of schizophrenic symptomatology in a small group of patients with a long-standing history of Parkinson's disease (7). Thus, studies of the neurochemical pathology of Parkinson's disease not only contribute to our understanding of this particular brain disorder but may also shed some light on other neurochemically as yet poorly understood disturbances of brain function.

REFERENCES

1. Ariëns Kappers, C. U., and Theunissen, W. F. (1907): Die Phylogenese des Rhinencephalons, des Corpus Striatum und der Vorderhirnkommissuren. *Folia Neurobiol.*, 1:173–288.
2. Bartholini, G., Stadler, H., Gadea-Ciria, M., and Lloyd, K. G. (1975): The effect of antipsychotic drugs on the release of neurotransmitters in various brain areas. In: *Antipsychotic Drugs, Pharmacodynamics and Pharmacokinetics,* edited by G. Sedvall, pp. 105–116. Pergamon Press, New York.
3. Bernheimer, H., Birkmayer, W., Hornykiewicz, O., Jellinger, K., and Seitelberger, F. (1973): Brain dopamine and the syndromes of Parkinson and Huntington. *J. Neurol. Sci.*, 20:415–455.
4. Björklund, A., and Lindvall, O. (1977): The mesencephalic dopaminergic projec-

tions to the limbic areas. In: *Symposium on the Limbic System*, edited by K. Livingston and O. Hornykiewicz. Plenum Press, New York (*in press*).

5. Brownstein, M., Saavedra, J. M., and Palkovits, M. (1974): Norepinephrine and dopamine in the limbic system of the rat. *Brain Res., 79*:431–436.

6. Costa, E., and Gessa, G. L. (Eds.) (1977): Dopamine in the limbic regions of the human brain: Normal and abnormal. *Adv. Biochem. Psychopharmacol., 16*:57–70.

7. Crow, T. J., Johnstone, E. C., and McClelland, H. A. (1976): The coincidence of schizophrenia and Parkinsonism: Some neurochemical implications. *Pschol. Med., 6*:227–233.

8. Farley, I. J., and Hornykiewicz, O. (1976): Noradrenaline in subcortical brain regions of patients with Parkinson's disease and control subjects. In: *Advances in Parkinsonism*, edited by W. Birkmayer and O. Hornykiewicz, pp. 178–185. Editiones Roche, Baseil.

9. Farley, I. J., and Hornykiewicz, O. (1977): Noradrenaline distribution in subcortical areas of the human brain. *Brain Res., 126*:53–62.

10. Farley, I. J., Price, K. S., and Hornykiewicz, O. (1977): Dopamine in the limbic regions of the human brain: Normal and abnormal. *Adv. Biochem. Psychopharmacol., 16*:57–64.

11. Fuxe, K., Hökfelt, T., and Ungerstedt, U. (1970): Morphological and functional aspects of central monoamine neurons. *Int. Rev. Neurobiol., 13*:93–126.

12. Hassler, R. (1938): Zur Pathologie der Paralysis Agitans und des postenzephalitischen Parkinsonismus. *J. Psychol. Neurol. (Lpz.), 48*:387–476.

13. Hornykiewicz, O. (1973): Dopamine in the basal ganglia: Its role and therapeutic implications (including the clinical use of L-dopa). *Br. Med. Bull., 29*:172–178.

14. Hornykiewicz, O., Lisch, H.-J., and Springer, A. (1968): Homovanillic acid in different regions of the human brain: Attempt at localizing central dopamine fibres. *Brain Res., 11*:662–671.

15. Iversen, S. (1977): Behavioral implications of dopaminergic neurons in the mesolimbic system. *Adv. Biochem. Psychopharmacol., 16*:209–214.

16. MacLean, P. (1970): The limbic brain in relation to the psychoses. In: *Physiological Correlates of Emotion*, edited by P. Black, pp. 129–146. Academic Press, New York.

17. Matthysse, S. (1974): Schizophrenia: Relationships to dopamine transmission, motor control and feature extraction. In: *The Neurosciences, Third Study Program*, edited by F. O. Schmitt and F. G. Worden, pp. 733–737. MIT Press, Cambridge, Mass.

18. Moore, R. Y., Bhatnagar, R. K., and Heller, A. (1971): Anatomical and chemical studies of a nigro-neostriatal projection in the cat. *Brain Res., 30*:119–135.

19. Pijnenburg, A. J. J., Honig, W. M. M., Van Der Heyden, J. A. M., and Van Rossum, J. M. (1976): Effects of chemical stimulation of the mesolimbic dopamine system upon locomotor activity. *Eur. J. Pharmacol., 35*:45–58.

20. Portig, P. J., and Vogt, M. (1969): Release into the cerebral ventricles of substances with possible transmitter function in the caudate nucleus. *J. Physiol., 204*:687–715.

21. Riddell, D., and Szerb, J. C. (1971): The release in vivo of dopamine synthesized from labelled precursors in the caudate nucleus of the cat. *J. Neurochem., 18*:989–1006.

22. Snyder, S. H. (1974): Catecholamines as mediators of drug effects in schizophrenia. In: *The Neurosciences, Third Study Program*, edited by F. O. Schmitt and F. G. Worden, pp. 721–732. MIT Press, Cambridge, Mass.

Advances in Biochemical Psychopharmacology, Vol. 19,
edited by P. J. Roberts et al.
Raven Press, New York © 1978.

Dopamine and Schizophrenia

T. J. Crow, E. C. Johnstone, A. Longden, and F. Owen

*Division of Psychiatry, Clinical Research Centre, Northwick Park Hospital,
Harrow Middlesex HA1 3UJ, England*

Much of the credit for drawing attention to the possible role of dopaminergic mechanisms in the phenomena of schizophrenia should be attributed to Randrup and his colleagues (23,24) who, in the early 1960s, initiated a program of research which established the role of dopamine in the behavioral actions of the amphetamines. The close similarity of amphetamine psychosis to acute paranoid schizophrenia had been earlier recognized by Connell (7), and Carlsson and Lindqvist (6) had described the actions of various neuroleptic drugs on dopamine turnover and suggested that the effects might be related to these drugs' ability to block a dopamine receptor. van Rossum (25) suggested that dopamine receptor blockade was related to the antipsychotic potency of these compounds, and Randrup and Munkvad (24) demonstrated a selective reversal by neuroleptic drugs of the behavioral changes induced in animals by the amphetamines.

From these observations developed what may be referred to as the "dopamine hypothesis" of schizophrenia—that some (or perhaps all) of the symptoms of schizophrenia arise from excessive activity of dopaminergic mechanisms, and that the effects of this excess (and thus the symptoms of schizophrenia) can be reduced by the dopamine receptor blockade induced by neuroleptic drugs. It should be noted that there are really two separate and logically distinct hypotheses here—the "dopamine overactivity" hypothesis of schizophrenia, and the "dopamine receptor blockade" hypothesis of the antipsychotic effect. As will be noted below, although current evidence—with some reservations—favors the latter hypothesis, there are increasingly substantial reasons for questioning the former.

AMPHETAMINE PSYCHOSIS

Recent clinical (14) and experimental (3) observations on amphetamine intoxication have supported Connell's conjecture that the psychotic states induced by amphetamine are often indistinguishable from acute paranoid schizophrenia. Griffith et al. (17) demonstrated that psychotic changes could be induced in most, if not all, volunteer subjects if sufficiently large doses were given, and these changes often occurred before sleep deprivation could have been a serious factor. Therefore, the changes are likely to be due to a direct pharmacological action of the drug. CSF sampling techniques have been used (3) to show that dopamine turnover is increased following administration of psychotogenic doses of amphetamine in man, and there is some evidence (2,18) that the psychotic changes can be reversed by drugs interfering with dopaminergic transmission.

There are therefore grounds for believing that the amphetamine psychosis is associated with, and may possibly be of a consequence of, abnormally increased dopaminergic transmission.

ANTIPSYCHOTIC EFFECT

Mechanism

The belief that the antipsychotic effects of neuroleptic drugs are associated with their ability to block dopaminergic transmission has been strengthened by the discovery of *in vitro* assays for the dopamine receptor. These drugs inhibit the dopamine-induced activation of striatal adenylate cyclase, and their potency in this respect is quite well correlated with their clinical efficacy in schizophrenia (21). However, the potency of the butyrophenones is less than might be expected from clinical observations, but when assessed in an *in vitro* assay of the receptor based on haloperidol binding, the effectiveness of this class of compounds falls more readily into place (9,26).

A direct test of the dopamine blockade hypothesis in the clinical situation was made possible by the observation that the two stereoisomers of the thiaxanthene flupenthixol differ widely in their ability to block both the dopamine-sensitive adenylate cyclase (21) and haloperidol binding (15), the α- or *cis* isomer being several orders of potency more active than the β- or *trans* isomer in either case. In a double-blind controlled trial (12) the clinical efficacies of these two isomers were compared with that of placebo in the

Flupenthixol trial

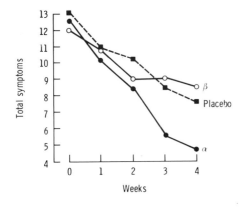

FIG. 1. The effects of α- and β-flupenthixol and placebo on the symptoms of acute schizophrenia (12) over the first 4 weeks of treatment.

TABLE 1. *Relative potencies of the two isomers of flupenthixol*

$\alpha = \beta$ or $\alpha \simeq \beta$	$\alpha \gg \beta$
Norepinephrine receptor: Inhibition of norepinephrine-sensitive adenylate cyclase	Dopamine receptor: Inhibition of dopamine or haloperidol binding; inhibition of dopamine-sensitive adenylate cyclase
Cholinergic receptor: Inhibition of QNB binding and ACh antagonism	
Opiate receptor: Inhibition of naloxone and dihydromorphine binding	Serotonin receptor: Inhibition of 5-HT and LSD binding; 5-HT antagonism
Inhibition of dopamine uptake	
Inhibition of GABA uptake	

For data and references see: 12, 15, 21.

treatment of 45 patients with acute schizophrenia diagnosed by Present State Examination criteria.

Patients were rated by standardized clinical interview at weekly intervals, and the findings revealed (Fig. 1) that in terms of total symptom scores patients on α-flupenthixol improved to a significantly greater extent than those on placebo, while those on β-flupenthixol obtained no benefit from drug treatment.

These findings are consistent with the hypothesis that dopamine blockade is a significant, and possibly the sole, component in the therapeutic effect. However, the extent to which other mechanisms can be ruled out depends on whether it can be demonstrated that the two isomers do not differ with respect to such actions. Some findings on the relative efficacy of the two isomers are summarized in Table 1.

It is apparent that although the two isomers differ in their effects on the dopamine receptor, they also differ, in the same direction and to approximately the same extent, in their ability to block the serotonin (5-HT) receptor. Therefore 5-HT receptor blockade cannot be ruled out on the basis of this trial, but since the correlation between 5-HT receptor blocking potency, assessed by receptor binding techniques (4), and antipsychotic potency is very low, by contrast with the correlation between dopamine receptor blockade and therapeutic potency, it seems highly unlikely that the former action is relevant. The evidence is therefore highly consistent with the dopamine blockade hypothesis.

Relevance to the Symptoms of Schizophrenia

In this trial it was also possible (11) to examine the selectivity of the antipsychotic effect with respect to particular features of the illness. For

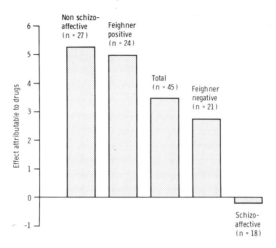

FIG. 2. The magnitude of the therapeutic improvement attributable to drug therapy in patient groups defined by different diagnostic criteria. All patients were selected from the total group (N = 45) of patients included in the trial of the isomers of flupenthixol. Improvement attributable to drug therapy is calculated as the mean change in total ratings in patients on α-flupenthixol minus the mean of change in patients on β-flupenthixol and placebo (11).

example, it was possible to examine the magnitude of the drug effect, calculated as the improvement on α-flupenthixol as compared to the mean improvement on β-flupenthixol and placebo, in groups of patients defined by different diagnostic criteria (Fig. 2).

This analysis reveals that when the patient group is subdivided either by the Feighner criteria (which stipulate an element of progressive deterioration as a feature of schizophrenia) or by the presence of affective symptoms, the drug effect is greater in those with the more typically schizophrenic illnesses (i.e., Feighner positive or nonschizoaffective psychoses) in each case.

Analysis of individual symptoms assessed at weekly interviews revealed that the improvement which could be attributed to drugs occurred principally on those symptoms (delusions, hallucinations, and thought disorder) which have sometimes been described as positive symptoms, and was little evident with respect to nonpsychotic symptoms (depression or anxiety) or on the negative features (flattening of affect, mutism, retardation of speech) of the disease.

Time Course

Prolactin secretion is controlled by the inhibitory influence of the tuberoinfundibular dopamine system, and the well-established increase in prolactin release following neuroleptic drugs can be used as an index of drug-induced dopamine receptor blockade. In the trial of the isomers of flupenthixol, it was demonstrated that prolactin secretion increased by over 300% in patients

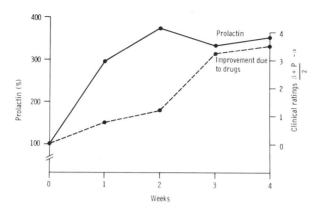

FIG. 3. The time course of prolactin increase on α-flupenthixol compared with the time course of the clinical change attributable to drug therapy (8).

on α-flupenthixol but was virtually unchanged in those on β-flupenthixol or placebo (8). By subtracting the clinical ratings of patients on α-flupenthixol from the mean ratings on β-flupenthixol and placebo, it was possible to estimate the extent of the improvement which could be attributed to drug therapy and to compare the time course of this effect with the time course of dopamine receptor blockade as reflected in increased prolactin secretion (Fig. 3).

The results reveal a surprising discrepancy. Whereas increased prolactin secretion is well established at the end of the first week and may be present well before this, the improvement attributable to drug therapy appears mainly in the third week of treatment. This suggests that the therapeutic change is not a direct effect of dopamine receptor blockade, such as might be expected, for example, if a simple neurohumoral imbalance were being reversed, but rather that dopamine receptor blockade permits other and longer term changes to take place, and that these latter changes are reflected in clinical state.

Site of Action

It has long been recognized that although many, if not all, neuroleptic drugs induce extrapyramidal symptoms, these changes are not directly related to the antipsychotic action. It is generally accepted that the extrapyramidal effects are due to dopamine receptor blockade in the corpus striatum, and if, as suggested above, the antipsychotic effect is also due to dopamine receptor blockade, it remains to be explained how these actions can be dissociated. One possibility, as suggested by Andén (1), is that the antipsychotic effect occurs at an extrastriatal dopaminergically innervated site such as the nucleus accumbens. This possibility has recently been assessed (10) in animal experiments in which three drugs, chlorpromazine, fluphenazine, and thiorida-

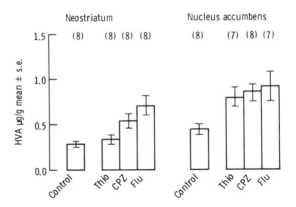

FIG. 4. The effects of three drugs—thioridazine (Thio), chlorpromazine (CPZ), and fluphenazine (Flu)—on HVA levels in neostriatum and nucleus accumbens. The dose ratios (1:1:0.05) were selected to correspond to therapeutically equivalent daily dosages. Figures in parenthesis represent number of animals studied.

zine, known to differ in incidence of extrapyramidal side effects, were compared in their actions on dopamine turnover in nucleus accumbens and corpus striatum at equivalent antipsychotic doses (Fig. 4).

The results revealed that, at least at intermediate dose levels, there were quite striking differences in the relative potencies of the three drugs in the two areas. Whereas in the corpus striatum the effects on dopamine turnover were widely different and the drugs' had varying abilities to induce extrapyramidal side effects (i.e., fluphenazine > chlorpromazine > thioridazine), in the nucleus accumbens the effects were closely similar, and therefore, since equivalent antipsychotic doses were used, were much more closely related to the antipsychotic effect. The results are entirely consistent with the hypothesis that the antipsychotic effect is secondary to dopamine receptor blockade in the nucleus accumbens, although they do not exclude a site elsewhere within the mesolimbic dopamine system, e.g., frontal cortex.

ARE DOPAMINERGIC NEURONS OVERACTIVE IN SCHIZOPHRENIA?

In spite of the evidence which suggests that dopamine receptor blockade is necessary for the antipsychotic effects, there are substantial objections to the dopamine overactivity hypothesis of schizophrenia:

1. CSF studies of HVA following probenecid administration (5,22) have yielded no evidence of increased dopamine turnover even though with this technique it is possible to demonstrate such an effect in amphetamine psychosis (3). Moreover, there is a suggestion that with increasing severity of symptoms there is a decrease in dopamine turnover (22).

2. Studies of prolactin secretion in unmedicated acute (20) and chronic (19) schizophrenic patients have revealed no evidence of the decrease in

prolactin secretion, which might be expected if there were increased dopamine release from the tuberoinfundibular system.

3. Schizophrenic illnesses can occur in patients with long-standing Parkinson's disease (13), and there appears to be no particular modification of the symptoms of the one disease by the other. The significance of this coincidence is enhanced by the observation that dopamine is as depleted in mesolimbic regions as in the corpus striatum in Parkinson's disease (16). This suggests that increased dopamine release is not necessary for typically schizophrenic symptoms to be expressed.

POSTMORTEM FINDINGS

Direct observations on dopaminergic processes in schizophrenic brain are possible only on postmortem material, and by the time patients with schizophrenia die it is entirely possible that the pathological process responsible for the original illness is no longer active. Nevertheless, dopamine turnover can be assessed by measuring the levels of the metabolite HVA, and this method has produced meaningful results in the case of Parkinson's disease.

Recently we have assessed HVA, as an index of dopamine turnover, and glutamic acid decarboxylase (GAD), as an index of GABA neurons, in dopaminergically innervated areas of schizophrenic and control brain. The findings (Table 2) show no significant differences between schizophrenic and control brain with respect to either transmitter in either area.

However, a comparison of the relationship between the two parameters in the two areas (Table 3) revealed an interesting difference. Whereas in control brains and in the striatum in schizophrenics there was a strong positive correlation between GAD and HVA values, in the nucleus accumbens in the schizophrenics this relationship was absent.

Two explanations are possible. Either the action of psychotropic drugs may disrupt the interaction between GABA and dopaminergic mechanisms specifically in the nucleus accumbens, or there may in schizophrenia be a primary disturbance of this relationship which is in some way related to the

TABLE 2. HVA and GAD in dopaminergically innervated brain areas

	Controls (N = 10)	Schizophrenics (N = 10)
Putamen		
HVA	4.1 ± 2.1 (SD)	4.7 ± 2.8
(μg/g)		
GAD	4.1 ± 3.0	4.3 ± 2.8
(μmoles/g/hr)		
Accumbens		
HVA	4.3 ± 2.1	4.4 ± 2.4
GAD	5.0 ± 2.9	4.0 ± 3.0

TABLE 3. Correlation of GAD and HVA

	Controls (N = 10)	Schizophrenics (N = 10)
Putamen	0.77 (p < 0.01)	0.70 (p < 0.05)
Accumbens	0.77 (p < 0.01)	−0.01 (ns)

manifestation of the disease. A comparison of the patient group on $(N = 4)$ and off neuroleptic drugs before death suggested that the effect might not be drug related, but the numbers involved are small. With either explanation the localization of the effect to the nucleus accumbens seems of particular interest.

CONCLUSIONS

The findings of a recent trial of the isomers of flupenthixol are entirely consistent with the dopamine receptor blockade hypothesis of neuroleptic action and rule out some other possible mechanisms. However, the time course of the therapeutic effect suggests that dopamine receptor blockade, if necessary, is not directly related to the clinical improvement but is perhaps a necessary condition for other slower changes to take place which are themselves reflected in the change in clinical state. Moreover, the anti-psychotic effect may be relevant only to the positive symptoms (delusions, hallucinations, and thought disorder) of schizophrenia, and not to the negative symptoms which are the central features of the defect state.

CSF and neuroendocrine findings have cast doubt on the dopamine over-activity hypothesis of schizophrenia, and the observation that schizophrenic and parkinsonian symptoms can coexist suggests that increased dopamine release is not necessary for the expression of a schizophrenic illness. Pre-liminary studies of postmortem material from schizophrenic and control patients provide no evidence of increased dopaminergic activity but suggest the possibility of a disturbance of the relationship between GABA and dopamine neurons in the nucleus accumbens.

REFERENCES

1. Andén, N.-E. (1972): Dopamine turnover in the corpus striatum and the limbic system after treatment with neuroleptic and antiacetylcholine drugs. *J. Pharm. Pharmacol.*, 24:905–906.
2. Angrist, B., Lee, H. K., and Gershon, S. (1974): The antagonism of amphetamine-induced symptomatology by a neuroleptic. *Am. J. Psychiatry*, 131:817–819.
3. Angrist, B., Sathananthan, G., Wilk, S., and Gershon, S. (1974): Amphetamine psychosis: Behavioural and biochemical aspects. *J. Psychiatr. Res.*, 11:13–23.
4. Bennett, J. P., and Snyder, S. H. (1975): Stereospecific binding of D-lysergic acid diethylamide (LSD) to brain membranes: Relationship to serotonin receptors. *Brain Res.*, 94:523–544.

5. Bowers, M. B. (1974): Central dopamine turnover in schizophrenic syndromes. *Arch. Gen. Psychiatry,* 31:50–54.
6. Carlsson, A., and Lindqvist, M. (1963): Effect of chlorpromazine and haloperidol on formation of 3-methoxy-tyramine and normetanephrine in mouse brain. *Acta Pharmacol. Toxicol.,* 20:140–144.
7. Connell, P. H. (1958): Amphetamine psychosis. Maudsley Monograph No. 5. Chapman & Hall, London.
8. Cotes, P. M., Crow, T. J., and Johnstone, E. C. (1978): Serum prolactin as an index of dopamine receptor blockade in acute schizophrenia. *Br. J. Clin. Pharmacol.,* 4:651.
9. Creese, I., Burt, D. R., and Snyder, S. H. (1976): Dopamine receptor binding predicts clinical and pharmacological potencies of antischizophrenic drugs. *Science,* 192:481–483.
10. Crow, T. J., Deakin, J. F. W., and Longden, A. (1977): The nucleus accumbens— A possible site of antipsychotic action of neuroleptic drugs. *Psychol. Med.,* 7:213–221.
11. Crow, T. J., Frith, C. D., and Johnstone, E. C. (1978): The clinical effects of the isomers of flupenthixol—The consequences of dopamine receptor blockade in acute schizophrenia. *Br. Clin. Pharmacol.,* 4:648.
12. Crow, T. J., and Johnstone, E. C. (1977): Stereochemical specificity in the antipsychotic effects of flupenthixol in man. *Br. J. Pharmacol.,* 59:466P.
13. Crow, T. J., Johnstone, E. C., and McClelland, H. A. (1976): The coincidence of schizophrenia and Parkinsonism: Some neurochemical implications. *Psychol. Med.,* 6:227–233.
14. Ellinwood, E. H. (1967): Amphetamine psychosis: I. Description of the individuals and process. *J. Nerv. Ment. Dis.,* 144:274–283.
15. Enna, S. J., Bennett, J. P., Burt, D. R., Creese, I., and Snyder, S. H. (1976): Stereospecificity of interaction of neuroleptic drugs with neurotransmitters and correlation with clinical potency. *Nature,* 263:338–347.
16. Farley, I. J., Price, K. S., and Hornykiewicz, O. (1977): Dopamine in the limbic regions of the human brain: Normal and abnormal. In: *Non-Striatal Dopamine,* (edited by E. Costa and G. L. Gessa). Raven Press, New York.
17. Griffith, J. D., Cavanaugh, J., Held, J., and Oates, J. A. (1972): Dextroamphetamine: Evaluation of psychomimetic properties in man. *Arch. Gen. Psychiatry,* 26:97–100.
18. Gunne, L. M., Ängåard, E., and Jönsson, L. E. (1972): Clinical trials with amphetamine blocking drugs. *Psychiatr. Neurol. Neurochir.,* 75:225–226.
19. Johnstone, E. C., Crow, T. J., and Mashiter, K. (1977): Anterior pituitary hormone secretion in chronic schizophrenia—an approach to neurohumoural mechanisms. *Psychol. Med.,* 7:223–228.
20. Meltzer, H. Y., Sachar, E. J., and Frantz, A. G. (1974): Serum prolactin levels in unmedicated schizophrenic patients. *Arch. Gen. Psychiatry,* 31:564–569.
21. Miller, R. J., Horn, A. S., and Iversen, L. L. (1974): The action of neuroleptic drugs on dopamine-stimulated adenosine cyclic 3', 5'-monophosphate production in neostriatum and limbic forebrain. *Mol. Pharmacol.,* 10:759–766.
22. Post, R. M., Fink, E., Carpenter, W. T., and Goodwin, F. K. (1975): Cerebrospinal fluid amine metabolites in acute schizophrenia. *Arch. Gen. Psychiatry,* 32:1013–1069.
23. Randrup, A., and Munkvad, I. (1967): Stereotyped activities produced by amphetamine in several animal species and man. *Psychopharmacologia,* 11:300–310.
24. Randrup, A., and Munkvad, I. (1965): Special antagonism of amphetamine-induced abnormal behaviour. Inhibition of stereotyped activity with increase of some normal activities. *Psychopharmacologia,* 7:416–422.
25. van Rossum, J. M. (1966): The significance of dopamine receptor blockade for the mechanism of action of neuroleptic drugs. *Arch. Int. Pharmacodyn. Ther.,* 160:492–494.
26. Seeman, P., Lee, T., Chau-Wong, M. and Wong, K. (1976): Antipsychotic drug doses and neuroleptic/dopamine receptors. *Nature,* 261:717–719.

Advances in Biochemical Psychopharmacology, Vol. 19,
edited by P. J. Roberts et al.
Raven Press, New York © 1978.

Dopamine Receptor Mechanisms: Behavioral and Electrophysiological Studies

Urban Ungerstedt, Tomas Ljungberg, and *Wolfram Schultz

Department of Histology, Karolinska Institut, S-104 01 Stockholm, 60 Sweden

The mechanisms involved in dopamine (DA) neurotransmission have lately received considerable attention as a number of features of the DA synapse are being revealed. This chapter gives an account of two aspects of DA neurotransmission that have interested us in particular: (a) the supersensitivity developing after degeneration of the presynaptic DA nerve terminals, and (b) the postulated existence of different DA receptors.

DOPAMINE RECEPTOR SUPERSENSITIVITY

Evidence for development of supersensitivity after degeneration of the presynaptic DA nerve terminals was first shown reproducibly with the "6-hydroxydopamine rotational model" (20). 6-Hydroxydopamine was injected locally into the ascending bundle of DA axons in the mesencephalon. This caused an essentially complete degeneration of all ascending neurons. The animals developed a typical motor asymmetry deviating in their posture and movements toward the DA-denervated side. When such animals were treated with a DA releasing drug, such as amphetamine, they developed a strong rotational behavior toward the lesioned side (21). In contrast, apomorphine, which is considered to be a DA receptor stimulating drug (7), caused strong rotational behavior in the opposite direction, i.e., toward the intact side. We interpreted this (20) as an expression of DA receptor supersensitivity that had developed in DA-denervated areas as a consequence of the terminal degeneration.

The fact that animals rotated after systemic apomorphine injections indicated that the lesioned side was more sensitive than the innervated. However, it was not possible to quantify the degree of supersensitivity with the rotational method in the way it was originally used. Other investigators using various ways of injecting 6-hydroxydopamine (6,8,17,18,22) were, however, able to show a difference in motor activity between normal and denervated animals given apomorphine. Such studies indicated a 2- to 10-fold increased response as a consequence of the DA neuronal degeneration. However, motor

---

* Present address: Physiologisches Institut Der Universität Freiburg Schweiz.

activity measurements suffer from several problems such as nonlinearity and difficulties in discriminating between different behavioral patterns that may be elicited after the drug. We therefore made an attempt to modify the rotational method in order to achieve an estimation of the increased sensitivity to apomorphine after degeneration.

Animals with a unilateral 6-hydroxydopamine-induced lesion of the ascending DA axons were tested for rotational behavior after apomorphine. The animals were then subjected to electrocoagulations in various areas of the internal capsule and the lateral hypothalamus. The animals were subsequently retested on the same dose of apomorphine, and the change in rotational behavior, as a consequence of the electrocoagulation, was determined. The detailed anatomical mapping of the extent of the various lesions revealed a critical area in the crus cerebri, which was common to all lesions that reduced the apomorphine-induced rotation by more than 85% (Fig. 1) (15). The localization corresponds well with the area where striatal efferent fibers may be expected. We have therefore suggested that the strionigral pathway may serve not as a feedback pathway as originally thought but rather as the output pathway responsible for the neuronal changes causing rotational behavior in this model (15).

On the basis of these anatomical findings it is possible to create a rotational model where the sensitivity of normal DA receptors can be compared with the sensitivity of denervated DA receptors (14). We thus compared two groups of animals in which we had eliminated striatal efferent pathways on one side of all animals by electrocoagulation. Any rotational behavior would thus express only the DA receptor stimulation on the side opposite the electrocoagulation. On this side the animals were either lesioned with

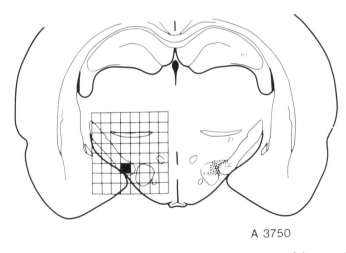

A 3750

FIG. 1. Frontal section of the rat brain showing the critical area in the crus cerebri common to all lesions reducing the apomorphine-induced rotational behavior after an ipsilateral dopamine system degeneration by more than 85%.

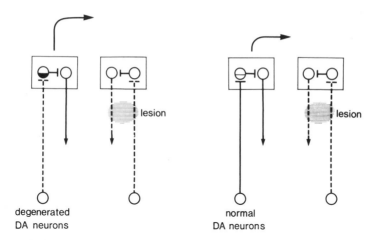

FIG. 2. Principle diagram explaining the model used to quantify the degree of supersensitivity. The two squares on the left symbolize the left and right striopallidal system in an animal with a left-sided degeneration of dopamine neurons. The two squares on the right symbolize the left and right striopallidal systems in an animal with a normal dopamine innervation on the left side. In both animals the right striopallidal systems are eliminated by a lesion which includes the critical area in Fig. 1. The difference in rotational behavior between the two types of animals is dependent only on the difference in sensitivity to apomorphine on the left side of the animals.

6-hydroxydopamine or normally innervated (Fig. 2). It was possible to directly compare the degree of rotational behaviors elicited from a normal innervated DA receptor and from a DA-denervated receptor. The comparison of the dose-response curves indicated a 10- to 40-fold difference in sensitivity (Fig. 3). This is considerably more than any other figure published. We have

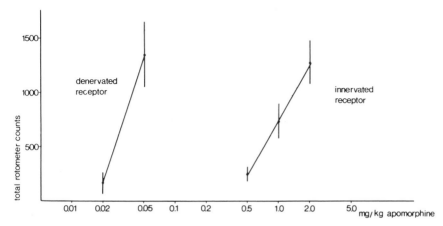

FIG. 3. Dose-response curves of the rotational behavior in dopamine-denervated and dopamine-innervated animals given different doses of apomorphine. The animals were lesioned according to the principle in Fig. 2. There is a strong shift to the left after dopamine neuron degeneration indicating a 10–40-fold difference in sensitivity to apomorphine.

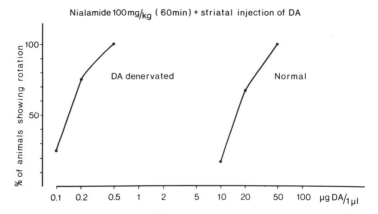

FIG. 4. Guide cannulas were implanted in normal animals and in dopamine-denervated animals ipsilateral to the denervation. After pretreatment with the monoamine oxidase inhibitor nialamide, the animals were injected into the caudate nucleus with different doses of dopamine in a total volume of 1 μl. Each animal was used only once. The diagram shows the percent of animals showing rotation at each dose tested. Each point represents 4–6 animals. There is a 100-fold increase in sensitivity to dopamine after denervation.

therefore tried to confirm these findings by studying the effects of local injections of DA into the striatum after pretreatment with a monoamine oxidase inhibitor. Figure 4 shows the percent of animals showing rotational behavior after various doses of DA. This study clearly confirms our previous study and indicates an almost 100-fold difference in sensitivity to the locally injected DA.

Apart from behavioral studies there are several reports in the literature of changes in adenylate cyclase activity after DA neuronal degeneration. However, none of these studies shows an increase in adenylate cyclase activity that corresponds to our behavioral findings. At the most there seems to be a doubling of adenylate cyclase activity (10,16). Even in studies where DA receptor binding has been compared to rotational behavior the maximum increase of ^{3}H-haloperidol binding after DA degeneration is not more than two-fold (5).

The astonishing difference between supersensitivity measured in behavioral models and supersensitivity expressed as changes in adenylate cyclase activity or receptor binding raises the question whether supersensitivity is a phenomenon occurring on the level of the neuron carrying the DA receptor or in a chain of neurons that "translates" a minor increase in DA receptor sensitivity to a strong behavioral "supersensitivity." In order to investigate this problem we studied the influence of systemically administered apomorphine on single units recorded in the striatum in normal and DA-denervated animals (19).

Striatal cells show very low spontaneous activity. When cells are isolated solely with the help of this low activity, there will be a considerable bias in that only relatively fast firing cells are discovered. In order to avoid this bias we used iontophoresis of sodium glutamate in order to excite cells.

When a single unit was isolated a base-line firing rate was established during 10 to 20 min of continuous glutamate iontophoresis. Apomorphine was then administered subcutaneously during the iontophoresis of glutamate, and the change in firing rate was noticed. Figure 5 shows the number of responding and nonresponding cells in normal as well as DA-denervated animals after various doses of apomorphine (s.c.). When comparing the two groups of animals it is apparent that there is a 10- to 80-fold increased sensitivity in the denervated animals, again confirming our findings in behavioral models. In fact, when comparing rotational behavior after a particular dose of apomorphine with the response of single cells in the striatum in the later electrophysiological analysis of the same animal, there is a surprising correspondence in the duration of the behavioral and electrophysiological change (Fig. 6). Although our electrophysiological data fit with the hypothesis that the supersensitivity response occurs at the level of the DA-denervated neuron, our lack of knowledge whether every recorded neuron carried DA receptors makes it impossible to arrive at a final conclusion concerning the "site" of supersensitivity. A major reason for the discrepancy between our findings and those reported from studies of adenylate cyclase activity or receptor binding may even be the principle by which supersensitivity is defined. In our behavioral as well as electrophysiological studies, we determine supersensitivity by looking at threshold doses for eliciting a particular response and preferably the threshold for producing any response. In the biochemical studies, however, the degree of supersensitivity is expressed as the maximal increase in the amplitude of the response. It is obvious that more research

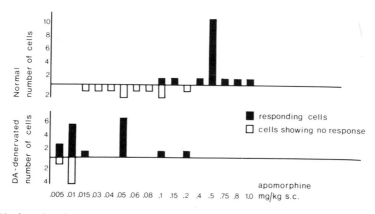

FIG. 5. Number of single units responding or not responding by decreased firing in normal striatum and denervated striatum after various doses of apomorphine. In the normally innervated striatum all cells responded after doses of apomorphine that were higher than 0.4 mg/kg. In the dopamine-denervated striatum all cells responded after doses higher than 0.015 mg/kg apomorphine. We have estimated that the denervated striatum is 10–80-fold more sensitive to apomorphine than the normal striatum (see ref. 19). The recordings from normally innervated striatum were performed in normal animals without any lesion, whereas the recordings from dopamine-denervated striatum were performed on unilaterally 6-hydroxydopamine-lesioned animals.

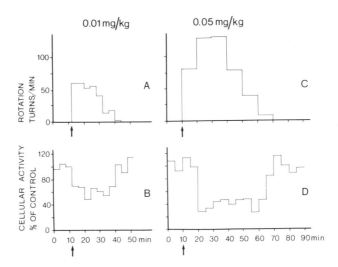

FIG. 6. Diagrams A and C show the apomorphine-induced rotational behavior after two doses of apomorphine in two different animals. Diagrams B and D show the change in firing of single units in the denervated striatum of the same animals and after the same doses of apomorphine. The electrophysiological experiments were conducted about 1 week after the behavioral experiments.

is needed before it is possible to determine which of the two definitions is most relevant in terms of neuronal functioning.

EVIDENCE FOR DIFFERENT DA SYNAPTIC MECHANISMS

The finding that degeneration of the presynaptic DA nerve terminals gives rise to supersensitive responses to DA agonists indicates that the DA receptor may exist in different states of sensitivity. The dynamics of such sensitivity changes are still largely unknown, but it seems reasonable that the receptor may exist in hypo- as well as hypersensitive states depending on the intensity of stimulation. Future investigations of the speed by which this change takes place will obviously be of considerable importance for the understanding of DA neurotransmission.

Apart from the indications that the DA receptor may exist in different states of sensitivity, several recent studies have indicated the existence of different DA receptors. The modulatory influence of DA agonists on DA release and synthesis and on electrical activity of DA neurons has led to the postulation of presynaptic DA receptors, often referred to as autoreceptors (1,2). Studies with local injections into the brain with different DA agonists and antagonists have furthermore led to the suggestion that there may exist different kinds of postsynaptic DA receptors (3).

From these considerations of different DA receptors it seems obvious that the behavior that results from the injection of a DA receptor-stimulating drug such as apomorphine (7) may be highly complex and express the inter-

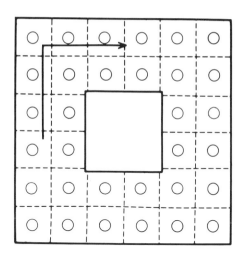

FIG. 7. Outline of the automatic testbox seen from above. The size is 69 × 69 cm. The dotted lines show the localization of photobeams detecting the movements of the animal. "Activity" was defined as the total number of photobeam interruptions. "Locomotion" was defined as the number of times the animal walked the distance corresponding to the solid arrow. The gnawing behavior was almost always performed on the edges of the holes in the bottom of the cage. This behavior was detected by a vibration sensory system which was adjusted so that one "gnaw" gave one count. For a detailed description of the box see ref. 11.

play of many different mechanisms. In order to receive a greater resolution of the behavioral recording, we have recently designed a computerized behavioral test system where we can record eight components of behavior over time (11). The design of the box and the choice of the recording parameters have been worked out empirically by observing the stereotyped behavior induced by drugs such as amphetamine and apomorphine (Fig. 7). When analyzing the behavioral patterns induced by high doses of apomorphine in habituated animals, we have recognized two behavioral components with peaks that are separated in time and that can be measured separately, i.e., locomotion and gnawing (12).

Our continued investigations of the behavior induced by low doses of apomorphine led to the astonishing finding that the locomotion pattern of behavior or the gnawing pattern of behavior could be preferentially induced depending on the site of apomorphine injection (12). When apomorphine was injected subcutaneously into the flank of the rat the gnawing pattern was induced, whereas the locomotion pattern was induced when apomorphine was injected subcutaneously in the neck of the animal (Fig. 8). The locomotion behavior, which dominates after an injection into the neck, continues to dominate with increasing doses of apomorphine, and the same is true for gnawing behavior when the injection is made into the flank. One pattern of behavior is thus not changed into another pattern of behavior as the dose is increased; instead, the patterns follow different dose-response curves. This shows that it is probably not correct to rate stereotyped behavior according to the commonly used rating scales as these scales are based on the assumption that the stereotyped behavior is transformed from a locomotor pattern to a gnawing pattern as the apomorphine dose is increased (4).

The observation that the peak of the locomotion behavior after an injection into the neck occurred before the peak of the gnawing behavior after an injection into the flank (Fig. 8) suggested to us that the effect was related

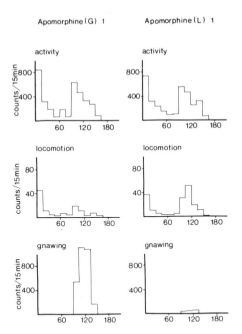

FIG. 8. Recordings of "activity," "locomotion," and "gnawing" in the automatic test box. The left part of the figure shows the gnawing (G) type of behavior after an injection of apomorphine 1 mg/kg s.c. into the flank of an animal that has habituated to the test box for 90 min. A small locomotion peak is followed by a strong gnawing peak.

The right part of the figure shows the locomotion (L) type of behavior after apomorphine 1 mg/kg s.c. into the neck. There is a relatively high locomotion peak which, however, is not followed by a gnawing peak. Note that the "activity" recordings that correspond to the most commonly used activity boxes do not distinguish between these distinctly different behavioral patterns.

to the speed of resorption from the subcutaneous injection site. We therefore prolonged the time of resorption from a neck injection by using propylene glycol as injection vehicle, and this did, in fact, induce the gnawing type of behavior instead of the locomotion type which was induced when apomorphine was injected in saline. In order to test the reversed condition, i.e., a very fast resorption, animals were lightly anesthetized with ether and in-

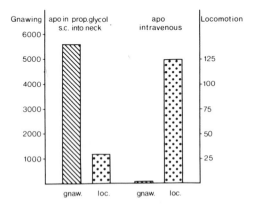

FIG. 9. Experiment designed to vary the speed by which a particular dose of apomorphine reaches the brain. When apomorphine 2 mg/kg is injected s.c. into the neck in a propylene glycol vehicle, which causes slow resorption, the animals show strong gnawing behavior and relatively little locomotion. However, the same dose of apomorphine injected i.v. into the tail vein induces a strong locomotion behavior without any gnawing. There is a significant difference (p < 0.01) for both locomotion and gnawing when the two treatments are compared.

jected into the tail vein. These animals showed strong locomotor behavior (Fig. 9). The fact that the same dose of apomorphine (2 mg/kg) induces gnawing when resorbed slowly and locomotion when injected intravenously does obviously not support the previous assumption that low doses of apomorphine induce locomotion whereas high doses induce gnawing.

It is well known that different neuroleptic drugs, i.e., different DA receptor blocking drugs, differ in their clinical properties, for example, as regards the incidence of extrapyramidal side effects (9). We therefore tested a series of neuroleptic drugs with different pharmacological profiles for their ability to inhibit the apomorphine-induced behavior. We found pronounced differences among the neuroleptic drugs in their ability to inhibit the gnawing component or the locomotion component after apomorphine 5 mg/kg s.c. In Table 1 the drugs are rated according to their relative potencies in inhibiting locomotion versus gnawing. This rating clearly separates the atypical neuroleptic drugs sulpiride, clozapine, and thioridazine from drugs such as chlorpromazine, haloperidol, and metoclopramide. When comparing this rating to the clinical experience of these drugs (9), drugs known to induce various types of extrapyramidal side effects are rated on one end of the scale while those possessing antipsychotic potency and showing low incidences of extrapyramidal side effect are on the other end of the scale.

Our studies with apomorphine show some of the complexities of DA neurotransmission. The degeneration-induced supersensitivity indicates that a change of receptor "state" may be possible. However, the factors contributing to this change are still obscure. Although our behavioral and electrophysiological studies indicate that an almost 100-fold increase in sensitivity occurs after denervation, the increase in receptor binding and adenylate cyclase activity does not seem to account for this large increase. The mechanism behind the translation of the receptor event to the behavioral output obviously remains to be explained.

TABLE 1. *Inhibition of apomorphine-induced behavior by different neuroleptics*

	Clinical profile		Animal data
	Antipsychotic	Extrapyramidal side effects	ED_{50} loc/ED_{50} gnaw[a]
Metoclopramide	No	only side effects	5.7 (17/3)
Haloperidol	Yes	+++	2.8 (0.45/0.16)
Chlorpromazine	Yes	++	1.0 (8/8)
Thioridazine	Yes	+	0.05 (1/20)
Clozapine	Yes	+	0.12 (3.5/30)
Sulpiride	Yes	+	< 0.25 (50/ > 200)

[a] The neuroleptic drugs are arranged according to the ratio ED_{50} loc/ED_{50} gnaw, which is the ratio between the ED_{50} doses for inhibiting the locomotion and the gnawing, respectively, after apomorphine 5 mg/kg s.c. (see ref. 13). This way of classifying the drugs corresponds closely to their individual properties as regards extrapyramidal side effects and antipsychotic activity.

The analysis of the behavioral patterns induced by apomorphine in normal, habituated animals reveals another interesting feature of DA neurotransmission. Depending on the speed of apomorphine resorption, an early locomotion peak or a later gnawing peak is the dominating behavioral component. The fact that the locomotion pattern does not change into the gnawing pattern when the dose is changed, and vice versa, suggests that the two behavioral responses reflect different DA synaptic mechanisms. This is further supported by the strongly different properties of neuroleptic drugs in inhibiting apomorphine-induced locomotion or gnawing. From our present knowledge of DA neurotransmission it seems reasonable to assume that the induction and the inhibition of locomotion and gnawing reflect an action on different pre- and/or postsynaptic DA receptors. Our finding that the speed of apomorphine resorption seems to have a qualitative effect on DA neurotransmission indicates that we in future studies on DA receptor mechanisms have to take into account not only the structural aspects but also the dynamics of the change in the intensity of receptor stimulation.

REFERENCES

1. Bunney, B. S., and Aghajanian, G. K. (1975): Evidence for drug actions on both pre- and postsynaptic catecholamine receptors in the CNS. In: *Pre- and Postsynaptic Receptors,* edited by E. Usdin and W. E. Bunney, Jr. Marcel Dekker Inc., New York.
2. Carlsson, A. (1975): Receptor-mediated control of dopamine metabolism. In: *Pre- and Postsynaptic Receptors,* edited by E. Usdin and W. E. Bunney, Jr. Marcel Dekker Inc., New York.
3. Cools, A. R., and van Rossum, J. M. (1976): Excitation-mediating and inhibition-mediating dopamine receptors: A new concept towards a better understanding of electrophysiological, biochemical, pharmacological, functional and clinical data. *Psychopharmacologia,* 45:243.
4. Costall, B., and Naylor, R. J. (1973): The role of telencephalic dopaminergic systems in the mediation of apomorphine-stereotyped behaviour. *Eur. J. Pharmacol.,* 24:8–24.
5. Creese, I., Burt, D. R., and Snyder, J. H. (1977): Dopamine receptor binding enhancement accompanies with lesion-induced behavioral supersensitivity. *Science,* 197:596–598.
6. Creese, I., and Iversen, S. D. (1973): Blockage of amphetamine induced motor stimulation and stereotypy in the adult rat following neonatal treatment with 6-hydroxydopamine. *Brain Res.,* 55:369–382.
7. Ernst, A. M. (1967): Mode of action of apomorphine and dexamphetamine on gnawing compulsion in rats. *Psychopharmacologia,* 10:316–323.
8. Kelly, P. H., Seviour, P. W., and Iversen, S. D. (1975): Amphetamine and apomorphine responses in the rat following 6-OHDA lesions of the nucleus accumbens septi and corpus striatum. *Brain Res.,* 94:507–522.
9. Klein, D. F., and Davis, J. (1969): *Diagnosis and Drug Treatment of Psychiatric Disorders.* Williams and Wilkins, Baltimore.
10. Krueger, B. K., Forn, J., Walters, J. R., Roth, R. H., and Greengard, P. (1976): Stimulation by dopamine of adenosine cyclic 3,5-monophosphate formation in rat caudate nucleus: Effect of lesions of the nigro-neostriatal pathway. *Mol. Pharmacol.,* 12:639–648.
11. Ljungberg, T., and Ungerstedt, U. (1978): A new method for simultaneous registration of 8 behavioral parameters related to monoamine neurotransmission. *Pharmacol. Biochem. Behav.,* 8:483–489.

12. Ljungberg, T., and Ungerstedt, U. (1977): Different behavioural patterns induced by apomorphine: Evidence that the method of administration determines the behavioural response to the drug. *Eur. J. Pharmacol.*, 46:41–50.
13. Ljungberg, T., and Ungerstedt, U. (1978): Classification of neuroleptic drugs according to their ability to inhibit apomorphine induced locomotion and gnawing. Evidence for two different mechanisms of action. *Psychopharmacology*, 56:239–247.
14. Marshall, J. F., and Ungerstedt, U. (1977): Supersensitivity to apomorphine following destruction of the ascending dopamine neurons: Quantification using the rotational model. *Eur. J. Pharmacol.*, 41:361–367.
15. Marshall, J. F., and Ungerstedt, U. (1977): Striatal efferent fibers play a role in maintaining rotational behavior in the rat. *Science*, 198:62–64.
16. Mishra, R. K., Gardner, E. L., Katzman, R., and Makman, M. H. (1974): Enhancement of dopamine-stimulated adenylate cyclase activity in rat caudate after lesions in substantia nigra: Evidence for denervation supersensitivity. *Proc. Natl. Acad. Sci. U.S.A.*, 7:3883–3887.
17. Nahorski, S. R. (1975): Behavioural supersensitivity to apomorphine following cerebral dopaminergic denervation by 6-hydroxydopamine. *Psychopharmacologia*, 42:159–162.
18. Schoenfeld, R., and Uretsky, N. (1972): Altered response to apomorphine in 6-hydroxydopamine-treated rats. *Eur. J. Pharmacol.*, 19:115–118.
19. Schultz, W., and Ungerstedt, U. (1978): Striatal cell supersensitivity in dopamine lesioned rats correlated to behavior. *Neuropharmacology (in press)*.
20. Ungerstedt, U. (1971): Postsynaptic supersensitivity after 6-hydroxydopamine induced degeneration of the nigro-striatal dopamine system. *Acta Physiol. Scand.* [*Suppl.*], 367:69–93.
21. Ungerstedt, U. (1971): Striatal dopamine release after amphetamine or nerve degeneration revealed by rotational behavior. *Acta Physiol. Scand.* [*Suppl.*], 367:49–68.
22. Uretsky, N. J., and Schoenfeld, R. I. (1971): Effect of L-dopa on the locomotor activity of rats pretreated with 6-hydroxydopamine. *Nature* [*New Biol.*], 234:157–159.

Advances in Biochemical Psychopharmacology, Vol. 19,
edited by P. J. Roberts et al.
Raven Press, New York © 1978.

Interactions of 5-Hydroxytryptamine and γ-Aminobutyric Acid with Dopamine

*C. J. Pycock, **R. W. Horton, and *C. J. Carter

Departments of Pharmacology, *The Medical School, University of Bristol,
Bristol BS8 1TD, England; and **Institute of Psychiatry, Denmark Hill,
London SE5 8AF, England

Both 5-hydroxytryptamine (5-HT) and γ-aminobutyric acid (GABA) are accepted as neurotransmitter substances in the central nervous system (32,56). Electrophysiological studies suggest that 5-HT causes predominantly inhibitory responses on those neurones clearly identified as having a 5-HT input, although some cells have been shown to exhibit excitatory responses to iontophoretically applied 5-HT (1). Similarly, GABA possesses powerful inhibitory actions on the majority of central neurons tested (39).

Examination of the regional distribution of a potential transmitter candidate may provide an insight into those areas in which it may serve a neurotransmitter role. Unlike dopamine (DA), both 5-HT and GABA are widely distributed in many regions of the brain (23,26). Central 5-HT-containing pathways are now well established, with the major 5-HT cell bodies being located in the raphe nuclei of the rostral brainstem (12,22). Whereas many

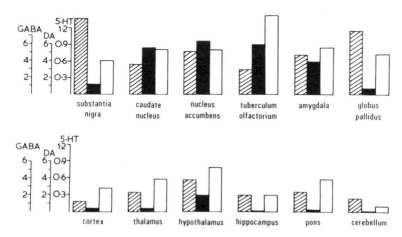

FIG. 1. Regional distribution of GABA (striped columns), DA (closed columns) and 5-HT (open columns) in rat brain. GABA is expressed as μmoles/g whereas DA and 5-HT are given as μg/g brain. (Values derived from refs. 3, 23, 26, 34, 57, and personal observations.)

brain regions are known to contain high concentrations of GABA, evidence for exact GABA-mediated neuronal pathways is less well defined. It is interesting to note that high concentrations of 5-HT and GABA are found in those areas known to contain DA (Fig. 1). Such a correlation may suggest a functional interrelationship between these two neurotransmitters and DA. These proposed interactions have been investigated in the following experiments.

5-HYDROXYTRYPTAMINE

Apart from the high concentrations of 5-HT found in those areas of the brain rich in DA terminals, there is evidence of 5-HT-mediated inputs in the region of DA cell bodies. A projection from the raphe to the substantia nigra has been demonstrated electrophysiologically in the rat (24), whereas autoradiographic studies show inputs from the raphe to the area of the nucleus interpeduncularis in the cat (8).

This evidence suggests that 5-HT-mediated inputs are potentially capable of modifying activity in the nigroneostriatal and mesolimbic pathways, which on the basis of the electrophysiological evidence is likely to be inhibitory.

5-Hydroxytryptamine-Dopamine: Biochemical Interactions

There is little reported work on a functional biochemical interaction between the monoamine neurotransmitters DA and 5-HT. The experimental work of Grabowska (29) suggests that DA receptor stimulation following apomorphine results in increased 5-HT levels, whereas DA receptor blockade reduces 5-HT concentrations (10).

In this study the possible relationship between DA and 5-HT in the nucleus accumbens of the rat has been investigated. The concentrations of the DA metabolites homovanillic acid (HVA) and dihydroxyphenylacetic acid (DOPAC) were measured (70) following bilateral focal injections of 5-HT into the nucleus accumbens, and, conversely, the concentrations of 5-HT and its metabolite 5-hydroxyindoleacetic acid (5-HIAA) were estimated (21) after injection of DA. DA (range 5 to 50 μg in 2 μl) or 5-HT (oxalate salt 5 and 25 μg in 2 μl) was injected bilaterally into the nucleus accumbens of rats implanted with guide cannulas 2 days previously. The stereotaxic coordinates used in this and all subsequent cannulations were derived from the atlas of König and Klippel (42).

Injection of DA caused no significant changes in the concentrations of 5-HT or 5-HIAA in either the striatum or nucleus accumbens (Fig. 2), although 5-HT concentrations tended to decrease and 5-HIAA levels to increase in the limbic area with the higher concentrations of DA injected, suggesting an increased 5-HT turnover. Conversely, injection of 5-HT into

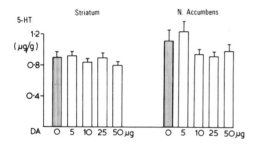

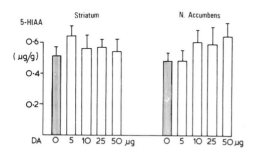

FIG. 2. Effect of DA (5–50 μg) injected bilaterally into the nucleus accumbens on the concentrations of 5-HT (*upper trace*) and 5-HIAA (*lower trace*) in striatum and accumbens. Rats were killed 1 hr after injection. Results are the mean of 6 observations: vertical bars represent SE.

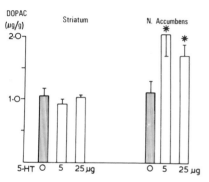

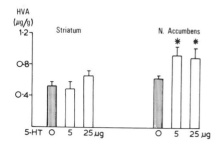

FIG. 3. Effect of 5-HT (5 and 25 μg) injected bilaterally into the nucleus accumbens on the concentrations of HVA (*upper trace*) and DOPAC (*lower trace*) in striatum and accumbens. Rats were killed 1 hr after injection. Results are the mean of 6 observations: vertical bars represent SE. *$p < 0.05$.

the nucleus accumbens was associated with significant increases in the concentrations of DOPAC and HVA indicative of an enhanced turnover of DA in this brain region (Fig. 3). Striatal DA metabolite levels were not significantly altered.

Systemic administration of various drugs which modify cerebral 5-HT mechanisms was also accompanied by changes in DA turnover (Fig. 4). The putative 5-HT receptor blocking drug metergoline (28) (5 mg/kg) caused significant decreases of HVA and DOPAC concentrations in limbic and striatal areas, although no changes were observed in the region of the substantia nigra. Quipazine (25 mg/kg), a proposed 5-HT agonist (33), tended to increase HVA and DOPAC levels in limbic and striatal regions, although no points were of statistical significance (Fig. 4). Neither ORG 6582 (20 mg/kg) (Organon Laboratories), a proposed 5-HT uptake blocking compound (65), nor fenfluramine (20 mg/kg), an amphetamine derivative with a preferential releasing effect on 5-HT terminals (14), significantly altered DA metabolite levels in any of the regions assayed.

The results of these experiments suggest that enhancing 5-HT function is associated with increased DA turnover, whereas blocking 5-HT mechanisms decreases DA turnover. However, such changes in transmitter turnover as reported above must be viewed with caution since many drugs have a broad

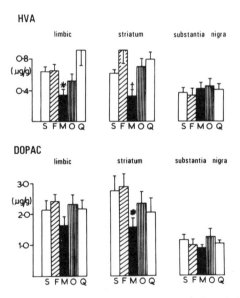

FIG. 4. Effect of fenfluramine (F) (20 mg/kg), metergoline (M) (5 mg/kg), ORG 6582 (O) (20 mg/kg), and quipazine (Q) (25 mg/kg) on concentrations of HVA (upper trace) and DOPAC (lower trace) in limbic (nucleus accumbens + tuberculum olfactorium), striatal, and nigral regions (left to right) of rat brain. All drugs were administered intraperitoneally: animals were killed 1 hr after drug injection. Control animals received saline (S). Results are the mean of 6 observations: vertical bars represent SE. *$p < 0.05$; †$p < 0.01$.

spectrum of pharmacological activity. A direct effect of the drug, rather than a secondary alteration in turnover of one transmitter in response to a primary pharmacological manipulation of another transmitter, cannot be entirely excluded.

5-Hydroxytryptamine-Dopamine: Behavioral Interactions

Manipulation of central DA mechanisms results in three main behavioral states—hyperactivity and stereotypy following DA receptor stimulation and catalepsy associated with DA receptor blockade. Each of these can be modified or, in some cases, initiated by altering central 5-HT function.

It has been shown that depletion of cerebral 5-HT levels either by administration of p-chlorophenylalanine (PCPA) or following lesion of the raphe nuclei induces hyperactivity (37,60,63). Conversely, injection of 5-HT into discrete brain regions can abolish the hyperactive response induced by DA agonists (18).

These general concepts are supported in the following experiments. 5-HT (range 1 to 25 μg) injected bilaterally into the nucleus accumbens exerted a powerful inhibitory action on the hyperactive response in the rat induced by the systemic administration of amphetamine (1 mg/kg) (Fig. 5). The suppression has a rapid onset and a dose-dependent duration.

Bilateral injection of DA into nucleus accumbens of nialamide-pretreated rats evokes a dose-related hyperactive response (54). Bilateral injection of methysergide (range 1 to 10 μg in 2 μl saline), a proposed 5-HT receptor antagonist (6), potentiated the locomotor activity of rats previously injected with a threshold dose of DA (5 μg) (Fig. 6). The effect lasted approximately 1 hr.

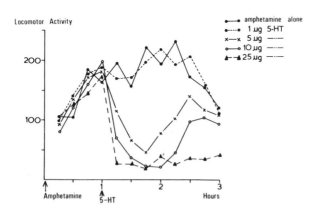

FIG. 5. Effect of 5-HT (range 1–25 μg) injected bilaterally into the nucleus accumbens on the hyperactive response induced by amphetamine (1 mg/kg, i.p.) in rats. Locomotor activity was assessed with each animal placed individually in a photocell box. The units represent the number of interruptions of a single light beam in each 15-min period. Each point is the mean of 6–8 observations. SEs were in the range 10%–15% and are omitted for clarity.

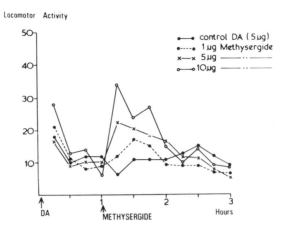

FIG. 6. Effect of methysergide (1–10 μg) injected bilaterally into the nucleus accumbens 1 hr after injection of 5 μg DA bilaterally into the same site. Rats were pretreated 2 hr previous to the DA injection with nialamide (50 mg/kg; i.p). Each point is the mean of 6 observations as in the legend to Fig. 5.

Catalepsy is the maintenance of an abnormal position or posture. This behavioral state is usually an index of decreased DA transmission, but can be reduced by lesions of the raphe nuclei (15) or pretreatment with PCPA (44). Similarly, 5-HT antagonists have been reported to antagonize the effects of neuroleptic-induced catalepsy (49), whereas we have observed a potentiation of the cataleptic response to haloperidol following systemic administration of proposed 5-HT agonists, uptake blocking agents, and the 5-HT precursor 5-hydroxytryptophan (5-HTP) (11). Figure 7 shows the enhanced cataleptic response to haloperidol (1 mg/kg) following quipazine

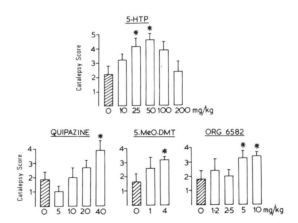

FIG. 7. Effect of 5-HTP, quipazine, 5-MeO-DMT, and ORG 6582 on the cataleptic response induced in rats by haloperidol (1 mg/kg). Catalepsy was assessed according to a numerical scoring system (ref. 15) 1 hr after haloperidol. All agents were administered intraperitoneally; 5-HTP 1 hr prior to, ORG 6582 simultaneously, and quipazine and 5-MeO-DMT 30 min after haloperidol. Each column is the mean of 6 observations: vertical bars represent SE. *$p < 0.05$.

(40 mg/kg), 5-methoxy-N,N-dimethyltryptamine (5-Meo-DMT)(31) (1 and 4 mg/kg), ORG 6582 (5 and 10 mg/kg), and 5-HTP (25 and 50 mg/kg).

Hyperactivity and catalepsy represent opposite ends of a behavioral spectrum. Classically this spectrum is interpreted in terms of DA receptor function. The above results suggest a reciprocal relation for 5-HT receptor activity in these behavioral states. Such a system is expressed simplistically in Fig. 8.

Although catalepsy and hyperactivity may represent a balanced DA:5-HT system (Fig. 8), stereotyped behavior is less easily interpreted. Various authors report enhanced stereotypy to DA agonists following blockade of cerebral 5-HT function (7,68,69) or reduced stereotypy following pretreatment with 5-HTP (68,69). Conversely, other workers note decreased stereotypy following lesions of the raphe nuclei (16). In preliminary studies we have found that stereotypy to apomorphine (0.25 to 1 mg/kg) can be potentiated by low doses of quipazine (1.2 and 2.5 mg/kg) and ORG 6582 (1 mg/kg) and antagonized by metergoline (2 and 4 mg/kg) (Fig. 9). Interestingly, the higher doses of the 5-HT agonists had no effect nor reduced the stereotypic intensity in keeping with original observations (68,69).

At present it is difficult to assess the complete role of 5-HT (and, indeed, of other central neurotransmitters) in stereotyped behaviors. Certainly the classic stereotypic agents apomorphine and amphetamine are known to affect 5-HT mechanisms, and the above experimental data emphasize its importance. The different types of behaviors (sniffing, hyperactivity, gnawing) observed following focal injection of DA or putative DA agonists into various DA-containing regions may be interpreted in terms of different DA receptors (52). However, it is possible that such effects may in part reflect a differential

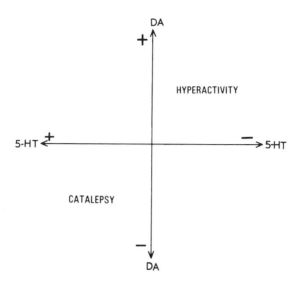

FIG. 8. Hypothetical representation of the interaction between DA and 5-HT in the behavioral states of hyperactivity and catalepsy (see text).

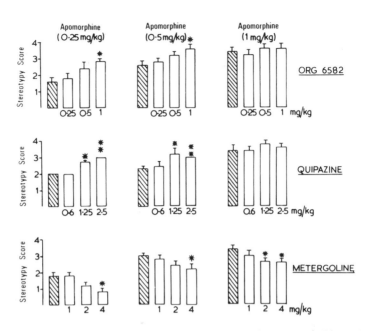

FIG. 9. Effect of ORG 6582 (0.25–1 mg/kg) (*upper trace*), quipazine (0.6–2.5 mg/kg) (*central trace*), and metergoline (1–4 mg/kg) (*lower trace*) on apomorphine-induced stereotypy in rats. Apomorphine (0.25–1 mg/kg) was given subcutaneously and stereotypy was assessed according to a numerical scoring system (ref. 16). All 5-HT drugs were administered intraperitoneally simultaneously with apomorphine. Each column is the mean of 6 observations: vertical bars represent SE. *p < 0.05; **p < 0.005.

DA:5-HT interaction. Injection of DA into tuberculum olfactorium results in mild locomotor stimulation and stereotyped sniffing and biting, whereas injection into the nucleus accumbens is associated with hyperactivity (17). Such behavioral differences may be related to the fact that the tuberculum olfactorium contains approximately twice the concentration of 5-HT as the nucleus accumbens (57).

5-Hydroxytryptamine-Dopamine: A Functional Relationship

From the behavioral aspects it is apparent that 5-HT activity can modify various DA-dependent behaviors. For example, drugs facilitating 5-HT transmission enhance neuroleptic catalepsy or potentiate stereotypy seen to DA agonists, whereas 5-HT antagonists cause the reverse. However, it is probably important that the functional status of the DA receptor already be defined, i.e., it must, for example, be partially blocked by the neuroleptic drug before 5-HT agonists cause potentiation of the behavioral response.

Biochemically a DA:5-HT relationship also exists. DA receptor stimulation usually results in hyperactivity, decreased DA turnover, and increased 5-HT turnover. The reverse is true for DA receptor blockade which induces catalepsy. 5-HT agonists tend to increase DA turnover, potentiate catalepsy, and inhibit hyperactivity. 5-HT antagonists decrease DA turnover, reduce catalepsy, and enhance hyperactivity. These results support the reciprocal 5-HT:DA relationship illustrated in Fig. 8.

GABA

On biochemical and neuroanatomical evidence, a functional relationship between GABA and DA has been proposed (35). However, the extent and exact sites for such an interaction are still the subject of much research and speculation. There is strong experimental evidence to support a GABA-mediated pathway from the striatopallidal complex to the substantia nigra (40,48). Such a pathway is believed to exert an inhibitory influence on the nigroneostriatal DA tract (48).

GABA-Dopamine: Biochemical Interactions

To date there are few reports investigating the biochemical interactions between GABA and DA in the brain. Direct DA receptor stimulation with apomorphine increases GABA turnover (53), whereas DA receptor blockade is reported as decreasing GABA levels in substantia nigra, striatum,

Table 1. *Effect of EOS on regional GABA concentrations and DA turnover and of reserpine and haloperidol on GABA concentrations in rat brain*

Treatment	Transmitters and metabolites assayed	Striatum	Brain regions Limbic (nucleus accumbens + tuberculum olfactorium)	Ventral mid-brain (including substantia nigra)
Control	DA	2.88 ± 0.23	2.77 ± 0.35	0.36 ± 0.12
	HVA	0.42 ± 0.04	0.31 ± 0.01	0.34 ± 0.04
	DOPAC	1.17 ± 0.14	1.25 ± 0.10	0.61 ± 0.15
	GABA	1.43 ± 0.13	2.37 ± 0.08	1.70 ± 0.19
EOS	DA	3.86 ± 0.97 (134%)	3.01 ± 0.56 (109%)	0.39 ± 0.09 (108%)
	HVA	0.36 ± 0.04 (84%)	0.28 ± 0.02 (91%)	0.29 ± 0.02 (85%)
	DOPAC	0.94 ± 0.17 (80%)	0.82 ± 0.15 (68%)[a]	0.63 ± 0.07 (103%)
	GABA	6.15 ± 0.40 (430%)[b]	9.44 ± 1.99 (398%)[b]	5.00 ± 0.61 (294%)[b]
Reserpine	GABA	1.55 ± 0.08 (108%)	2.35 ± 0.09 (99%)	1.84 ± 0.14 (108%)
Haloperidol	GABA	1.53 ± 0.22 (107%)	2.15 ± 0.14 (91%)	1.69 ± 0.13 (99%)

For treatment times and doses see text. DA and its metabolites expressed as $\mu g/g$: GABA is given as $\mu moles/g$. Each value is the mean of 6 results ± SEM.
[a] $p < 0.05$.
[b] $p < 0.005$ (Student's t-test).

and limbic structures (41,50). Conversely, focal injections of GABA into substantia nigra elevate brain DA levels (2).

We have investigated the effect of elevated cerebral GABA concentrations on DA turnover in discrete brain areas using ethanolamine O-sulfate (EOS), an active-site-directed inhibitor of the GABA-metabolizing enzyme GABA transaminase (GABA-T) (27). Rats received an injection of EOS (100 μg in 1.5 μl saline) into the lateral ventricle and were killed after 24 hr. In different series of rats, GABA (30), DA (47), HVA, and DOPAC (70) concentrations were estimated in striatum, limbic areas (nucleus accumbens and tuberculum olfactorium), and ventral mid-brain including substantia nigra. EOS caused a three to fourfold increase in GABA concentrations in all regions and a 34% rise in striatal DA levels ($p > 0.05$) (Table 1). EOS caused a general decrease of HVA and DOPAC concentrations in both striatal and limbic regions, limbic DOPAC levels being significantly lowered ($p < 0.05$). Although not outstandingly striking, EOS pretreatment tends to decrease DA turnover, a result in agreement with the recent work of Huot et al. (36) who showed a similar pattern following treatment with γ-acetylenic GABA, another catalytic inhibitor of GABA-T (38).

Alternatively, we could demonstrate no effect on GABA concentration following manipulation of central DA mechanisms. Neither reserpine (10 mg/kg, 12 hr) nor haloperidol (3 mg/kg, 2 hr) affected GABA levels in striatal, limbic, or ventral mid-brain regions, although we are unable to comment on the effectiveness of such treatments on the turnover rate of intraneuronal GABA.

GABA-Dopamine: Behavioral Interactions

Electrophysiological studies support the hypothesis that GABA exerts an inhibitory influence on DA neurons (5,19,62). The current evidence suggests the existence of a GABAergic (inhibitory)-dopaminergic link in striatum (4,13,46) and substantia nigra (19,48).

Behavioral data add weight to the postulated GABA-mediated control of the nigroneostriatal DA pathway. For example, rotational behavior can be elicited by manipulating GABA mechanisms in the region of one substantia nigra (25,52,67). In this section we have focused our interest toward the possible GABA-mediated control of DA function within the mesolimbic system and in particular in the nucleus accumbens. Previous work has suggested such a control exists (55,64), and we have previously demonstrated that EOS-induced elevation of GABA concentrations within the region of the nucleus accumbens inhibits both the hyperactivity response following bilateral DA injection into this site and the increased locomotor activity normally seen after systemically administered amphetamine (55). Apomorphine-induced stereotyped behavior patterns, however, were not significantly changed (55). Further support for a GABA:DA interaction within

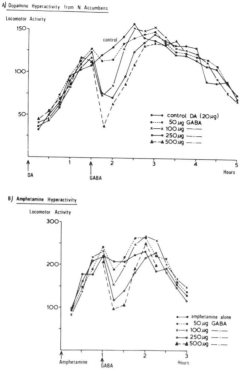

FIG. 10. Effect of GABA (50–500 μg) injected bilaterally into the nucleus accumbens on (A) DA-induced hyperactivity following focal injection of DA (20 μg) bilaterally into this site 90 min previously, and (B) amphetamine-induced hyperactivity (1 mg/kg, i.p., 1 hr previously). Rats were pretreated with nialamide (50 mg/kg, i.p.) 2 hr previous to the DA injection. Each point is the mean of 6 observations as in the legend to Fig. 5.

the nucleus accumbens is provided by Scheel-Krüger and colleagues (59) who demonstrated an antagonism of ergometrine-induced locomotor activity by the potent GABA agonist muscimol, and from Huot et al. (36) using γ-acetylenic GABA.

We now report that GABA itself, when injected bilaterally into the nucleus accumbens in concentrations of 100 to 500 μg, causes a dose-dependent depression of both the effect of locally applied DA (20 μg) and that of systemically administered amphetamine (1 mg/kg) (Fig. 10). The effect was rapid in onset and short in duration, lasting a maximum of 30 to 40 min. The brevity of the effect presumably reflects the high-affinity uptake mechanisms for the removal of GABA. During the period of the GABA effect on the locomotor activity, animals appeared normal and did not become cataleptic. A similar result was obtained using the putative GABA agonist 3-aminopropane sulfonic acid (3-APS) (20). When injected bilaterally into the nucleus accumbens, 3-APS (range 10 to 40 μg) inhibited, in a dose-dependent manner, the hyperactive response seen following DA (20 μg)

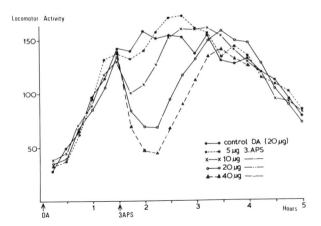

FIG. 11. Effect of 3-APS (10–40 μg) injected bilaterally into the nucleus accumbens 90 min after injection of 20 μg DA bilaterally into the same site. Rats were pretreated 2 hr previous to the DA injection with niala-mide (50 mg/kg, i.p.). Each point is the mean of 7 observations as in the legend to Fig. 5.

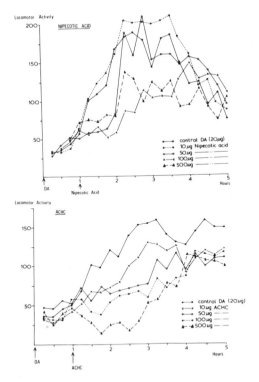

FIG. 12. Effect of two putative blocking agents of GABA uptake—nipecotic acid (10–500 μg) (upper trace) and ACHC (10–500 μg) (lower trace)—injected bilaterally into the nucleus accumbens 1 hr after injection of 20 μg DA bilaterally into the same site. Rats were pretreated 2 hr previous to the DA injection with nialamide (50 mg/kg, i.p.). Each point is the mean of 6–8 observations as in the legend to Fig. 5.

administration to this site (Fig. 11). 3-APS proved to be approximately 10-fold as effective as GABA in this model with a longer duration, lasting approximately 1.5 hr.

A class of compounds now being widely applied to various aspects of GABA pharmacology is the GABA uptake blocking compounds (66). We have investigated two such compounds—nipecotic acid and cis-1,3-aminocyclo-hexane carboxylic acid (ACHC)—in our model of nucleus accumbens DA function. Both compounds caused a depression of the DA-dependent hyper-active response elicited from the nucleus accumbens (Fig. 12). Nipecotic acid (range 10 to 500 μg) was most effective at the 100-μg dose resulting in a significant depression of activity for about 3 hr. The higher dose of 500 μg was not as effective. In a similar way ACHC caused a dose-related depression of activity, the range 50 to 500 μg being significantly effective, indicating a more potent action than that of nipecotic acid.

From these studies it is not possible to predict whether these putative uptake-blocking compounds are having a direct effect on central GABA (or any other) receptors or that the behavioral changes observed are purely the result of an enhanced action of endogenously released GABA. Nipecotic acid is a powerful noncompetitive inhibitor of GABA uptake (45) which is probably effective on both neuronal and glial mechanisms (9). ACHC is reported to be a selective inhibitor of neuronal GABA uptake (9) with some possible intrinsic receptor action since iontophoretically applied ACHC inhibits the firing of central neurons (61). It is indeed likely that these com-pounds are, at least in part, acting by inhibiting GABA reuptake. The fact

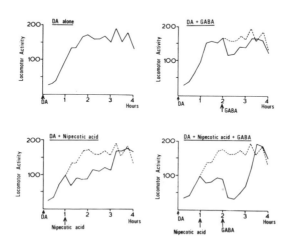

FIG. 13. Effect of nipecotic acid (100 μg) and GABA (100 μg) injected bilaterally into the nucleus ac-cumbens 1 and 2 hr, respectively, after injection of 20 μg bilaterally into the same site. Rats were pre-treated 2 hr previous to the DA injection with nialamide (50 mg/kg, i.p.). Each point is the mean of 6 observations as in the legend to Fig. 5.

that ACHC was apparently more effective on our system than nipecotic acid might imply that neuronal uptake of GABA is of more significance than glial uptake in this region of the brain, although no positive statements regarding the predominance of glial or neuronal uptake can be made at this stage.

In an additional experiment we were able to show that nipecotic acid was able to potentiate and prolong the effects of GABA in the DA hyperactivity model (Fig. 13). Alone both nipecotic acid (100 μg) and GABA (100 μg) resulted in some depression of the locomotor response seen following bilateral injection of DA (20 μg) into the region of the nucleus accumbens. Together the effects were potentiated suggesting a result mediated by blockade of the major GABA inactivation mechanism (reuptake).

Blockade of GABA receptors (picrotoxin, bicuculline) in the region of the nucleus accumbens leads to increased arousal, myoclonic jerks, and a potentiation of the DA-dependent hyperactive response mediated from this site (C. J. Pycock, R. W. Horton, and C. J. Carter, *unpublished observations*).

GABA-Dopamine: A Functional Relationship

The results presented above together with other reported work provide biochemical and behavioral support for an inhibitory role of GABA on DA mechanisms at various sites in the brain (e.g., substantia nigra, striatum, and limbic areas). The behavioral and electrophysiological evidence provides convincing data that GABA receptor stimulation directly inhibits the results of DA receptor stimulation. The biochemical data are less strong as the available results seem conflicting. For example, it has been shown that elevated GABA concentrations decrease DA turnover, whereas blocking DA receptors with neuroleptic drugs decreases GABA turnover.

In general, the studies of central GABA pharmacology implicate a reciprocal GABA:DA relationship in the brain. However, some anomalies have been shown to exist which might disrupt our general hypothesis. For example, behavioral excitation has been reported following either injection of the GABA agonist muscimol into the region of the substantia nigra (58) or chronically elevated nigral GABA concentrations after repeated EOS injection (43). As emphasized by Scheel-Krüger and colleagues (58), the interpretation of such results may be more complex than to just suppose a single GABA-DA inhibitory link at that site in the brain. It is possible that several regulatory GABA systems may be involved, or that we must contemplate the existence of changes in GABA receptor sensitivity following chronic elevation of cerebral GABA concentrations. Whatever mechanisms are involved, further research is required to establish fully the extent of the GABA:DA relationship within the central nervous system.

CONCLUSIONS

Manipulation of DA mechanisms in laboratory animals produces profound alterations in behavior which are not directly seen after modifying other neurotransmitter systems. These behaviors are consistently reproducible and quantifiable and therefore provide a useful basis on which to investigate other neurotransmitter functions. The techniques used in this study have employed both systemic administration and direct injections of drugs. Although open to the criticisms of additional factors such as structural damage and spread of drugs, intracerebral injection methods are one of the few brain research techniques available for studying the biochemical and behavioral aspects of local transmitter actions. It is also the method for applying putative transmitter substances rather than synthetic drugs which often have a broad spectrum of pharmacological activity.

The general conclusion is that both 5-HT and GABA exert inhibitory influences on DA function with the postulate of a reciprocal balance between 5-HT and DA and GABA and DA in the brain. In this respect 5-HT and GABA would appear similar, although one has an apparently organized system of neuronal pathways and the other, a ubiquitous distribution. In support of similar actions on DA, it is interesting to observe that GABA function would equally well fit into the hypothetical balance designed for 5-HT (Fig. 8). Such functional interactions offer the possibilities of treating those neurological disorders primarily related to DA dysfunction (Parkinson's disease, dyskinesias, psychoses) with agents other than the classic dopaminergic drugs. At present, few known compounds specifically interact with either 5-HT or GABA transmitter mechanisms, but the hunt is on.

ACKNOWLEDGMENTS

C. J. P. and R. W. H. thank the National Fund for Crippling Diseases for financial support. C. J. C. acknowledges support from the Medical Research Council. We thank Dr. N. Bowery for generous supplies of ACHC, Dr. G. A. R. Johnston for nipecotic acid, Dr. J. Watkins for 3-APS, and Dr. M. Sugrue for ORG 6582. We thank Farmitalia for supplies of metergoline, Sandoz Ltd. for methysergide, Miles Laboratories for quipazine, Smith Kline & French for dexamphetamine sulfate, and Searle for haloperidol. The expert technical assistance of Mrs. Shirley Burns is gratefully acknowledged.

REFERENCES

1. Aghajanian, G. K., Haigler, H. J., and Bennett, J. L. (1975): Amine receptors in CNS. III. 5-Hydroxytryptamine in brain. In: *Handbook of Psychopharmacology, Vol. 6,* edited by L. L. Iversen, S. D. Iversen, and S. H. Snyder, pp. 63–96. Plenum Press, New York.

2. Andén, N.-E., and Stock, G. (1973): Inhibitory effect of gammahydroxybutyric acid and gammaaminobutyric acid on the dopamine cells in the substantia nigra. *Naunyn-Schmiedebergs Arch. Pharmacol.,* 279:89–92.
3. Balcom, G. J., Lenox, R. H., and Meyerhoff, J. L. (1975): Regional γ-aminobutyric acid levels in rat brain determined after microwave fixation. *J. Neurochem.,* 24:609–613.
4. Bartholini, G., and Stadler, H. (1977): Evidence for an intrastriatal GABA-ergic influence on dopamine neurones of the cat. *Neuropharmacology,* 16:343–347.
5. Bernardi, G., Marciani, M. G., Morocutti, C., and Giacomini, P. (1976): The action of picrotoxin and bicuculline on rat caudate neurones inhibited by GABA. *Brain Res.,* 102:379–384.
6. Bieger, D., Larochelle, L., and Hornykiewicz, O. (1972): A model for the quantitative study of central dopaminergic and serotoninergic activity. *Eur. J. Pharmacol.,* 18:128–136.
7. Blum, K., Wallace, J. E., Meyer, E., and Schwertner, H. A. (1977): Intensification of amphetamine-induced excitation by methysergide, a serotonergic receptor blocker. *Experientia,* 33:213–215.
8. Bobillier, P., Seguin, S., Petitjean, F., Salvert, ·D., Touret, M., and Jouvet, M. (1976): The raphé nuclei of the cat brain stem: A topographical atlas of their efferent projections as revealed by autoradiography. *Brain Res.,* 113:449–486.
9. Bowery, N. G., Jones, G. P., and Neal, M. J. (1976): Selective inhibition of neuronal GABA uptake by cis-1,3-aminocyclohexane carboxylic acid. *Nature,* 264:281–283.
10. Bürki, H. R., Ruch, W., and Asper, H. (1975): Effects of clozapine, thioridazine, perlapine and haloperidol on the metabolism of the biogenic amines in the brain of the rat. *Psychopharmacologia,* 41:27–33.
11. Carter, C. J., and Pycock, C. J. (1977): Possible importance of 5-hydroxytryptamine in neuroleptic-induced catalepsy. *Br. J. Pharmacol.,* 60:267–268P.
12. Conrad, L. C. A., Leonard, C. M., and Pfaff, D. W. (1974): Connections of the median and dorsal raphé nuclei in the rat: An autoradiographic and degeneration study. *J. Comp. Neurol.,* 156:179–206.
13. Cools, A. R., and Janssen, H.-J. (1976): γ-Aminobutyric acid: The essential mediator of behaviour triggered by neostriatally applied apomorphine and haloperidol. *J. Pharm. Pharmacol.,* 28:70–74.
14. Costa, E., Groppetti, A., and Revuelta, A. (1971): Action of fenfluramine on monoamine stores of rat tissues. *Br. J. Pharmacol.,* 41:57–64.
15. Costall, B., Fortune, D. H., Naylor, R. J., Marsden, C. D., and Pycock, C. (1975): Serotonergic involvement with neuroleptic catalepsy. *Neuropharmacology,* 14:859–868.
16. Costall, B., and Naylor, R. J. (1974): Stereotyped and circling behaviour induced by dopaminergic agonists after lesions of the midbrain raphé nuclei. *Eur. J. Pharmacol.,* 29:206–222.
17. Costall, B., and Naylor, R. J. (1975): The behavioural effects of dopamine applied intracerebrally to areas of the mesolimbic system. *Eur. J. Pharmacol.,* 32:87–92.
18. Costall, B., Naylor, R. J., Marsden, C. D., and Pycock, C. J. (1976): Serotoninergic modulation of the dopamine response from the nucleus accumbens. *J. Pharm. Pharmacol.,* 28:523–526.
19. Crossman, A. R., Walker, R. J., and Woodruff, G. N. (1973): Picotoxin antagonism of γ-aminobutyric acid inhibitory responses and synaptic inhibition in the rat substantia nigra. *Br. J. Pharmacol.,* 49:696–698.
20. Curtis, D. R., and Watkins, J. C. (1961): Analogues of glutamic acid and γ-amino-n-butyric acid having potent actions on mammalian neurones. *Nature,* 191:1010–1011.
21. Curzon, G., and Green, A. R. (1970): Rapid method for the determination of 5-hydroxytryptamine and 5-hydroxyindoleacetic acid in small regions of rat brain. *Br. J. Pharmacol.,* 39:653–655.
22. Dahlström, A., and Fuxe, K. (1964): Evidence for the existence of monoamine-containing neurons in the central nervous system. I. Demonstration of monoamines

in the cell bodies of brain stem neurons. *Acta Physiol. Scand.* [*Suppl. 232*], 62:1–55.

23. Deguchi, T., and Barchas, J. (1972): Regional distribution and developmental change of tryptophan hydroxylase activity in rat brain. *J. Neurochem.*, 19:927–929.

24. Dray, A., Gonye, T. J., Oakley, N. R., and Tanner, T. (1976): Evidence for the existence of a raphé projection to the substantia nigra in rat. *Brain Res.*, 113:45–57.

25. Dray, A., Oakley, N. R., and Simmonds, M. A. (1975): Rotational behaviour following inhibition of GABA metabolism unilaterally in the rat substantia nigra. *J. Pharm. Pharmacol.*, 27:627–629.

26. Fahn, S. (1976): Regional distribution studies of GABA and other putative neurotransmitters and their enzymes. In: *GABA in Nervous System Function*, edited by E. Roberts, T. N. Chase, and D. B. Tower, pp. 169–186. Raven Press, New York.

27. Fowler, L. J. (1973): Analysis of the major amino acids of rat brain after *in vivo* inhibition of GABA transaminase by ethanolamine O-sulphate. *J. Neurochem.*, 21:437–440.

28. Fuxe, K., Agnati, L., and Everitt, B. (1975): Effects of methergoline on central monoamine neurons. Evidence for a selective blockade of central 5-HT receptors. *Neurosci. Lett.*, 1:283–290.

29. Grabowska, M. (1976): The involvement of serotonin in the mechanism of central action of apomorphine. *Pol. J. Pharmacol. Pharm.*, 28:389–394.

30. Graham, L. T., and Aprison, M. H. (1966): Fluorometric determination of aspartate, glutamate and γ-aminobutyrate in nerve tissue using enzymic methods. *Anal. Biochem.*, 15:487–497.

31. Grahame-Smith, D. G. (1971): Inhibitory effect of chlorpromazine on the syndrome of hyperactivity produced by L-tryptophan or 5-methoxy-N,N-dimethyltryptamine in rats treated with a monoamine oxidase inhibitor. *Br. J. Pharmacol.*, 43:856–864.

32. Green, A. R., and Grahame-Smith, D. G. (1975): 5-Hydroxytryptamine and other indoles in the central nervous system. In: *Handbook of Psychopharmacology, Vol. 3*, edited by L. L. Iversen, S. D. Iversen, and S. H. Snyder, pp. 169–245. Plenum Press, New York.

33. Hong, E., Sancilia, L., Vargas, R., and Pardo, E. G. (1969): Similarities between the pharmacological actions of quipazine and serotonin. *Eur. J. Pharmacol.*, 6:274–280.

34. Hornykiewicz, O. (1966): Dopamine (3-hydroxytryptamine) and brain function. *Pharmacol. Rev.*, 18:925–964.

35. Hornykiewicz, O., Lloyd, K. G., and Davidson, L. (1976): The GABA system, function of the basal ganglia, and Parkinson's disease. In: *GABA in Nervous System Function*, edited by E. Roberts, T. N. Chase, and D. B. Tower, pp. 479–485. Raven Press, New York.

36. Huot, S., Lippert, B., Palfreyman, M. G., and Schechter, P. J. (1977): Inhibition of dopaminergic activity in the extrapyramidal and limbic systems by γ-acetylenic GABA. *Br. J. Pharmacol.*, 60:264–265P.

37. Jacobs, B. L., Wise, W. D., and Taylor, K. M. (1974): Differential behavioural and neurochemical effects following lesions of the dorsal or medium raphé nuclei in rats. *Brain Res.*, 79:353–361.

38. Jung, M. J., Lippert, B., Metcalfe, B. W., Schechter, P. J., Böhlen, P., and Sjoerdsma, A. (1977): The effect of 4-amino hex-5-ynoic acid (γ-acetylenic GABA, γ-ethynyl GABA), a catalytic inhibitor of GABA transaminase, on brain GABA metabolism *in vivo*. *J. Neurochem.*, 28:717–723.

39. Kelly, J. S., and Beart, P. M. (1975): Amino acid receptors in CNS. II. GABA in supraspinal regions. In: *Handbook of Psychopharmacology, Vol. 4*, edited by L. L. Iversen, S. D. Iversen, and S. H. Snyder, pp. 129–209. Plenum Press, New York.

40. Kim, J. S., Bak, I. J., Hassler, R., and Okada, Y. (1971): Role of γ-aminobutyric acid (GABA) in the extrapyramidal motor system: 2. Some evidence for the existence of a type of GABA-rich strionigral neurons. *Exp. Brain Res.*, 14:95–104.

41. Kim, J.-S., and Hassler, R. (1975): Effects of acute haloperidol on the gamma-aminobutyric acid system in rat striatum and substantia nigra. *Brain Res.*, 88:150–153.

42. König, J. F. R., and Klippel, R. A. (1963): *The Rat Brain*. Williams & Wilkins, Baltimore.
43. Koob, G. F., Del Fiacco, M., and Iversen, S. D. (1977): Dissociable properties of dopamine neurons in the nigrostriatal and mesolimbic dopamine systems. *Adv. Biochem. Psychopharmacol.*, 16:589–595.
44. Kostowski, W., Gumulka, W., and Czlonkowski, A. (1972): Reduced cataleptogenic effects of some neuroleptics in rats with lesioned midbrain raphé and treated with *p*-chlorophenylalanine. *Brain Res.*, 48:443–446.
45. Krogsgaard-Larsen, P., and Johnston, G. A. R. (1975): Inhibition of GABA uptake in rat brain slices by nipecotic acid, various isoxazoles and related compounds. *J. Neurochem.*, 25:797–802.
46. Ladinsky, H., Consolo, S., Bianchi, S., and Jori, A. (1976): Increase in striatal acetylcholine by picrotoxin in the rat: Evidence for a GABAergic-dopaminergic-cholinergic link. *Brain Res.*, 108:351–361.
47. Laverty, R., and Sharman, D. F. (1965): The estimation of small quantities of 3,4-dihyproxyphenylethylamine in tissues. *Br. J. Pharmacol.*, 24:538–548.
48. McGeer, P. L., McGeer, E. G., and Hattori, T. (1977): Dopamine-acetylcholine-GABA neuronal linkages in the extrapyramidal and limbic systems. *Biochem. Psychopharmacol.*, 16:397–402.
49. Maj, J., Mogilnicka, E., and Przewlocka, B. (1975): Antagonistic effect of cyproheptadine on neuroleptic-induced catalepsy. *Pharmacol. Biochem. Behav.*, 3:25–27.
50. Marco, E., Mao, C. C., Cheney, D. L., Revuelta, A., and Costa, E. (1976): The effects of antipsychotics on the turnover rate of GABA and acetylcholine in rat brain nuclei. *Nature*, 264:363–365.
51. Neumeyer, J. L., Dafeldecker, W. P., Costall, B., and Naylor, R. J. (1977): Aporphines. 21. Dopaminergic activity of aporphine and benzylisoquiniline derivatives. *J. Med. Chem.*, 20:190–196.
52. Oberlander, C., Dumont, C., and Boissier, J. R. (1977): Rotational behaviour after unilateral intranigral injection of muscimol in rats. *Eur. J. Pharmacol.*, 43:389–390.
53. Pérez de la Mora, M., Fuxe, K., Hökfelt, T., and Ljungdahl, Å. (1975): Effect of apomorphine on the GABA turnover in the DA cell group rich area of the mesencephalon. Evidence for the involvement of an inhibitory GABAergic feedback control of the ascending DA neurons. *Neurosci. Lett.*, 1:109–114.
54. Pijnenburg, A. J. J., and van Rossum, J. M. (1973): Stimulation of locomotor activity following injection of dopamine into the nucleus accumbens. *J. Pharm. Pharmacol.*, 25:1003–1005.
55. Pycock, C. J., and Horton, R. W. (1976): Possible GABA-mediated control of dopamine-dependent behavioural effects from the nucleus accumbens of the rat. *Psychopharmacology*, 49:173–179.
56. Roberts, E. (1974): γ-Aminobutyric acid and nervous system function—a perspective. *Biochem. Pharmacol.*, 23:2637–2649.
57. Saavedra, J. M., Brownstein, M., and Palkovits, M. (1974): Serotonin distribution in the limbic system of the rat. *Brain Res.*, 79:437–441.
58. Scheel-Krüger, J., Arnt, J., and Magelund, G. (1977): Behavioural stimulation induced by muscimol and other GABA agonists injected into the substantia nigra. *Neurosci. Lett.*, 4:351–356.
59. Scheel-Krüger, J., Cools, A. R., and Honig, W. (1977): Muscimol antagonizes the ergometrine-induced locomotor activity in nucleus accumbens: Evidence for a GABA-dopaminergic interaction. *Eur. J. Pharmacol.*, 42:311–313.
60. Segal, D. S. (1976): Differential effects of para-chlorophenylalanine on amphetamine-induced locomotion and stereotypy. *Brain Res.*, 116:267–276.
61. Segal, M., Sims, K., and Smissman, E. (1975): Characterisation of an inhibitory receptor in rat hypothalamus: A microiontophoretic study using conformationally restricted amino acid analogues. *Br. J. Pharmacol.*, 54:181–188.
62. Spehlmann, R., Norcross, K., and Grimmer, E. J. (1977): GABA in the caudate nucleus: A possible synaptic transmitter of interneurones. *Experientia*, 33:623–625.
63. Srebro, B., and Lorens, S. A. (1975): Behavioral effects of selective midbrain raphé lesions in the rat. *Brain Res.*, 89:303–325.

64. Stevens, J., Wilson, K., and Foote, W. (1974): GABA blockade, dopamine and schizophrenia. Experimental studies in the cat. *Psychopharmacologia,* 39:105–119.
65. Sugrue, M. F., Goodlet, I., and Mireylees, S. E. (1976): On the selective inhibition of serotonin uptake *in vivo* by Org 6582. *Eur. J. Pharmacol.,* 40:121–130.
66. Tapia, R. (1975): Biochemical pharmacology of GABA in CNS. In: *Handbook of Psychopharmacology, Vol. 4,* edited by L. L. Iversen, S. D. Iversen, and S. H. Snyder, pp. 1–58. Plenum Press, New York.
67. Tarsy, D., Pycock, C., Meldrum, B., and Marsden, C. D. (1975): Rotational behaviour induced in rats by intranigral picrotoxin. *Brain Res.,* 89:160–165.
68. Weiner, W. J., Goetz, C., and Klawans, H. L. (1975): Serotonergic and antiserotonergic influences on apomorphine-induced stereotyped behaviour. *Acta Pharmacol. Toxicol.,* 36:155–160.
69. Weiner, W. J., Goetz, C., Westheimer, R., and Klawans, H. L. (1973): Serotonergic and antiserotonergic influences on amphetamine-induced stereotyped behaviour. *J. Neurol. Sci.,* 20:373–379.
70. Westerink, B. H. C., and Korf, J. (1976): Regional rat brain levels of 3,4-dihydroxyphenylacetic acid and homovanillic acid: Concurrent fluorometric measurement and influence of drugs. *Eur. J. Pharmacol.,* 38:281–291.

Advances in Biochemical Psychopharmacology, Vol. 19,
edited by P. J. Roberts et al.
Raven Press, New York © 1978.

GABA-Dopamine Interaction in Substantia Nigra and Nucleus Accumbens—Relevance to Behavioral Stimulation and Stereotyped Behavior

J. Scheel-Krüger, *J. Arnt, C. Bræstrup, **A. V. Christensen,
†A. R. Cools, and G. Magelund

*Psychopharmacological Research Laboratory, Dept. E., Sct. Hans Hospital Roskilde, Den-mark: *Department of Pharmacology, The Royal Danish School of Pharmacy, Copenhagen, Denmark; **Department of Pharmacology, H. Lundbeck & Co., Copenhagen, Denmark; and †Department of Pharmacology, University of Nijmegen, Nijmegen, The Netherlands*

Recently we found that muscimol (1 to 10 ng) and several other GABA-ergic drugs, baclofen (0.1 μg), imidazole acetic acid (10 μg), and GABA (10 to 100 μg), injected unilaterally into the caudal substantia nigra, pars reticulata (SNR), induced a strong contralateral turning in rats. The bilateral injection of muscimol (10 to 100 ng) induced strong stereotyped behavior—head movements, sniffing, licking, and gnawing (4).

The contralateral turning and behavioral stimulation of muscimol was found independent of dopamine receptor activity, since haloperidol, perphena-zine, or reserpine plus α-methyltyrosine did not antagonize. Muscimol bi-laterally injected into the SNR (2 × 10 ng) immediately antagonized the neuroleptic-induced catalepsy (4). Neither did a 6-OH-dopamine (8 μg in-jection into the SNR) lesion of the nigrostriatal dopamine pathway antag-onize the muscimol-induced contralateral turning. However, the muscimol-induced turning was antagonized by locally injected bicuculline methiodide (0.1 μg) or picrotoxin (0.25 μg) (J. Arnt and J. Scheel-Krüger, *unpublished observations*). These data are against the traditionally considered hypothesis that GABA within the substantia nigra only inhibits dopamine neuronal ac-tivity but emphasizes another and/or an additional role of GABA in this area.

However, muscimol influenced biochemically the nigrostriatal dopamine pathway: The neostriatal levels of the dopamine metabolites HVA and DOPAC were significantly ($p < 0.05$) increased 30 min after muscimol, 25 ng injected into the right SNR, 139% and 142%, respectively, compared to the control side (1 μl saline into the left SNR). The dopamine level was increased 60 min after muscimol (143% $p < 0.01$), and the DOPAC and HVA levels further increased (170% and 150%, $p < 0.01$). The L-DOPA accumulation measured 30 min after NSD 1015 (100 mg/kg i.p.) was significantly increased (196% compared to the saline side, $p < 0.01$) by muscimol, 25 ng injected in the SNR 5 min before NSD 1015.

These data indicate increased dopamine synthesis in neostriatum after muscimol injected into the SNR. All these results may agree with the hypothesis that muscimol, like GABA, inhibits the impulse flow in the nigrostriatal dopamine pathway. However, the behavioral effects of the highly potent and specific GABA agonist muscimol (see 3,4) are mediated by a nondopaminergic mechanism involving GABA. The nucleus accumbens in the rat represents another brain area with high levels of the neurotransmitters dopamine and GABA (7). We have therefore been interested in the possible modulatory influence of GABA within this area on two dopamine-dependent behavioral effects, the locomotor activity and the stereotyped behavior induced by ergometrine or apomorphine. The locomotor activity induced by the dopamine agonist ergometrine 1 μg bilaterally injected into the nucleus accumbens was completely antagonized for up to 3 hr following the injection of muscimol, 10 ng bilaterally into the accumbens (7). By direct inspection of the rats in the photocell activity cages, it was seen that these rats were calm and silent without stereotypies.

In another series of experiments muscimol (10 and 100 ng) was injected bilaterally into the nucleus accumbens and 10 min later a dose of 0.25 mg/kg apomorphine was injected subcutaneously into the neck. Muscimol especially in the 100-ng dose induced a strong increase in continuous licking and gnawing already seen 5 to 10 min after 0.25 mg/kg apomorphine. Walking and rearing after apomorphine were strongly depressed by muscimol (8). Muscimol (10 ng) injected bilaterally into the accumbens of naive rats induced *per se* no gross behavioral changes, whereas 100 ng induced sedation increasing to catalepsy 1 hr after the injection. These results indicate that a

TABLE 1. *Muscimol facilitates stereotyped gnawing*

Treatment	Distribution of gnawing activity (%)			
	0	+	++	+++
NaCl + apomorph. (10)	85	10	5	0
Musc. + apomorph. (10)	20	73	0	7
NaCl + meth.phen. (10)	90	5	5	0
Musc. + meth.phen. (10)	10	0	10	80

Muscimol HBr 1 mg/kg s.c. was given 15 min before apomorphine (10 mg/kg s.c.) or methylphenidate (10 mg/kg s.c.). The mice were placed in the gnawing cages immediately after apomorphine or methylphenidate for 1 hr, 2 mice in each cage. At least 10 groups of 2 mice were used for each schedule. The gnawing was measured on corrugated paper placed in the bottom of the cages. The gnawing activity is shown as the percentage distribution of gnawing activity obtained for each cage as classified according to the following rank scale: 0, +, ++, +++.

GABAergic mechanism within nucleus accumbens differentially influences two dopamine-dependent behavioral effects—locomotor activity and stereotyped behavior.

The same profile of action was found in mice after nonsedative doses of muscimol given in combination with high stimulant doses of dopaminergic drugs such as apomorphine, cocaine, or methylphenidate. All drugs were given systemically (6): The pretreatment with muscimol HBr 1 mg/kg s.c. 15 min before apomorphine 1.5 mg/kg s.c. or cocaine 10 mg/kg i.p. induced a remarkable state of sedation in the mice, also measured in the Motron activity cages as a highly significant reduction in activity compared with the controls, which received only saline or muscimol. However, muscimol HBr 1 mg/kg s.c. given 15 min before higher doses of cocaine 30 mg/kg i.p. or methylphenidate (10 mg/kg s.c.) induced a remarkable facilitation of stereotyped gnawing in the mice (Table 1). The profile of action of muscimol is thus clearly different from that of antipsychotic neuroleptic drugs with dopamine receptor blocking properties, since these drugs antagonize both motility and stereotypy (5). The nucleus accumbens has for some time mainly been associated with dopamine-dependent motility (5). However, recently Cools (1) found a modifying influence on apomorphine stereotyped behavior after the injection of ergometrine or DPI into the nucleus accumbens, and he interpreted the results as related to an influence on functionally different types of dopamine receptors and/or different dopamine systems. Costall et al. (2) have injected several dopamine derivatives into the accumbens and suggested the presence of different dopamine mechanisms within this nucleus involved in the regulation of locomotor activity and stereotyped behavior.

The present results with muscimol given either systemically or locally into the accumbens invite the hypothesis that this GABA agonist differentially is able to modify various dopamine systems and/or receptors involved in dopamine-dependent locomotor activity and stereotyped behavior.

REFERENCES

1. Cools, A. R. (1977): Two functionally and pharmacologically distinct dopamine receptors in the rat brain. *Adv. Biochem. Psychopharmacol.*, 16:215–225.
2. Costall, B., Naylor, R. J., Cannon, J. G., and Lee, T. (1977): Differentiation of the dopamine mechanisms mediating stereotyped behaviour and hyperactivity in the nucleus accumbens and caudate-putamen. *J. Pharm. Pharmacol.*, 29:337–342.
3. Naik, S. R., Guidotti, A., and Costa, E. (1976): Central GABA receptor agonists: Comparison of muscimol and baclofen. *Neuropharmacology*, 15:479–484.
4. Scheel-Krüger, J., Arnt, J., and Magelund, G. (1977): Behavioural stimulation induced by muscimol and other GABA agonists injected into the substantia nigra. *Neurosci. Lett.*, 4:351–356.
5. Scheel-Krüger, J., Bræstrup, C., Nielsen, M., Golembiowska, K., and Mogilnicka, E. (1977): Cocaine: Discussion on the role of dopamine in the biochemical mechanism of action. *Adv. Behav. Biol.*, 21:373–407.
6. Scheel-Krüger, J., Christensen, A. V., and Arnt, J. (1978): Muscimol differentially facilitates stereotypy but antagonizes motility induced by dopaminergic drugs: A complex GABA-dopamine interaction. *Life Sci.*, 22:75–134.

7. Scheel-Krüger, J., Cools, A. R., and Honig, W. (1977): Muscimol antagonizes the ergometrine-induced locomotor activity in nucleus accumbens: Evidence for a GABA-dopaminergic interaction. *Eur. J. Pharmacol.* 42:311–313.

8. Scheel-Krüger, J., Cools, A. R., and van Wel, P. M. (1977): Muscimol a GABA-agonist injected into the nucleus accumbens increases apomorphine stereotypy and decreases motility. *Life Sci.,* 21:1697–1702.

Advances in Biochemical Psychopharmacology, Vol. 19,
edited by P. J. Roberts et al.
Raven Press, New York © 1978.

Neurochemical and Behavioral Correlates of Chronic Apomorphine Administration in the Rat

Marie Kenny and B. E. Leonard

Pharmacology Department, University College, Galway, Republic of Ireland

The systemic administration of apomorphine produces stereotyped behavior in several animal species. Following acute apomorphine administration, this behavior is often characterized by compulsive sniffing, licking, and gnawing at the wire mesh of the cage, and occasionally by stereotyped fighting (1,2,4). Strömbom (3) has shown that whereas low doses (< 0.2 mg/kg) of apomorphine depress motor activity in rodents, higher doses (> 0.2 mg/kg) have the opposite effect. The aim of the present study was therefore to investigate the effects of various doses of apomorphine given daily for up to 14 days on the nature of the stereotyped response. The study was extended to see if it was possible to correlate the different types of stereotypy which occur immediately following the subcutaneous injection of the drug with the behavior of the animals in an "open field" apparatus some 9 hr after injection when stereotypy is absent. Lastly, the changes in the concentrations of the catecholamines, serotonin, and γ-aminobutyric acid (GABA) were studied in four brain regions of rats given low (0.1 mg/kg) and high (0.75 mg/kg) chronic doses of the dopamine agonist to see if there was an obvious correlation between the behavioral and neurochemical changes. We also studied the changes in the concentrations of these neurotransmitters in groups of rats showing the "sniffing" and "fighting" stereotypy after 1 mg/kg apomorphine.

In the first experiment, the effect of 1 mg/kg (given twice daily) s.c. of apomorphine was studied. Initially, most rats showed a characteristic sniffing and burrowing behavior; some animals reared and licked the cage walls. However, 3 days after the commencement of the experiment, some 30% of the animals started stereotyped fighting, and the intensity of this response increased with each succeeding drug treatment to such an extent that the dose of drug was reduced first to 0.5 mg/kg once daily (from days 5 through 9) and then to 0.25 mg/kg once daily (from days 9 through 14) in order to maintain the animals in good health. Although the dose of drug was reduced, the intensity and time of onset of the stereotyped fighting were unaffected even though the duration of the response was decreased. Approximately 20%

of the rats showed the sniffing-burrowing responses throughout the period of drug treatment, whereas the remaining 50% exhibited irritability and fighting which alternated with intense rearing and chewing stereotypy. From this experiment, it would appear that in an apparently homogeneous group of Wistar rats (male; 160 to 180 g), there are two distinct types of stereotyped responses ("sniffing" and "fighting") which occur with the same dose of drug. Furthermore, a sensitivity develops a few days after the commencement of drug administration to apomorphine in those animals showing the stereotyped fighting response but not those showing the sniffing and burrowing response. When rats showing only "sniffing" or "fighting" stereotypy were later studied in the "open field" apparatus, it was found that the "fighters" had a higher rearing score and the "sniffers" a lower rearing score than the saline-injected controls; both groups showed increased grooming activity throughout the period of drug treatment. Only the "sniffers" differed appreciably from the controls with respect to the ambulation score—this was decreased particularly toward the end of the drug treatment period and for at least 1 week after drug withdrawal.

In the second experiment, various doses of apomorphine (0.1, 0.5, 0.75, and 1.0 mg/kg s.c. twice daily) were given to groups of rats for 7 days and the nature of their stereotypy assessed in their home cages for 90 min after injection. In general, there was a qualitative relationship between the type of behavior and the dose of the agonist administered with stereotyped fighting being more pronounced with doses above 0.5 mg/kg and hypersexuality (male-male mounting) occurring mainly with the lowest dose studied. Sniffing and burrowing was also more prominent in groups given 0.75 mg/kg of apomorphine. Thus there appears to be some correlation between the chronic dose administered and the nature of the stereotyped response.

In the biochemical study, changes in the concentrations of serotonin, norepinephrine, dopamine, and GABA were determined in the olfactory tubercle, striatum, mid-brain, and brainstem after the administration of 0.1 or 0.75 mg/kg s.c. (twice daily) for 7 days. Animals were killed 15 hr after the last dose. Striatal serotonin, norepinephrine, and GABA concentrations were significantly raised in the lowest dose group; the only change in the group given 0.75 mg/kg of the drug was a reduction in norepinephrine.

In the olfactory tubercle, the concentration of dopamine was raised in the 0.75 mg/kg group but unchanged in the 0.1 mg/kg group, whereas the GABA concentration rose in this brain region after the lowest dose but was unchanged after the highest dose. No changes in the concentration of these neurotransmitters occurred in the brainstem or mid-brain regions. In an attempt to assess the effect of these chronic doses of apomorphine on catecholamine turnover in the four brain regions, we determined the extent of amine depletion after α-methylparatyrosine administration. In the striatum, the lowest dose of apomorphine had no effect on turnover whereas the highest dose increased dopamine turnover. In the midbrain, the 0.1 mg/kg dose decreased dopamine turnover whereas the highest dose had no effect. No change occurred in norepinephrine turnover in any brain region, neither was there a significant change in dopamine turnover in the olfactory tuberculum.

In the second biochemical study, changes in the concentrations of the four neurotransmitters were determined in the same four brain regions in groups of rats which showed the two distinct types of stereotypy ("sniffing" and "fighting") after 1 mg/kg apomorphine. Striatal dopamine, olfactory tubercle norepinephrine, and brainstem GABA concentrations were significantly increased in the "sniffing" group whereas no changes were observed in any of these parameters in the four brain areas of the "fighting" groups.

From these studies it would appear that no direct correlation exists between the nature of the stereotyped response to chronic apomorphine and the changes in neurotransmitter concentrations in those brain regions which have been functionally implicated in drug-induced stereotypy. The increased striatal dopamine turnover after the chronic administration of 0.75 mg/kg apomorphine may correlate with the greater frequency of rearing seen in these animals in the "open field" apparatus. Clearly, more detailed investigations must be undertaken before any satisfactory correlations may be found between the complex behavior and discrete neurochemical changes which occur after chronic apomorphine administration.

ACKNOWLEDGMENT

The authors wish to thank Organon International B.V., The Netherlands, for financial assistance.

REFERENCES

1. Ernst, A. M. (1965): Relation between the action of dopamine and apomorphine and their O-methylated derivatives upon the CNS. *Psychopharmacologia,* 7:391–399.
2. Rossum, J. M. van (1970): Mode of action of psychomotor stimulant drugs. *Int. Rev. Neurobiol.,* 12:307–383.
3. Strömbom, U. (1975): On the functional role of pre- and postsynaptic catecholamine receptors in brain. *Acta Physiol. Scand. [Suppl.],* 431:1–43.
4. Ther, L., and Schramm, H. (1962): Apomorphine-synergismus (Zwangsnagen bei Mäusen) als Test zur Differenzienung psychotroper Substanzen. *Arch. Int. Pharmacodyn. Ther.,* 138:302–310.

Advances in Biochemical Psychopharmacology, Vol. 19,
edited by P. J. Roberts et al.
Raven Press, New York © 1978.

Dopamine-mimetic Activity of Some Aminotetralins, as Revealed by the Production of Cyclic AMP in Rabbit Retina *In Vitro*

*Michel Schorderet and ** John McDermed

*Department of Pharmacology, School of Medicine, Geneva, Switzerland; and
**Department of Chemistry, Wellcome Research Laboratories,
Research Triangle Park, North Carolina 27709

Previous work performed with isolated retina of calf, rat (1,2), and rabbit (3,4,9,10) has shown that this preparation is very suitable for detecting dopamine activity of various drugs, as revealed by the production of cyclic AMP. Derivatives of aminotetralins have recently been synthesized (7,8) and their ability to activate dopamine receptors tested *in vivo* (5,7,8). Since several parameters at the pharmacokinetic and/or pharmacodynamic level may complicate the interpretation of data from such investigations *in vivo* (5,7,8), each of several aminotetralins was applied on the retinal system in order to gain better insight into the structural requirements of such compounds for dopamine agonist activity and thereby to infer whether the structure of dopamine receptors in the retina is similar to or different from that of receptors in other tissues, such as brain (G. N. Woodruff; P. Seeman; *this volume*) or kidney (L. I. Goldberg, *this volume*).

The methods employed for the dissection and isolation of the rabbit retina have been described elsewhere (3,4,9,10). Following a preincubation period of 40 min at 35°C, a final 10-min incubation was performed at the same temperature in a Krebs-Ringer medium (pH 7.4) containing 5 mM theophylline. Cyclic AMP and proteins were then measured as described (9). For each experiment, a pool of 20 half-retinas was used with at least 5 kept as controls. A comparison to the potency of dopamine was then made with each of the potential agonists at concentrations from 10^{-4} to 5×10^{-7} M. Dopamine was used as a positive control in each experiment. Agonist activity of a compound was considered to be absent when cyclic AMP levels in the experimental half-retinas were not significantly different from those of the untreated controls (Student's *t*-test). Compounds which were found to be ineffective at 10^{-4} M concentration were not tested at lower concentrations. It has been previously shown that the rabbit retina contains a homogeneous population of catecholamine-containing cells, namely, the dopamine cells located in the inner nuclear layer (6). At maximally (10^{-4} M) and half-maximally (10^{-6} M) effective concentrations, a dopamine analogue (epinine) and a dopamine-mimetic drug (apomorphine) are as potent as dopamine in stimulating cyclic AMP accumulation (3,4,9,10). In contrast, although epinephrine and norepinephrine are also as potent as dopamine at 10^{-4} M concentration, they have no stimulating effects at 10^{-6} M (11). This and other evidence suggest that the occurrence of α- and β-adrenergic receptors in rabbit retina is very unlikely (11).

Table 1 shows the results obtained with intact retinas exposed to several aminotetralins. Compounds 1 to 4 are as potent as dopamine at 10^{-4} M concentration. However, when the same compounds are tested at lower concentrations (e.g., 5×10^{-6} M, Table 1), it is found that compound 1 is ineffective, consonant with experiments *in vivo* using three different pharmacological tests (8). The latter compound has been shown to be 10 to 100 times less potent than the other analogues such as 2, 3, and 4 (8). At concentrations lower than 10^{-4} M (e.g., 5×10^{-6} M), compounds 2, 3, and 4 are still as potent as dopamine in experiments *in vitro*. Of these three dihydroxy compounds the substitution at nitrogen in compound 4 appears to be optimum for activity *in vivo* (8). Unexpectedly, however, it was found that compound 4 at 5×10^{-7} M was ineffective, in contrast to small agonist effects of compound 3. This single discrepancy between experiments *in vivo* (8) and *in vitro* (*this study*) is unexplained and needs further investigation.

A second class of aminotetralins includes compounds 5, 6, and (+)-7, which are totally devoid of dopamine agonist activity at the highest concentration used (10^{-4} M). Compounds 5 and (+)-7 failed to stimulate emesis in dogs at relatively high doses (8). The inactivity of compound 6 *in vitro* (Table 1) suggests that its activity *in vivo* (8) may be due to demethylation after subcutaneous injection. The lack of stimulating effects *in vitro* with compound 5 (Table 1) is notable. This seems to confirm the observations *in vivo* (8) that cyclization of the nitrogen substituents in 2-aminotetralins abolishes their dopamine-mimetic activity, regardless of the substitution pattern in the aromatic ring. Finally, it may be noted that compound ($\pm$)-7 is a noncatechol derivative whose effectiveness depends on its stereoconfiguration, since the dextro enantiomer is inactive, whereas the racemate and the levo enantiomer induce a significant accumulation of cyclic AMP (Table 1). Comparable results have been obtained in binding studies (P. Seeman, *this volume*) where the dextro enantiomer was shown to be poorly active, in contrast to the levo enantiomer. In retina, the levo enantiomer is still effective at 5×10^{-6} M concentration, although the cyclic AMP increases induced by ($\pm$)- or ($-$)-7 are 70% lower than those of dopamine (Table 1). Still, these results would support an earlier conclusion that catechol group in 2-aminotetralins is not indispensable for dopamine-mimetic activity (7,8).

Taken together, these investigations *in vitro* confirm that some aminotetralins are potent dopamine agonists (5,7,8). Whether this simple test *in*

TABLE 1. *The effects of some aminotetralins (AMT) on cyclic AMP concentrations (pmoles per mg protein) compared with those of dopamine (DA) in intact retina of rabbit*

	Concentration of AMT or DA (C = control retinae)		
	5×10^{-7}	5×10^{-6}	10^{-4} M
1	N.T.	C = 16.9 ± 1.4(5) DA = 65.7 ± 6.3(5)* 1 = 20.4 ± 0.6(5)**	C = 21.8 ± 2.1(5) DA = 74.8 ± 17.3(3)* 1 = 88.4 ± 12.1(5)*
2	C = 13.9 ± 1.3(5) DA = 35.5 ± 7.6(5)* 2 = 14.0 ± 1.6(5)**	C = 16.9 ± 1.4(5) DA = 65.7 ± 6.3(5)* 2 = 53.8 ± 6.3(5)*	C = 12.6 ± 1.0(5) DA = 43.5 ± 2.7(3)* 2 = 35.4 ± 4.8(5)*
3	C = 17.0 ± 1.1(8) DA = 46.9 ± 3.2(10)* 3 = 25.2 ± 2.0(10)+	C = 18.3 ± 1.3(5) DA = 63.3 ± 8.9(5)* 3 = 72.1 ± 11.(5)*	C = 21.5 ± 1.5(5) DA = 45.7 ± 9.5(3)* 3 = 63.6 ± 12.9(5)*
4	C = 15.6 ± 1.1(5) DA = 44.5 ± 5.7(5)* 4 = 19.5 ± 1.9(5)**	C = 18.3 ± 1.3(5) DA = 63.3 ± 8.9(5)* 4 = 79.9 ± 10.4(5)*	C = 16.4 ± 0.9(5) DA = 38.1 ± 6.4(5)* 4 = 55.2 ± 9.8(5)**
5	N.T.	N.T.	C = 15.7 ± 0.6(10) DA = 42.9 ± 4.8(10)* 5 = 17.9 ± 1.0(10)**

Table 1. Continued

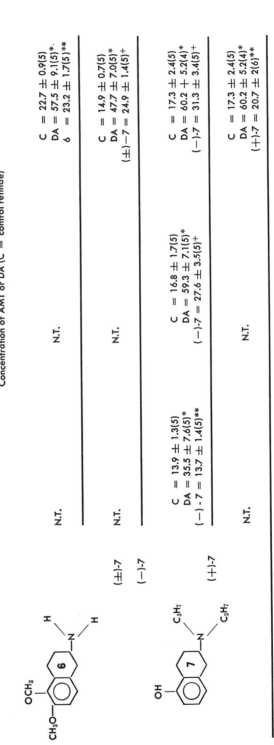

	Concentration of AMT or DA (C = control retinae)		
6	N.T.	N.T.	C = 22.7 ± 0.9(5) DA = 57.5 ± 9.1(5)*. 6 = 23.2 ± 1.7(5)**
(±)-7	N.T.	N.T.	C = 14.9 ± 0.7(5) DA = 47.7 ± 7.0(5)* (±)-7 = 24.9 ± 1.4(5)+
(−)-7	C = 13.9 ± 1.3(5) DA = 35.5 ± 7.6(5)* (−)-7 = 13.7 ± 1.4(5)**	C = 16.8 ± 1.7(5) DA = 59.3 ± 7.1(5)* (−)-7 = 27.6 ± 3.5(5)+	C = 17.3 ± 2.4(5) DA = 60.2 + 5.2(4)* (−)-7 = 31.3 ± 3.4(5)+
7 (+)-7	N.T.	N.T.	C = 17.3 ± 2.4(5) DA = 60.2 ± 5.2(4)* (+)-7 = 20.7 ± 2(6)**

The data are means ± SEM for the number of experiments given in parentheses. Statistical analysis is performed according to Student's t- test: * different from control (p < 0.05); ** not different from control (p > 0.05); † different from control and from DA (p < 0.05). N.T. = not tested.

vitro using isolated retina may be satisfactory for rapid screening of any agent interacting with pre- and/or postsynaptic receptors needs further studies.

ACKNOWLEDGMENTS

This work was supported by grant number 3.544.075 from the Swiss National Science Foundation. The authors express thanks to Mrs. C. Kolakofsky-Blank for excellent technical assistance.

REFERENCES

1. Brown, J. H., and Makman, M. H. (1972): Stimulation by dopamine of adenylate cyclase in retinal homogenates and of adenosine-3':5'-cyclic monophosphate formation in intact retina. *Proc. Natl. Acad. Sci. U.S.A.*, 69:539–543.
2. Brown, J. H., and Makman, M. H. (1973): Influence of neuroleptic drugs and apomorphine on dopamine-sensitive adenylate cyclase of retina. *J. Neurochem.*, 21: 477–479.
3. Bucher, M. B., and Schorderet, M. (1974): Apomorphine-induced accumulation of cyclic AMP in isolated retinas of the rabbit. *Biochem. Pharmacol.*, 23:3079–3082.
4. Bucher, M. B., and Schorderet, M. (1975): Dopamine- and apomorphine-sensitive adenylate cyclase in homogenates of rabbit retina. *Naunyn-Schmiedeberg's Arch. Pharmacol.*, 288:103–107.
5. Costall, B., Naylor, R. J., Cannon, J. G., and Lee, T. (1977): Differential activation by some 2-aminotetralin derivatives of the receptor mechanisms in the nucleus accumbens of rat which mediate hyperactivity and stereotyped biting. *Eur. J. Pharmacol.*, 41:307–319.
6. Häggendal, J., and Malmfors, T. (1965): Identification and cellular localization of the catecholamines in the retina and the choroid of the rabbit. *Acta Physiol. Scand.*, 64:58–66.
7. McDermed, J. D., McKenzie, G. M., and Freeman, H. S. (1976): Synthesis and dopaminergic activity of (±)-, (+)-, and (−)-2-dipropylamino-5-hydroxy-1,2,3,4-tetrahydronaphthalene. *J. Med. Chem.* 19:547–549.
8. McDermed, J. D., McKenzie, G. M., and Phillips, A. P. (1975): Synthesis and pharmacology of some 2-aminotetralins. Dopamine receptor agonists. *J. Med. Chem.*, 18:362–367.
9. Schorderet, M. (1975): The effects of dopamine, piribedil (ET-495) and its metabolite S-584 on retinal adenylate cyclase. *Experientia*, 31:1325–1326.
10. Schorderet, M. (1976): Direct evidence for the stimulation of rabbit retina dopamine receptors by ergot alkaloids. *Neurosci. Lett.*, 2:87–91.
11. Schorderet, M. (1977): Pharmacological characterization of the dopamine mediated accumulation of cyclic AMP in intact retina of rabbit. *Life Sci.*, 20:1741–1748.

Advances in Biochemical Psychopharmacology, Vol. 19,
edited by P. J. Roberts et al.
Raven Press, New York © 1978.

Some Characteristics of Mutant Han-Wistar Rats which Exhibit Paresis and Paralysis

Neville N. Osborne and Karl-H. Sontag

Forschungsstelle Neurochemie & Abteilung Biochemische Pharmakologie, Max Planck Institute, Göttingen, Germany

A strain of Han-Wistar rats characterized by spastic paresis and partial paralysis has recently been described (6). Genetic analysis of a small colony of these rats established that the disease is due to an autosomal recessive gene (6). These mutants are unusual, since the occurrence of neural disorders in rats is very rare in comparison with mice. Robertson (7), for example, quotes only three proven cases of mutants in rats, and they do not exhibit spastic paresis.

The first abnormal signs in the animals (male and female) can be observed at the age of about 4 to 5 weeks. At a later stage the animals become hyperactive and display ataxic movements when walking, although the sensory responses are normal. From the 35th day, ataxia and incoordination are progressively obvious; both fore and hind limbs are affected. Between the 42nd and 50th day the spasticity and paralysis are more evident, i.e., the limbs are rigid and extended and show a more or less permanent palmar and plantar flexion (Fig. 1). Thereafter, the ability to stand upright is almost lost and any movement by the animal is achieved through the use of the fore-limbs, with the hind limbs dragging. This development is accompanied by a mild to severe tremor in the muscles of the head and limbs. During the whole process, that is, from the 4th to the 5th week of age, the body weight of the spastic animals increases more slowly than that of the unaffected animals, so that at about the 63rd day the affected animals' body weights are about 75% of the controls' (6). This is also evident from Fig. 1. Moreover, as the degree of spasticity increases, the animal's ability to feed or drink is gradually and progressively impaired, until the animal eventually dies unless fed by hand.

Electromyographic studies on the gastrocnemius-soleus muscle have also been carried out in order to analyze the motor activity of the spastic animals (2,6). In these experiments the animals were placed in ventilated perspex boxes and the hind legs allowed to hang freely through slots in the bottom of the box. The muscular activity of the gastrocnemius-soleus muscles was then recorded electromyographically, as described by Wand et al. (8). The gastrocnemius-soleus muscle of the spastic animals showed spontaneous and

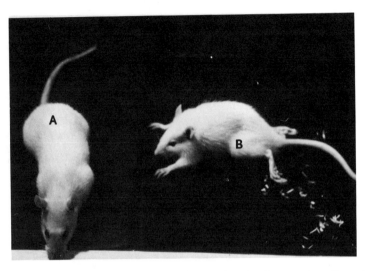

FIG. 1. Normal (A) and mutant (B) 3-month-old twin rats. It is clear that the mutant is smaller and drags its hind limbs. The back of the mutant is typically bent and the musculature rigid.

sustained motor unit discharges which were not observed under the same conditions in normal, healthy rats. In healthy animals, sudden phases in the activity of the muscle due to movements such as sniffing or biting were sometimes observed, but these were never sustained. It has therefore been suggested that the sustained firing activity which originates from spinal alpha-motoneurons is the cause of the rigidity in the hind legs of the spastic animals (6). Moreover, the spastic paresis is almost certainly due to a supraspinal defect, since interruption of the connections influencing the spinal cord removes the facilitation of the spontaneous firing of spinal motoneurons (*unpublished data*). The spontaneous and sustained unit discharges observed in the gastrocnemius-soleus muscle of spastic animals can be eliminated by a previous injection of either L-DOPA (L-dihydroxyphenylalanine) or apomorphine, but not D-DOPA (ref. 2 and Fig. 2). This observation is of interest and suggests, together with the overall symptoms of the affected animals, that perhaps they might serve as models for the study of Parkinson's disease.

Since one characteristic of sufferers from Parkinson's disease is a decrease in dopamine in the striatum, levels of this amine and other putative transmitters or enzymes in the striata of spastic mutant rats were measured (5). In Parkinson's disease the "nigro-basal ganglia-nigral loop"—which involves cholinergic, dopaminergic, and GABA-ergic neurons—is of prime importance (1), and special emphasis was placed on their transmitter substances. In the biochemical experiments, 2- to 3-month-old twins consisting of one mutant and one normal (control) rat were used. The striata were rapidly dissected and their contents analyzed for dopamine, tyrosine hydroxylase,

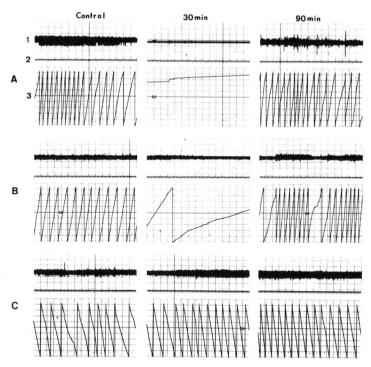

FIG. 2. Effect of 2 mg/kg apomorphine (A), 100 mg/kg L-DOPA (B), and 100 mg/kg D-DOPA on the electromyographic activity of the gastrocnemius-soleus muscle of spastic rats 30 and 90 min following i.p. injection. The spontaneous activity of the muscle before the effects of the drugs can be seen in the "control." 1, signal under investigation; 2, time scale; 3, integral of muscle activity as demonstrated in 1.

choline acetyltransferase (ChAc), and amino acids. As shown in Table 1, the activity of the dopamine-synthesizing enzyme tyrosine hydroxylase, in the mutant rat striata was significantly less than in the control animals. In the case of Parkinson's disease, there is also a decrease in the tyrosine hydroxylase activity in the striatum (3). However, the dopamine content in the mutants was significantly greater than in the controls, which contrasts with Parkinson's syndrome, where striatal dopamine is diminished (3). Furthermore, the increase in striatal dopamine content in the mutants (see Table 1) is related to the degree of paralysis (5). The fact that the dopamine content in the mutants is greater but the tyrosine hydroxylase activity lower in the mutants as compared with the controls may be due to a number of reasons. It is possible, for example, that the synthesis of dopamine in the controls is lower but that the release mechanism for the amine in the mutants does not function as efficiently as in the control rats. It may also be that the measurement of tyrosine hydroxylase activity *in vitro* is misleading in itself as this enzyme's activity *in vivo* may be very different where the intracellular concentrations of cofactor and substrate are determining factors. The ChAc activity in the mutant striata was also greatly enhanced, in contrast with the

TABLE 1. Concentrations of various substances, tyrosinehydroxylase (nmoles/mg wet wt/min), and choline acetyltransferase (µmoles/g wet wt/min) in striata of normal and mutant rats

Substance (nmoles/mg wet wt)	Normal	Mutant
Phosphoserine	0.099 ± 0.006	0.105 ± 0.010
Taurine[a]	7.960 ± 0.235	9.346 ± 0.419
Phosphoethanolamine	2.612 ± 0.126	2.933 ± 0.132
Urea[a]	29.780 ± 2.099	43.661 ± 1.838
Aspartate	2.459 ± 0.092	2.734 ± 0.180
Threonine	0.699 ± 0.027	0.656 ± 0.029
Serine	1.017 ± 0.059	1.104 ± 0.041
Glutamate[a]	9.938 ± 0.192	11.106 ± 0.632
Glutamine[a]	4.467 ± 0.199	5.509 ± 0.274
Glycine	1.118 ± 0.065	1.239 ± 0.103
Alanine	0.857 ± 0.057	0.902 ± 0.036
Citrulline[a]	0.059 ± 0.004	0.049 ± 0.002
α-Amino-N-butyric acid	0.080 ± 0.005	0.124 ± 0.032
Valine[a]	0.099 ± 0.009	0.121 ± 0.007
Methionine	0.073 ± 0.007	0.079 ± 0.004
Cystathionine[a]	0.056 ± 0.003	0.075 ± 0.002
Isoleucine[a]	0.048 ± 0.005	0.060 ± 0.004
Leucine[a]	0.090 ± 0.010	0.112 ± 0.007
Tyrosine	0.088 ± 0.004	0.083 ± 0.004
Phenylalanine	0.081 ± 0.005	0.087 ± 0.006
GABA	2.815 ± 0.221	2.834 ± 0.174
Unknown	0.154 ± 0.014	0.167 ± 0.010
NH_3	1.600 ± 0.114	1.323 ± 0.115
Lysine	0.316 ± 0.024	0.277 ± 0.006
Histidine	0.103 ± 0.004	0.095 ± 0.005
Arginine	0.199 ± 0.014	0.188 ± 0.010
Total NH_3	65.223 ± 2.811	83.625 ± 3.209
Dopamine[a]	0.033 ± 0.002	0.056 ± 0.003
Tyrosine hydroxylase[a]	0.1283 ± 0.01	0.0985 ± 0.01
Choline acetyltransferase[a]	12.9 ± 1.4	16.9 ± 1.4

Results are expressed as mean ± SEM for 8 experiments analyzed in triplicate.

[a] Significant at $p < 0.05$ (Student's t-test).

control animals and sufferers from Parkinson's disease, where the enzyme activity is almost normal (1,4). Of the other substances analyzed (see Table 1), the mutant striata contain more glutamate, taurine, cystathionine, valine, leucine, isoleucine, and urea but less citrulline than the controls. The GABA content is, however, normal, which is of interest since GABA-ergic neurons are involved in the "nigro-basal ganglia-nigral loop" (1).

In general, the present data demonstrate that a number of biochemical abnormalities are associated with the striata of the mutant rats. The balance between cholinergic, dopaminergic, and GABA-ergic neurons in the "nigro-basal ganglia-nigral loop" in the mutants is fundamentally different from the balance in controls and sufferers from Parkinson's disease. The significance of these differences is not clear, although they would appear from the biochemical data to eliminate any possibility of using the animals as a model for the study of Parkinson's disease. Nevertheless, they may be of great value for examining one particular phenomenon, such as the cause for the lower tyrosine hydroxylase activity and higher dopamine content, and experiments are now in progress to elucidate as much as possible the biochemistry, physiology, and morphology of the mutants.

REFERENCES

1. Bunny, B. S., and Aghajanian, G. K. (1976): Dopaminergic influence in the basal ganglia: Evidence for striata-nigral feedback regulation. In: *The Basal Ganglia*, edited by M. D. Yahr, pp. 249–267. Raven Press, New York.
2. Cremer, H., Sontag, K.-H., and Wand, P. (1977): Decrease in motor unit hyperactivity after administration of dopaminetics to spastic Han:Wistar rats (*in preparation*).
3. Hornykiewicz, O. (1973): Dopamine in the basal ganglia. *Br. Med. Bull.*, 29:172–178.
4. McGeer, S. L., Hatton, T., Singh, V. K., and McGeer, E. G. (1976): Cholinergic systems in extrapyramidal functions. In: *The Basal Ganglia*, edited by M. D. Yahr, pp. 213–226. Raven Press, New York.
5. Osborne, N. N., Coelle, E.-F., Neuhoff, V., and Sontag, K.-H. (1977): Mutant spastic Han:Wistar rats: Biochemical abnormalities in their striata. *Neurosci. Lett.*, 6: 251–254.
6. Pittermann, W., Sontag, K.-H., Wand, P., Papp, K., and Deerberg, F. (1976): Spontaneous occurrence of spastic paresis in Han:Wistar rats. *Neurosci. Lett.*, 2: 45–49.
7. Robertson, R. (1965): *Genetics of the Norway Rat*. Pergamon Press, Oxford.
8. Wand, P., Kuschinsky, K., and Sontag, K.-H. (1973): Morphine-induced muscular rigidity in rats. *Eur. J. Pharmacol.*, 24:189–193.

Advances in Biochemical Psychopharmacology, Vol. 19,
edited by P. J. Roberts et al.
Raven Press, New York © 1978.

Dopaminergic Receptor Activity in Substantia Nigra in the Mechanisms of Autoregulation of Striatal Dopamine Release

*A. Groppetti, *M. Parenti, F. Cattabeni, A. Maggi, L. De Angelis,
M. Monduzzi,'and G. Racagni

*Institute of Pharmacology and Pharmacognosy, and *Institute of Pharmacology,
University of Milan, Milan, Italy*

Changes in striatal dopamine (DA) metabolism and impulse flow have been explained by assuming the existence of different compensatory mechanisms involving neuronal loops projecting from the basal ganglia to DA cell bodies in substantia nigra (3,6,8,9,16,31,46). Support for this theory has been derived from biochemical and neurophysiological evidence demonstrating that pharmacological blockade of central DA receptors enhances DA synthesis (2,4,7,11,15,32,40) and neuronal activity of DA neurons (6,29) whereas drugs which stimulate these receptors reduce DA metabolism (2,7,8) and dopaminergic nerve impulse flow (5,29). In addition to this, intraneuronal end-product inhibition occurring at the tyrosine hydroxylase step has been postulated in order to account for changes in DA metabolism (10). In fact, increase of DA levels by monoamine oxidase inhibitors reduces tyrosine hydroxylase activity (4,10). The finding that apomorphine prevents the increase of DA synthesis produced by γ-butyrolactone (46) has been instead interpreted as a result of a stimulation of presynaptic receptors (9,46). In fact, such an effect cannot be explained by end-product inhibition since DA synthesis increases even if there is an accumulation of DA in the nerve terminals. The existence of presynaptic receptors or autoreceptors have been assumed also to explain the byphasic dose-response curve following apomorphine administration. Accordingly, in the lowest doses, apomorphine elicits inhibition, whereas higher doses stimulate locomotor activity (9,20,49).

Recent studies (27,36,39,43) have identified a pool of DA in the substantia nigra. The existence of a DA-sensitive adenylate cyclase (DA-AC) in the substantia nigra has been also demonstrated (34,42,48). These findings lead to the possibility that a further mechanism might occur in the regulation of striatal DA release.

This investigation has been undertaken with the aim: 1. to localize the

DA-AC in the substantia nigra and 2. to investigate whether the DA receptors in the substantia nigra might be a site of action of drugs which elicit increase or inhibition of DA release in the striatum.

RECEPTOR-MEDIATED CONTROL OF STRIATAL DA RELEASE BY HALOPERIDOL

The extrapyramidal effects due to phenothiazines and butyrophenones administration depend on the blockade of DA receptors (28). Studies on the transsynaptic regulation of cholinergic neurons by dopaminergic axons in striatum have shown that these receptors are located on cholinergic interneurons, which might participate in the compensatory feedback mechanisms regulating DA cell bodies in the substantia nigra (1,14,37,45).

Substantia nigra receives GABAergic (22) fibers which originate from striatum and globus pallidus. We have, therefore, investigated the functional interneuronal connections between DA and GABA which appear to be operative in strionigral loop. Table 1 shows that 3-methoxytyramine (3-MT) levels are markedly decreased when the GABA concentrations in substantia nigra are increased after the administration of ethanolamine-O-sulfate (EOS), an inhibitor of GABA-transaminase as previously described (13,23). On the other hand, levels of 3-MT are increased in striatum 12 days after lesion of crus cerebri (Table 1), a lesion which interrupts most of the GABAergic fibers from striatum (44) (Table 1). Since 3-MT can be taken as an index of DA release (11,21,35), these results indicate that the GABAergic system in substantia nigra can affect the activity of dopaminergic neurons in striatum. This finding raises the question whether the GABAergic strionigral pathway is necessary for the increase of DA turnover in striatum following haloperidol. It was, therefore, of interest to

TABLE 1. *GABA influence on the release of striatal dopamine*

	Striatum 3-methoxytyramine nmoles/g	Substantia nigra GABA nmoles/mg protein
Control	0.22 ± 0.04	77 ± 5.0
EOS	0.07 ± 0.01[a]	138 ± 14.0[a]
Crus cerebri lesion	0.40 ± 0.13[a]	33 ± 2.1[a]

Lesion of crus cerebri has been made using a stereotaxically placed fine retractable knife: a. 3.8; l. 2.3, according to the atlas of Pellegrino and Cushman (41). Rats were sacrificed with high-energy microwave radiation 3.5 hr after ethanolamine-O-sulf. GABA and 3-methoxytyramine were determined with mass fragmentographic methods recently described (12,25).
[a] $p < 0.01$ values are mean ± SEM of 5 determinations.

TABLE 2. *Effect of lesion of crus cerebri on haloperidol-induced increase of striatal DOPAC, HVA, and 3-methoxytyramine (3-MT)*

	Intact side		Lesioned side	
	Saline	Haloperidol	Saline	Haloperidol
	nmoles/g		nmoles/g	
DOPAC	6.96 ± 0.53	29.46 ± 0.58[a]	7.08 ± 0.49	25.12 ± 1.25[b]
HVA	3.08 ± 0.10	10.82 ± 0.42[a]	3.23 ± 0.11	8.62 ± 0.48[b]
3-MT	0.18 ± 0.01	0.33 ± 0.02[a]	0.28 ± 0.01[a]	0.41 ± 0.03[b]

Lesion of crus cerebri has been made as described in Table 1. Rats were sacrificed 12 days after the lesion. Values are the mean ± SEM of 5 determinations.
[a] p < 0.01 with respect to intact side of saline-treated animals.
[b] p < 0.01 with respect to lesioned side of saline-treated animals.

study the effect of haloperidol on striatal DA metabolism after interruption of the descending strionigral GABAergic pathway at the level of the crus cerebri. Table 2 shows that the effect of haloperidol on striatal 3,4-dihydroxyphenylacetic acid (DOPAC), homovanillic acid (HVA), and 3-MT concentrations persists even after the lesion. Recent studies have suggested that a site of action of haloperidol might be the substantia nigra. In fact it has been demonstrated that antipsychotics may antagonize the stimulation by DA of the DA-sensitive adenylate cyclase in substantia nigra (18,34,42). It seems therefore feasible to investigate whether DA-AC in substantia nigra is located on GABAergic terminals. The results (Table 3) demonstrate that a decrease of GABA in substantia nigra after crus cerebri lesion is not associated with a loss of DA-AC activity. Of course, other mechanisms, i.e., pre- or postsynaptic receptors within striatum, could explain the persisting increase of DA metabolites by haloperidol even after interrupting the GABA loop. Recently, it has been shown that kainic acid injected into striatum elicits a degeneration of perikarya with a decrement in the activity of DA-AC, whereas dopaminergic terminals remain intact (38,47). Table 4 shows that haloperidol (1 mg/kg i.p.) is able to increase DOPAC and HVA concentrations both in the kainic-injected and in the control striatum.

TABLE 3. *Effect of lesion of crus cerebri on DA-sensitive adenylate cyclase activity in homogenates of rat substantia nigra*

	Intact side	Lesioned side
None	86.4 ± 5.1	95.4 ± 6.0
DA 5 × 10⁻⁶	123.4 ± 9.7[a]	128.0 ± 8.4[a]
DA 5 × 10⁻⁵	151.3 ± 8.2[a]	163.8 ± 10.1[a]

Adenylate cyclase activity was measured following the method of Kebabian et al. (33). Lesion of crus cerebri was made as described in Table 1.
[a] p < 0.01. Values are mean ± SEM of 5 determinations.

TABLE 4. *Effect of kainic acid pretreatment on haloperidol-induced increase of 3-MT, DOPAC, and HVA in striatum*

	Saline		Kainic acid	
	Control	Haloperidol	Control	Haloperidol
3-MT	0.21 ± 0.01	0.40 ± 0.01[a]	0.42 ± 0.1[a]	0.27 ± 0.03
DOPAC	5.3 ± 0.2	21.2 ± 1.0[a]	8.6 ± 0.7[a]	28.8 ± 1.3[b]
HVA	3.3 ± 0.1	9.9 ± 0.5[a]	5.1 ± 0.2[a]	15.3 ± 1.3[b]

Kainic acid (5 nmoles/rat) was injected directly into striatum. Animals were killed 6 days after kainic acid treatment and 1 hr after haloperidol (1 mg/kg i.p.). Values are mean ± SEM of 5 determinations.
[a] $p < 0.01$ with respect to controls of saline-injected animals.
[b] $p < 0.01$ with respect to controls of kainic acid-injected animals.

On the contrary, in the lesioned striatum 3-MT levels are not enhanced by haloperidol (Table 4).

ROLE OF NIGRAL DA RECEPTORS IN APOMORPHINE-INDUCED INHIBITION OF STRIATAL DA RELEASE

Apomorphine is regarded as a direct dopaminergic stimulant agent at the receptor site (17). Apomorphine has been also reported to decrease the conversion of labeled tyrosine to DA (2,9) and the firing rate of neurons in striatum and substantia nigra (5). Postsynaptic strionigral negative feedback loop, involving GABA fibers (5,9), or local mechanisms within striatum mediated via pre- and postsynaptic receptors (9,46) have been proposed in order to explain the apomorphine-induced changes of DA metabolism and impulse flow.

However, the presence of nigral DA receptors suggests that mechanisms might be involved in apomorphine-induced inhibition of DA release in striatum.

TABLE 5. *3-MT concentrations in striatum of rats given apomorphine (Apo) systemically or in substantia nigra*

	3-MT nmoles/g
Saline	0.170 ± 0.010
Apo systemically	0.048 ± 0.002[a]
Apo in substantia nigra	0.060 ± 0.002[a]

The animals were killed by high energy microwave radiation 7 min after apomorphine (1 mg/kg s.c. 10μg/substantia nigra.
[a] $p < 0.01$. Each value represents the mean ± SEM of 5 determinations.

TABLE 6. Effect of apomorphine on cAMP levels in striatum and substantia nigra

	Striatum	Substantia nigra
	(pmoles/mg protein)	
Saline	5.7 ± 0.4	4.8 ± 0.3
Apomorphine	10.1 ± 1.0[a]	9.6 ± 0.7[a]

Animals were sacrificed 7 min after apomorphine (1 mg/kg s.c.) administration. Values are mean ± SEM of 5 determinations.
[a] $p < 0.01$.

Table 5 shows that striatal 3-MT concentrations, after injection of apomorphine in substantia nigra, are reduced in the same way as after systemic administration. This result suggests that one of the sites of action of apomorphine might be the substantia nigra. Accordingly, apomorphine increases *in vivo* the cAMP content in striatum as well as in substantia nigra (Table 6), indicating that dopaminergic receptors in substantia nigra have been activated.

CONCLUDING REMARKS

The existence of regulatory mechanisms different from the striatal postsynaptic ones which involve feedback loops projecting from striatum to substantia nigra has been postulated in order to explain the effects of DA agonists and antagonists (9,29,46). The results presented here provide neurochemical and pharmacological evidence for this hypotheses. Our data lead to the following considerations:

1. GABAergic neurons that connect striatum to substantia nigra do control striatal DA release. In fact, when GABA content in substantia nigra is increased after administration of EOS, a GABA transaminase blocker, the striatal 3-MT levels are markedly reduced (Table 1). Furthermore, after stereotaxic lesion of crus cerebri, GABA concentrations in substantia nigra are lowered and 3-MT levels in striatum are significantly increased (Table 1).

2. The results in Table 2 on the effect of haloperidol on DA metabolites after lesion of the descending GABAergic pathway are in agreement with those obtained by Garcia-Munoz et al. (26). On the other hand, apomorphine, injected directly into the substantia nigra, increases *in vivo* the cAMP concentrations in this nucleus (Table 6), indicating that DA receptors in the substantia nigra have been stimulated. As a consequence 3-MT content in striatum is reduced (Table 5). These results seem to be the biochemical correlate of the electrophysiological data (5). In fact, apomorphine has been found to decrease the activity of DA neurons when it is administered systemically or applied by microiontophoresis directly onto DA neurons.

Summarizing these results demonstrate that the alteration of DA synthesis by these compounds might be due also to a mechanism other than post-synaptic feedback involving a GABAergic pathway. For instance, the activation of nigral DA-AC by apomorphine or their blockade by haloperidol might be responsible for the changes of DA metabolism by these drugs. Moreover, other neurons than GABA of the striopallidonigral pathways could also be operative in controlling striatal DA.

3. A decrease of GABA content in substantia nigra after crus cerebri lesion is not associated with a loss of the nigral DA-AC. This suggests that DA receptors in substantia nigra are not located in GABAergic neurons. The exact location of these receptors remains to be established. Our present knowledge of nigral DA receptors derives from studies showing that DA-AC activity is resistant to destruction of nigral DA neurons by 6-OH-DA, whereas it disappears after brain hemisection (18,24). These findings indicate that DA-AC is localized on neuronal afferences originating from striatum. On the basis of the results shown in Table 3, we must assume that neuronal pathways, different from GABA, might be regulated by nigral DA receptors. Since it has been demonstrated that substance P in substantia nigra originates largely from striatum (30), work is in progress to investigate whether substance P controls the activity of DA neurons.

4. The experiments shown in Table 4 demonstrate that intrastriatal injection of kainic acid does not prevent the increase of striatal DOPAC and HVA elicited by haloperidol. On the contrary, the haloperidol-induced increase of 3-MT in striatum is not present. Since kainic acid causes degeneration of neurons whose cell bodies are in the nucleus where the injection is made (38,47), most of the strionigral pathways are destroyed. The alterations of DOPAC, HVA, and 3-MT in the lesioned side of saline-treated animals (Table 4) might occur as a result of increased impulse flow in the nigrostriatal DA pathway due to persistent depolarization. In fact, Schwarcz and Coyle (47) have reported activation of tyrosine hydroxylase after injection of kainic acid. The question then arises as to why haloperidol increases HVA and DOPAC levels whereas 3-MT content is not influenced (Table 4). Our present interpretation is that the 3-MT concentrations in striatum cannot be increased by haloperidol after kainic acid lesion since the strionigral pathways have been severed, and, therefore, the effect of haloperiodol on DA neuronal activity exerted via DA receptors in substantia nigra is no longer functioning. In fact, the activity of DA-AC in substantia nigra is reduced after kainic acid to the same extent as after brain hemisection (*unpublished observation*). Hence, 3-MT formation, which might be considered a reliable indicator of the functional fraction of DA which is released into the synaptic cleft, cannot be affected by pharmacological agents when the mechanisms which regulate the impulse flow of DA neurons are altered.

On the other hand, the increase of HVA and DOPAC by haloperidol in the kainic acid treated animals (Table 4) and the antagonism of this effect by apomorphine (19) indicate the existence of regulatory mechanisms which are independent of the integrity of neuronal impulse flow. Much additional research is needed before we can rule out any hypothesis on the nature and the functional role of these mechanisms exerting an inhibitory influence on DA neurons within striatum.

ACKNOWLEDGMENTS

We thank Miss Giusi Carini for her skillful technical assistance and Miss Aurora Maccalli for typing the chapter.

REFERENCES

1. Agid, Y., Guyenet, P., Glowinski, J., Beaujouan, C., and Javoy, F. (1975): Inhibitory influence of the nigro-striatal dopamine system on the striatal cholinergic neurons in the rat. *Brain Res.,* 86:488–492.
2. Andén, N. E., Corrodi, H., Fuxe, K., and Hökfelt, T. (1967): Increased impulse flow in bulbo spinal noradrenaline neurons produced by catecholamine receptor blocking agents. *Eur. J. Pharmacol.,* 1:59–64.
3. Andén, N. E., Roos, B. E., and Werdinius, B. (1964): Effect of chlorpromazine, haloperidol and reserpine on the levels of phenolic acids in rabbit corpus striatum. *Life Sci.,* 3:149–158.
4. Besson, M. G., Cheramy, A., and Glowinski, J. (1971): Effects of some psychotropic drugs on dopamine synthesis in the rat striatum. *J. Pharmacol. Exp. Ther.,* 177:196–205.
5. Bunney, B. S., Aghajanian, G. K., and Roth, R. H. (1973): Comparison effects of L-DOPA, amphetamine and apomorphine on firing rate of rat dopaminergic neurones. *Nature [New. Biol.],* 245:123–125.
6. Bunney, B. S., Walter, J. R., Roth, R. H., and Aghajanian, G. K. (1973): Dopaminergic neurons: Effect of antipsychotic drugs and amphetamine on single cell activity. *J. Pharmacol. Exp. Ther.,* 185:560–571.
7. Carenzi, A., Cheney, B. L., Costa, E., Guidotti, A., and Racagni, G. (1975): Action of opiates, antipsychotics, amphetamine and apomorphine on dopamine receptors in rat striatum: In vivo changes of cAMP content and acetylcholine turnover rate. *Neuropharmacology,* 14:927–939.
8. Carlsson, A. (1974): Pharmacological and biochemical aspects of striatal dopamine receptors. In: *Frontiers in Neurology and Neuroscience Research,* edited by P. Seeman and G. M. Brown, pp. 1–3. Neuroscience Institute, University of Toronto, Toronto.
9. Carlsson, A. (1975): Receptor mediated control of dopamine metabolism. In: *Pre- and Postsynaptic Receptors,* edited by E. Usdin and W. Bunney, pp. 49–63. Marcel Dekker, New York.
10. Carlsson, A., Kehr, W., and Lindqvist, M. (1974): Short-term control of tyrosine hydroxylase. In: *Neuropsychopharmacology of Monoamines and Their Regulatory Enzymes,* edited by E. Usdin, pp. 135–142. Raven Press, New York.
11. Carlsson, A., and Lindqvist, M. (1963): Effect of chlorpromazine or haloperidol on formation of 3-methoxy-tyramine in mouse brain. *Acta Pharmacol.,* 20:140–144.
12. Cattabeni, F., Galli, C. L., and Eros, T. (1976): A simple and highly sensitive mass fragmentographic procedure for GABA determinations. *Anal. Biochem.,* 72:1–7.
13. Cattabeni, F., Maggi, A., De Angelis, L., Bruno, F., and Racagni, G. (1977): A simple approach to study the effect of haloperidol on GABA functional activity in the nigrostriatal system. *J. Neurochem.,* 28:1407–1408.
14. Consolo, S., Ladinsky, M., and Garattini, S. (1974): Effect of several dopaminergic drugs and trihexylphenidyl on cholinergic parameters in rat striatum. *J. Pharm. Pharmacol.,* 26:275–277.
15. Corrodi, H., Fuxe, K. Y., and Hökfelt, T. (1967): The effect of some psychoactive drugs on central monoamine neurons. *Eur. J. Pharmacol.,* 1:363–368.

16. Costa, E., and Neff, W. H. (1966): Isotopic and non-isotopic measurements of the rate of catecholamine biosynthesis. In: *Biochemistry and Pharmacology of the Basal Ganglia,* edited by E. Costa, L. J. Cote, and M. D. Yahr, pp. 141–155. Raven Press, New York.

17. Costall, B., and Naylor, R. J. (1973): On the mode of action of apomorphine. *Eur. J. Pharmacol.,* 21:350–361.

18. DiChiara, G., Mereu, G. P., Vargiu, L., Porceddu, M. L., Mulas, M., Trabucchi, M., and Spano, P. F. (1977): Evidence for the existence of regulatory DA receptors in the substantia nigra. In: *Advances in Biochemical Psychopharmacology,* edited by E. Costa and G. L. Gessa, pp. 477–481. Raven Press, New York.

19. DiChiara, G., Porceddu, M. L., Spano, P. F., and Gessa, G. L. (1977): Haloperidol increases and apomorphine decreases striatal dopamine metabolism after destruction of striatal dopamine-sensitive adenylate cyclase by kainic acid. *Brain Res.,* 130: 374–382.

20. DiChiara, G., Porceddu, M. L., Vargiu, L., Argiolas, A., and Gessa, G. L. (1976): Evidence for dopamine receptors mediating sedation in the mouse brain. *Nature,* 264:564–567.

21. Di Giulio, A. M., Groppetti, A., Cattabeni, F., Maggi, A., and Algeri, S. (1975): Functional significance of striatal 3-methoxy-tyramine. Proceedings of the First Meeting of the European Society of Neurochemistry, Bath, England.

22. Fonnum, F., Grofova, I., Rinvik, E., Storm-Mathisen, J., and Walberg, F. (1974): Origin and distribution of glutamate decarboxylase in substantia nigra of the cat. *Brain Res.,* 71:77–92.

23. Fowler, L. J. (1973): Analysis of the major amino acids of rat brain after in vivo inhibition of GABA transaminase by ethanolamine-O-sulphate. *J. Neurochem.,* 21: 437–440.

24. Gale, K., Guidotti, A., and Costa, E. (1977): On the location of DA sensitive adenylate cyclase in substantia nigra. *Science,* 195:503–505.

25. Galli, C. L., Cattabeni, F., Eros, T., Spano, P. F., Algeri, S., Di Giulio, A. M., and Groppetti, A. (1976): A mass fragmentographic assay of 3-methoxy-tyramine in rat brain. *J. Neurochem.,* 27:795–798.

26. Garcia-Munoz, M., Nicolaou, N. M., Tulloch, I. F., Wright, A. K., and Arbuthnott, G. W. (1977): Feedback loop or output pathway in striato-nigral fibers. *Nature,* 265:363–365.

27. Geffen, L. B., Jessel, T. M., Cuello, A. C., and Iversen, L. L. (1976): Release of dopamine from dendrites in rat substantia nigra. *Nature,* 260:258–260.

28. Greengard, P. (1974): Biochemical characterization of the dopamine receptor in the mammalian caudate nucleus. *J. Psychiatr. Res.,* 11:87–90.

29. Groves, P. M., Wilson, C. J., Young, S. J., and Rebec, G. V. (1975): Self-inhibition by dopaminergic neurons. *Science,* 190:522–529.

30. Hong, J. S., Yang, H. Y. I., Racagni, G., and Costa, E. (1977): Projections of substance P containing neurons from neostriatum to substantia nigra. *Brain Res.,* 122: 541–544.

31. Javoy, F., Agid, Y., Bouvet, D., and Glowinski, J. (1972): Feedback control of DA synthesis in dopaminergic terminals of the rat striatum. *J. Pharmacol. Exp. Ther.,* 182:454–463.

32. Javoy, F., Hamon, M., and Glowinski, J. (1970): Disposition of newly synthesized amines in cell bodies and terminals of central catecholaminergic neurons. (1) Effect of amphetamine and thiopreperazine on the metabolism of CA in the caudate nucleus, the substantia nigra and the ventromedial nucleus of the hypothalamus. *Eur. J. Pharmacol.,* 10:178–188.

33. Kebabian, J. W., Petzold, G. L., and Greengard, P. (1972): Dopamine sensitive adenylate cyclase in the caudate nucleus of rat brain and its similarity to the dopamine receptors. *Proc. Natl. Acad. Sci. U.S.A.,* 69:2145–2149.

34. Kebabian, J. W., and Saavedra, J. M. (1976): Dopamine-sensitive adenylate cyclase occurs in a region of substantia nigra containing dopaminergic dendrites. *Science,* 193:683–685.

35. Kehr, W. (1976): 3-Methoxy-tyramine as an indicator of impulse-induced dopamine release in rat brain in vivo. *Naunyn-Schmiedebergs Arch. Pharmacol.,* 293:209–215.

36. Korf, J., Zieleman, M., and Westerink, B. H. C. (1976): Dopamine release in substantia nigra? *Nature,* 260:257–258.
37. McGeer, P. L., Grewaal, D. S., and McGeer, E. G. (1974): Influence of noncholinergic drugs on rat striatal acetylcholine levels. *Brain Res.,* 80:211–217.
38. McGeer, E. G., and McGeer, P. L. (1976): Duplication of biochemical changes of Huntington's chorea by intrastriatal injection of glutamic acid and kainic acids. *Nature,* 263:517–519.
39. Nieoullon, N. A., Cheramy, A., and Glowinski, J. (1977): Release of dopamine in vivo from cat substantia nigra. *Nature,* 266:375–377.
40. Nybäck, H., Sedvall, G., and Kopin, I. J. (1967): Accelerated synthesis of dopamine-C^{14} from tyrosine C^{14} in rat brain after chlorpromazine. *Life Sci.,* 6:2307–2311.
41. Pellegrino, L. J., and Cushman, A. J. (1967): *A Stereotaxic Atlas of the Rat Brain,* edited by R. M. Elliott, G. Lindzey, and K. McCorquodale. Meredith Publishing Co., New York.
42. Phillipson, O. T., and Horn, A. S. (1976): Substantia nigra of the rat contains a dopamine sensitive adenylate-cyclase. *Nature,* 261:418–420.
43. Racagni, G., Bruno, F., Cattabeni, F., Maggi, A., Di Giulio, A. M., and Groppetti, A. (1976): Interaction among dopamine, acetylcholine and GABA in the nigro-striatal systems. Proceedings of the Symposium on Interactions among Putative Neurotransmitters in the Brain, Milan, Italy.
44. Racagni, G., Bruno, F., Cattabeni, F., Maggi, A., Di Giulio, A. M., Parenti, M., and Groppetti, A. (1978): Functional interaction between rat substantia nigra and striatum: GABA and dopamine interrelation. *Brain Res. (in press).*
45. Racagni, G., Cheney, D. L., Trabucchi, M., and Costa, E. (1976): In vivo actions of clozapine and haloperidol on the turnover rate of acetylcholine in rat striatum. *J. Pharmacol. Exp. Ther.,* 196:323–332.
46. Roth, P. H., Walters, J. R., Murrin, L. C., and Morgenroth, V. H. (1975): Dopamine neurons: Role of impulse flow and presynaptic receptors in the regulation of tyrosine hydroxylase. In: *Pre and Postsynaptic Receptors,* edited by E. Usdin and W. E. Bunney, pp. 1–48. Marcel Dekker, New York.
47. Schwarcz, R., and Coyle, J. T. (1977): Striatal lesions with kainic acid: Neurochemical characteristics. *Brain Res.,* 127:235–249.
48. Spano, P. F., DiChiara, G., Tonon, G. C., and Trabucchi, M.(1976): A dopamine-stimulated adenylate cyclase in rat substantia nigra. *J. Neurochem.,* 27:1565–1568.
49. Strömbom, U. (1977): Antagonism by haloperidol of locomotor depression induced by small doses of apomorphine. *J. Neural Transm.,* 40:191–194.

Advances in Biochemical Psychopharmacology, Vol. 19,
edited by P. J. Roberts et al.
Raven Press, New York © 1978.

Dopamine Metabolism in the Rat Retina and Brain after Acute and Repeated Treatment with Neuroleptics

B. Scatton, J. Dedek, and J. Korf

Synthélabo, L.E.R.S, Department of Biology, Neurochemistry Unit, Bagneux, France

Repeated treatment with neuroleptics modifies dopamine (DA) turnover differently in various brain regions. Thus, compared to the effect of a single injection, repeated treatment with neuroleptics reduces the increase in DA metabolism in the striatum (tolerance) (1,2). In contrast, no tolerance to the increase in DA turnover appears to occur in the mesocortical system (7). In the mesolimbic dopaminergic system, some investigators observed tolerance (4,9), although others (2,7) did not. In the mentioned studies different experimental conditions were used. Therefore, we have systematically investigated the effects of different doses of, and of duration of treatment with, neuroleptics on DA turnover in several brain areas of the rat. Both a "classic" (haloperidol) and an "atypical" (sulpiride) neuroleptic were used. Similar experiments were carried out in the retina in order to clarify whether or not development of tolerance also occurs in extracerebral DA neurons.

BRAIN DOPAMINE METABOLISM

Male Charles River rats (200 g) were injected intraperitoneally once a day for 11, 21, or 40 days with saline (controls) or various doses of haloperidol (0.2 to 5 mg/kg) or sulpiride (12.5 to 100 mg/kg) (subacute treatment). Other animals received saline for 10, 20, or 39 days and a single injection of haloperidol or sulpiride on the following day (acute treatment). All animals were sacrificed 2 hr after the last injection, and homovanillic acid (HVA) and 3,4-dihydroxyphenylacetic acid (DOPAC) were measured (10) in the striatum, nucleus accumbens, tuberculum olfactorium, and frontal cortex.

High Doses

Repeated treatment with high doses of haloperidol (5 mg/kg) or sulpiride (100 mg/kg) for 11 days induced tolerance to the increases in HVA and DOPAC in all cerebral structures studied. However, in the various regions, tolerance developed differently, according to the dose. Thus, the threshold dose inducing tolerance in the striatum was lower than that affecting other

TABLE 1. *Threshold doses of, and minimal treatment duration with, haloperidol for induction of tolerance to the increase in DA turnover in brain regions of the rat*

	Striatum	Nucleus accumbens	Tuberculum olfactorium	Frontal cortex
Threshold dose[a] (mg/kg i.p.)	0.2	2	1	5
Minimal duration required[b] (days)	11	40	40	No tolerance at 40

[a] The lowest dose giving a significant attenuation of cerebral HVA increase when administered daily for 11 days, compared to the single dose.

[b] The shortest period of haloperidol treatment (0.2 mg/kg i.p.) resulting in a significant attenuation of HVA increase.

regions (Table 1). Tolerance development in the frontal cortex was confirmed by measuring the rate of disappearance of DA after injection of α-methyl-p-tyrosine (5).

Low Doses

Moreover, repeated administration of a low dose (0.2 mg/kg i.p.) of haloperidol induced an earlier tolerance in the striatum than in the mesolimbic areas, whereas no tolerance occurred in the frontal cortex (5) (Table 1).

In another set of experiments, the increase in HVA levels was compared in two differently treated groups of animals: (a) 10-day treatment with sulpiride (100 mg/kg i.p.) plus a single injection of haloperidol (0.2 mg/kg i.p.) on the 11th day; (b) 10-day treatment with saline followed by a single dose of haloperidol (0.2 mg/kg i.p.) on the 11th day. Haloperidol induced a less marked increase in HVA levels in striatum and mesolimbic areas of animals pretreated with sulpiride than in saline-pretreated rats, suggesting development of cross-tolerance between the two neuroleptics.

RETINAL DOPAMINE METABOLISM

Animals were injected acutely or once a day for 11 days with various doses of haloperidol or sulpiride as described above and were sacrificed 2 hr after the last injection for determination of HVA levels in the retina.

In this structure, subacute treatment with haloperidol and sulpiride even at the highest doses (5 and 100 mg/kg, respectively) does not induce tolerance. The results were confirmed by measuring DA utilization after α-methyl-p-tyrosine injection (6).

CONCLUSIONS

Repeated treatment with cataleptogenic as well as noncataleptogenic neuroleptics induces a regionally different development of tolerance to the increase in DA turnover as compared to that observed after single administration of these drugs. In this respect, the striatum is the most sensitive structure followed by mesolimbic and mesocortical DA areas. In the retina no tolerance occurs.

The tolerance is probably not connected to induction of drug-metabolizing enzymes, as both threshold dose and minimal duration of treatment required for inducing tolerance differ for the various nervous structures. Moreover, the occurrence of cross-tolerance between the two structurally different drugs sulpiride and haloperidol does not support enzyme induction. As suggested by pharmacological and electrophysiological studies (3,8,11), the tolerance to the neuroleptic-induced increase in DA turnover is possibly a biochemical correlate of supersensitivity of pre- and/or postsynaptic DA receptors. Thus, the reduction of DA turnover may reflect decreased impulse flow in DA neurons, which is probably triggered by changes in receptor sensitivity.

Finally, the different sensitivity of the DA-rich areas investigated to tolerance development may be connected to differences in the mechanisms regulating the activity of the DA systems. The lack of tolerance development in the retina may then be explained by the possibly different interneuronal organization within this structure.

REFERENCES

1. Asper, H., Baggiolini, M., Burki, H. R., Lauener, H., Ruch, W., and Stille, G. (1973): Tolerance phenomena with neuroleptics. Catalepsy, apomorphine stereotypies and striatal dopamine metabolism in the rat after single and repeated administration of loxapine and haloperidol. *Eur. J. Pharmacol.,* 22:287–294.
2. Bowers, M. B., Jr., and Rozitis, A. (1974): Regional differences in homovanillic acid concentrations after acute and chronic administration of antipsychotic drugs. *J. Pharm. Pharmacol.,* 26:743–745.
3. Gianutsos, G., Drawbaugh, R. B., Hynes, M. D., and Lal, H. (1974): Behavioral evidence for dopaminergic supersensitivity after chronic haloperidol. *Life Sci.,* 14: 887–898.
4. Peringer, E., Jenner, P., Donaldson, I. M., and Marsden, C. D. (1976): Metoclopramide and dopamine receptor blockade. *Neuropharmacology,* 15:463–469.
5. Scatton, B. (1977): Differential regional development of tolerance to increase in dopamine turnover upon repeated neuroleptic administration. *Eur. J. Pharmacol.,* 46:363–369.
6. Scatton, B., Dedek, J., and Kork, J. (1977): Effect of single and repeated administration of haloperidol and sulpiride on striatal and retinal dopamine turnover in the rat. *Brain Res.,* 136, 135:374–377.
7. Scatton, B., Glowinski, J., and Julou, L. (1976): Dopamine metabolism in the mesolimbic and mesocortical dopaminergic systems after single or repeated administrations of neuroleptics. *Brain Res.,* 109:184–189.
8. Tarsy, D., and Baldessarini, R. J. (1974): Behavioural supersensitivity to apomorphine following chronic treatment with drugs which interfere with the synaptic function of catecholamines. *Neuropharmacology,* 13:927–937.
9. Waldmeier, P. C., and Maître, L. (1976): Clozapine: Reduction of the initial dopamine turnover increase by repeated treatment. *Eur. J. Pharmacol.,* 38:197–203.
10. Westerink, B. H. C., and Korf, J. (1976): Regional rat brain levels of 3,4-dihydroxyphenylacetic acid and homovanillic acid: Concurrent fluorometic measurement and influence of drugs. *Eur. J. Pharmacol.,* 38:281–289.
11. Yarbrough, G. G. (1975): Supersensitivity of caudate neurons after repeated administration of haloperidol. *Eur. J. Pharmacol.,* 31:367–372.

Advances in Biochemical Psychopharmacology, Vol. 19,
edited by P. J. Roberts et al.
Raven Press, New York © 1978.

Monoamine Oxidase Activity During (−)-Deprenil Therapy: Human Brain Post-Mortem Studies

P. Riederer, *M. B. H. Youdim, W. Birkmayer, and K. Jellinger

*Ludwig-Boltzmann Institute of Clinical Neurobiology, Lainz Municipal Hospital, Vienna, Austria; and *Technion—Israel Institute of Technology, School of Medicine, Department of Pharmacology, Bat Galim, Haifa, Israel*

USE OF DEPRENIL IN PARKINSON'S DISEASE

The discovery of functionally different forms of monoamine oxidase (MAO) led to the suggestion (4,15) that selective MAO inhibitors such as clorgyline and deprenil could be used to produce specific neuropharmacological effects (8,9). (−)-Deprenil (MAO "type B" inhibitor), unlike the other selective and nonselective inhibitors (including clorgyline), has the property of not potentiating the hypertensive action of tyramine (9).

Recently we have demonstrated that (−)-deprenil potentiated the antiakinetic effect of L-DOPA in parkinsonian patients, with a significant reduction of their "on-off" phenomenon (3). These results led us to examine the long-term effects of L-DOPA and (−)-deprenil in a much larger group of parkinsonian patients. (−)-Deprenil and Madopar® (L-DOPA plus the peripherally acting decarboxylase inhibitor benserazide) were given orally, and the combination resulted in a statistically significant ($p < 0.001$) reduction in patients' functional disability compared with Madopar® therapy alone (1). The addition of (−)-deprenil resulted in a reduction of the daily dose requirements of L-DOPA: and this was especially evident in parkinsonian patients who were treated for the first time with this regimen of antiparkinson therapy. Furthermore, the introduction of (−)-deprenil into L-DOPA therapy reverses the deteriorating effect produced by long-term L-DOPA therapy. More recently these results have been confirmed by Lee et al. (10).

The aim of this investigation was to examine the *in vivo* effects of (−)-deprenil on the human brain monoamine metabolism in order to obtain a rational basis for the observed therapeutic effects.

PLATELET MAO ACTIVITY IN PARKINSONIAN PATIENTS

Human platelet MAO activity, which is considered to be of "type B" (11, 16), has been used as a possible peripheral marker for CNS MAO. *In vitro* studies have indicated that human brain MAO activity, for the most part, is also of "type B" enzyme (4,14) and that dopamine (DA) as a substrate in human brain is "type B" (6). During the recent studies on the treatment of parkinsonian patients with Madopar® and (−)-deprenil, platelet MAO activity was measured before and after either oral or intravenous administration of 10 mg (−)-deprenil (1). The results showed that this dose of (−)-deprenil is sufficient to inhibit MAO activity by more than 90% within 1 hr of application and that the enzyme inhibition is sustained for up to 24 hr. It is important to note that the patients began to show clinical improvement at the time at which maximum MAO inhibition was observed. However, these results do not indicate whether brain MAO activity is inhibited to the same degree nor whether the potentiation of L-DOPA is due to the inhibition of MAO.

The measurement of MAO activity in 15 specific areas of human brain (13) confirmed earlier results (4) that the hypothalamus has the highest activity followed by the basal ganglia (caudate nucleus, putamen, globus pallidus, and substantia nigra). A comparison of inhibitory potency of (−)-deprenil, D,L-tranylcypramine, clorgyline, and harmaline on human brain mitochondrial MAO in these 15 areas showed that in all areas examined (−)-deprenil was by far the most potent inhibitor of brain MAO. The I^P_{50} calculated graphically was between 0.15 and 0.96 nmoles. In comparison, a 5,000-fold higher concentration of clorgyline [MAO "type A" inhibitor (13)] is needed to produce a 50% inhibition. These results are in close agreement with the earlier findings of Youdim (14) and Glover et al. (6) which demonstrated that human brain MAO is predominantly (> 80%) of "type B."

BRAIN MAO ACTIVITY IN DEPRENIL-TREATED PARKINSONIAN PATIENTS

For the past 4 years 300 parkinsonian patients have been treated with the combined Madopar® and (−)-deprenil regimen (1,2). In this period 4 patients died during medication because of the progression of the disease.

Case 1

A post-encephalitic parkinsonian patient, who had originally responded to 10 mg deprenil daily, lost his response and no other medication improved his condition. (−)-Deprenil was increased to 100 mg daily and he responded. Nevertheless, the patient died "intercurrent." Application of 100 mg (−)-deprenil results in a complete inhibition of MAO in all the brain areas examined. There was a marked increase of DA in globus pallidus, nucleus amygdala, cinguli, raphe plus formatio reticularis, and nucleus ruber, when compared to the brains from the untreated parkinsonian group. How-

TABLE 1. MAO activity in human brain: parkinsonian patients post mortem

Brain area	Dopamine-MAO			Serotonin-MAO		
	Control (nmoles/g/hr)	Long-term deprenil-treated Parkinson's patient (nmoles/g/hr)	% of controls	Control (nmoles/g/hr)	Long-term deprenil-treated Parkinson's patient (nmoles/g/hr)	% of controls
Thalamus	11,117	749[a]	6.7	1,275	296	23.2
		2421[b]	21.8		712	56.3
		57[c]	0.5		N.D.	—
		1464[b]	10		444	20.1
Amygdala	14,637	129[c]	0.8	2,198	670	30.0
Globus pallidus	22,013	920[c]	4.1	2,703	318	11.8

[a] Case 2, last deprenil medication 15 hr before death.
[b] Case 3, last deprenil medication 23 hr before death.
[c] Case 4, last deprenil medication 35 hr before death.
All autopsies were performed 3–12 hr after death.

ever, no increase of DA could be observed in striatum and substantia nigra, which suggests the complete degeneration of the nigrostriatal dopaminergic fibers in this patient. However, 5-hydroxytryptamine (5-HT) showed a marked increase in all brain areas which were under study, indicating that high dosages of (−)-deprenil are able to inhibit also MAO "type A" in the brain.

Cases 2 Through 4

Three other patients who had been receiving 10 mg (−)-deprenil daily showed increased response to L-DOPA. However, they all developed akinetic crises and death followed.

Table 1 summarizes the preliminary results obtained so far. It is apparent that 10 mg daily dosage of deprenil is sufficient to inhibit almost all dopamine-MAO activity. However, substantial serotonin-MAO activity is still present. These *in vivo* results not only confirm earlier findings that human brain MAO is of "type B" and that dopamine is a "type B" substrate but also lend support to the view that platelet MAO activity can be used to monitor the action of deprenil in parkinsonian patients (1).

DISCUSSION

Intraneuronal concentrations of DA and 5-HT in the human brain can be elevated either by increasing their rate of synthesis from their precursors L-DOPA (L-3,4-dihydroxyphenylalanine) and 5-hydroxytryptophan (5-HTP), respectively, or by inhibiting the major metabolic enzyme, MAO. However, commonly available MAO inhibitors such as nialamide, tranylcypromine, and niamid are of less therapeutic value since they cause hypertensive crisis, gastrointestinal irritations, as well as psychotic episodes. Furthermore, these MAO inhibitors reach their optimal therapeutic efficacy at least 2 weeks after application, and after withdrawal they are still effective for a period varying from days to weeks. In 1968 Johnston (8) demonstrated that clorgyline was an irreversible inhibitor of MAO, but that the enzyme inhibitor was substrate dependent. When 5-HT was used as a substrate, much lower concentrations of the inhibitor were necessary to inhibit the enzyme activity than when the substrate benzylamine was used. Such behavior was interpreted as being due to the presence of two enzyme species, MAO "type A" and MAO "type B," respectively.

In animal experiments, "type A" enzyme oxidatively deaminates the substrates 5-HT and norepinephrine. DA is a substrate for both forms of the enzyme (7). However, findings have indicated that in the human brain DA is a preferred substrate for MAO "type B" (6). Neff et al. (12) and Dzoljic et al. (5) have shown that deprenil can selectively increase DA concentration in rat brain. Our recent observations suggest that the same may be true of human brain (13). These studies are in close agreement with clinical and biochemical findings (1–3) of L-DOPA or Madopar® potentiation by (−)-deprenil. (−)-Deprenil may exert its beneficial effect by inhibiting "type B" MAO (Table 1). Another possible explanation could be its amphetamine-like action, which is especially observed with (+)-deprenil (J. Knoll, *personal communication*). However, recent pharmacological observations have clearly shown that (−)-deprenil does not possess amphetamine-like properties (J. Knoll, *personal communication*). This is in close agreement with our recent findings that parkinsonian patients who have been on long-term treatment with this drug show no withdrawal symptoms after changing their therapy.

It is of interest to note that the MAO in nerve endings of the rat striatum is of pure "type B." This has led Knoll (*personal communication*) to suggest that MAO "type B" inhibitors will be of therapeutic value.

It is important to note that the therapeutic regimen should not exceed 5 to 10 mg of (−)-deprenil daily. With such a dosage only DA is increased and not 5-HT or norepinephrine (13). In our previous studies (1,3) we have established that with a dose of 15 mg or more (−)-deprenil there is a greater incidence of side effects. This may be related to total MAO inhibition and the increase not only in DA but in 5-HT as well as norepinephrine.

CONCLUSION

The present investigation indicates that a daily 10-mg regimen of (−)-deprenil is sufficient to inhibit brain "dopamine-MAO" activity by more than 90%. This figure agrees well with the results obtained previously using the platelet MAO as a peripheral marker of CNS MAO, suggesting that the therapeutic efficacy of the drugs lies in the inhibition of brain MAO.

ACKNOWLEDGMENTS

The authors are grateful for financial assistance from the "Jubiläumsfonds der Österreichischen Nationalbank." We also thank the Chinoin Drug Company, Budapest, Hungary, for deprenil.

REFERENCES

1. Birkmayer, W., Riederer, P., Ambrozi, L., and Youdim, M. B. H. (1977): Implications of combined treatment with 'Madopar' and L-deprenil in Parkinson's disease. *Lancet*, 1:439–443.
2. Birkmayer, W., Riederer, P., and Youdim, M. B. H. (1978): Distinction between benign and malign type of Parkinson's disease. *J. Clin. Neurol. Neurosurg.* (*submitted*).
3. Birkmayer, W., Riederer, P., Youdim, M. B. H., and Linauer, W. (1975): Potentiation of anti-akinetic effect after L-Dopa treatment by an inhibitor of MAO-B, deprenil. *J. Neural Transm.*, 36:303–323.

4. Collins, G. G. S., Sandler, M., Williams, E. D., and Youdim, M. B. H. (1970): Multiple forms of human brain mitochondrial monoamine oxidase. *Nature,* 225: 817–820.
5. Dzoljic, M., Bruinvels, J., and Bonta, I. L. (1977): Desynchronization of electrical activity in rats induced by Deprenyl—An inhibitor of monoamine oxidase B and relationship with selective increase of dopamine and phenylethylamine. *J. Neural Transm.,* 40:1–13.
6. Glover, V., Sandler, M., Owen, F., and Riley, G. J. (1977): Dopamine is a monoamine oxidase B substrate in man. *Nature,* 265:80–81.
7. Houslay, M. D., Tipton, K. F., and Youdim, M. B. H. (1976): Multiple forms of monoamine oxidase: Fact or artefact. *Life Sci.,* 19:467–481.
8. Johnston, J. P. (1968): Some observations upon a new inhibitor of monoamine oxidase in brain tissue. *Biochem. Pharmacol.,* 17:1285–1297.
9. Knoll, J., and Magyar, K. (1972): Some puzzling pharmacological effects of monoamine oxidase inhibitor. *Adv. Biochem. Psychopharmacol.,* 5:393–408.
10. Lee, A. J., Shaw, K. M., Kohout, L. J., Stern, G. M., Elsworth, J. D., Sandler, M., and Youdim, M. B. H. (1977): Deprenyl in Parkinson's disease. *Lancet,* ii:791–795.
11. Murphy, D. L., and Donnelly, C. H. (1974): Monoamine oxidase in man: Enzyme characteristics in platelets, plasma and other human tissues. *Adv. Biochem. Psychopharmacol.,* 12:71–86.
12. Neff, N. H., Yang, H. Y., and Fuentes, J. A. (1974): The use of selective monoamine oxidase inhibitor drugs to modify amine metabolism in brain. *Adv. Biochem. Psychopharmacol.,* 12:49–58.
13. Riederer, P., Birkmayer, W., Rausch, W., Pavlak, E., Seemann, D., Jellinger, K., and Youdim, M. B. H. (1978): Inhibition of dopamine sensitive MAO by $(-)$-deprenil and the clinical implications of *in vitro* and *in vivo* human brain studies. *Nature (submitted).*
14. Youdim, M. B. H. (1976): Tyramine and psychiatric disorders. In: *Neuroregulators and Hypothesis of Psychiatric Disorders,* edited by E. Usdin, D. Hamburg, and J. Barchas, pp. 57–67. Oxford University Press, Oxford.
15. Youdim, M. B. H., Collins, G. G. S., Sandler, M., Bevan Jones, A. B., Pare, C. M. B., and Nicholson, W. J. (1972): Human brain monoamine oxidase, multiple forms and selective inhibitors *Nature,* 236:225–228.
16. Youdim, M. B. H., Grahame-Smith, D. G., and Woods, H. F. (1976): Some properties of human platelet monoamine oxidase in iron deficiency anaemia. *Clin. Sci. Mol. Med.,* 50:479–485.

Advances in Biochemical Psychopharmacology, Vol. 19,
edited by P. J. Roberts et al.
Raven Press, New York © 1978.

Dopamine Agonists and Reflex Epilepsy

G. M. Anlezark, R. W. Horton, and B. S. Meldrum

*Department of Neurology, Institute of Psychiatry, Denmark Hill,
London, SE5 8AF, England*

Many studies indicate an involvement of cerebral norepinephrine and 5-hydroxytryptamine (5-HT) in experimentally induced seizures in animals (2,11,12), but a critical role for dopamine (DA) has not been emphasized. Some evidence is available to show that DA may modify experimental seizures. L-Dihydroxyphenylalanine (L-DOPA) reverses reserpine-induced enhancement of audiogenic seizures (4), and apomorphine raises the maximal electroshock seizure threshold in rats (13). We have tested drugs believed to act as agonists at central DA receptors in two models of reflex epilepsy: sound-induced (audiogenic) seizures in DBA/2 mice and photically induced seizures in the Senegalese baboon *Papio papio*. In DBA/2 mice, the relation between the time course of action of drugs against audiogenic seizures and their effects on the cerebral metabolism of DA and 5-HT [estimated by whole brain concentrations of their metabolites homovanillic acid (HVA) and 5-hydroxyindoleacetic acid (5-HIAA)] was examined.

The drugs used were the DA agonists n-N-propylnorapomorphine (NPA) and apomorphine, the ergot alkaloids ergocornine, bromocriptine (CB 154, 2-bromo-α-ergocryptine), ergometrine, and lysergic acid diethylamide (LSD), and the 5-HT agonist quipazine [2-(1-piperazinyl)-quinoline maleate]. These ergot alkaloids possess DA agonist properties in behavioral and biochemical tests (3,7,8,11,14) and interact with central 5-HT receptors (1,5). Quipazine acts directly on 5-HT receptors with only indirect effects on DA neurons (6,15).

AUDIOGENIC SEIZURES IN DBA/2 MICE

Groups of 10 DBA/2 mice (19 to 23 days old) were subjected to auditory stimulation (doorbell, 109 dB at mouse level) following intraperitoneal injection of drugs at the doses and times shown (Fig. 1). In preliminary experiments, the dose-response relations and ED_{50}'s (clonic phase) were determined for each drug, and all gave dose-related protection against seizures (2,3). The doses chosen were related to the ED_{50}'s and the order of potency was (ED_{50}'s in mg/kg in parentheses): NPA (0.1) > ergocornine (1) = apomorphine (1) > bromocriptine (5) > LSD (9) ≥ ergometrine (10)

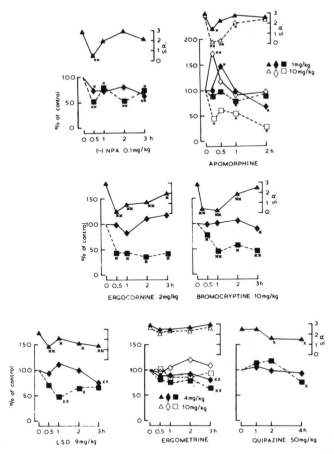

FIG. 1. Effects of (—)n-N-propylnorapomorphine (NPA), apomorphine, ergot alkaloids, and quipazine on audiogenic seizure response (S.R.) and whole brain concentrations of dopamine (DA) and homovanillic acid (HVA) in 19–23-day-old DBA/2 mice. S.R. ▲: right-hand axis, upper part of each diagram, graded as follows: O = no response; 1 = wild running; 2 = clonus; 3 = hindlimb tonus. Each point represents the mean maximum S.R. for 10 animals. Significant differences (p < 0.05) from control (Fisher's exact probability test) are denoted: x, incidence of tonic phase different from control; xx, incidence of clonic phase different from control. Biochemical measurements: ◆ DA; ■ HVA, left-hand axis, lower part of each diagram. Results are expressed as % of estimations in concurrent control animals treated with vehicle and exposed to auditory stimulation. Each point represents the mean of 5 determinations. Significant differences from control (Student's t-test) are denoted: x p < 0.05; xx p < 0.01. Time in hours on the lower axis.

> quipazine (50). Maximum seizure response for each mouse was recorded (see Fig. 1 legend). Mice were killed by decapitation after 60 sec of stimulation or during tonic extension. Estimations of whole brain concentrations of DA, 5-HT, HVA, and 5-HIAA were made as previously described (10).

The time course of changes in seizure susceptibility and DA metabolism is shown in Fig. 1. NPA reduced seizure response and cerebral concentrations of DA and HVA. Apomorphine (1 mg/kg) had a transient protective effect against seizures and reduced HVA whereas DA rose briefly. More profound and longer lasting effects occurred following 10 mg/kg. Ergocornine and bromocryptine reduced seizure response for 2 to 3 hr and induced profound decreases in HVA with little change in DA. LSD also reduced seizure response and HVA for 3 hr, but at a high dose. Quipazine diminished seizure response and HVA with a long latency of onset. DA concentrations were unchanged. The failure of ergometrine to influence seizure susceptibility and its weak action on DA metabolism were unexpected in view of its previously determined ability to protect against audiogenic seizures and DA agonist properties in behavioral tests.

PHOTICALLY INDUCED SEIZURES IN BABOONS

The experiments were performed on 11 adolescent Senegalese baboons. Stroboscopic stimulation (Dawe Strobotorch model 1202D, 15 to 35 flashes/sec) was applied in 5-min tests before and 0.25 to 5.5 hr, at hourly intervals, after intravenous drug administration. Myoclonic responses were graded: 0 = no response; 1 = eyelid myoclonus; 2 = myoclonus of head, neck, and upper limbs; 3 = whole body myoclonus; 4 = myoclonus continuing after termination of stimulation; S = generalized tonic-clonic seizure. Baboons varied in their responses, but most showed grade 2 or 3 in control tests. The drugs used were: ($\pm$) NPA, apomorphine, ergocornine, ergometrine, and bromocryptine. LSD (0.04 to 0.4 mg/kg) had already been shown to potently diminish photically induced myoclonus in baboons (17) so this was not repeated.

NPA and Apomorphine

Apomorphine (1 mg/kg) abolished myoclonic responses to photic stimulation 15 min after administration. Control responsiveness returned after 1 to 2 hr. ($\pm$) NPA (0.05 to 0.2 mg/kg) reduced responses for up to 4 hr.

Ergot Alkaloids

Ergometrine (0.15 to 1 mg/kg) was the most effective of the three ergot alkaloids and abolished or reduced myoclonic responses for 1 to 2 hr. Ergocornine (0.5 to 2 mg/kg) had a longer time course of action, photically induced responses being reduced or absent for up to 3 hr, but was more toxic inducing sedation and large-amplitude slow waves on the EEG. Bromocryptine (0.5 to 4 mg/kg) had a weak action against myoclonic responses, but this had prolonged time course with responsiveness slightly reduced for up to 6 hr following the higher doses.

The order of potency of these drugs, based on the dose giving a consistent reduction in myoclonic responsiveness, was: LSD $\geq$ NPA > ergometrine > apomorphine = ergocornine > bromocriptine.

COMPARISON OF DRUG ACTIONS IN MICE AND BABOONS

Comparing the orders of potency of drugs to reduce seizure activity in mice and baboons, it can be seen that apomorphine and ergocornine are as potent as each other in both models. NPA is more effective and bromocryptine less effective than either. However, both LSD and ergometrine are more effective in reducing photically induced myoclonus than in altering audiogenic seizure susceptibility. Obviously, different anatomical pathways are involved in the mediation of seizure activity in each model, and the dependence in the baboon on transmission in the visual pathway may explain the differing potencies of the two ergot alkaloids. The ergot alkaloids differ in their abilities to interact with central 5-HT neurons as assessed by their action on cerebral concentrations of 5-HIAA in DBA/2 mice. They all reduced cerebral 5-HIAA. Ergocornine (2 mg/kg) and bromocriptine (10 mg/kg) had a longer-lasting and more profound effect on HVA than on 5-HIAA (maximal decreases in 5-HIAA 46% of control after 2 hr and 73% of control after 0.5 hr, respectively). LSD (9 mg/kg) was almost equally effective in reducing cerebral 5-HT metabolism as in reducing DA turnover, whereas ergometrine (4 and 10 mg/kg) significantly diminished cerebral 5-HIAA at all times after administration (maxima: 4 mg/kg, 65% of control after 1 hr; 10 mg/kg, 57% of control after 0.5 hr) in contrast to its weak action on DA metabolism.

In neurophysiological experiments, LSD potently inhibits the firing rate of 5-HT neurons in the lateral geniculate body (9), a relay in the visual pathway. In photosensitive baboons, the drug modifies visual evoked responses in the lateral geniculate body, and this correlates well with the reduction in photosensitivity (16). A similar mechanism may operate for ergometrine as it is structurally similar to LSD. The results presented here strongly suggest that drugs which interact with central 5-HT receptors are potent inhibitors of reflex epilepsy in the baboon. DA agonist action is also effective as shown by the reduction in myoclonic responses following NPA and apomorphine. In DBA/2 mice, the potency of NPA, apomorphine, and the ergot alkaloids to reduce audiogenic seizures is similar to their potencies in behavioral tests of central DA function (3). Thus, DA agonist action is probably the mechanism by which these drugs reduce audiogenic seizure susceptibility. This is supported by the finding that the protective effects of ergocornine and apomorphine are blocked by the DA antagonist haloperidol (3), and that ergometrine which had little effect on DA metabolism was ineffective in reducing audiogenic seizures. However, a central 5-HT agonist action of ergot alkaloids in protection against audiogenic seizures cannot be excluded.

ACKNOWLEDGMENTS

We are grateful to the Wellcome Trust and the British Epilepsy Association for financial support, and to Professor J. L. Neumeyer for generous gifts of NPA.

REFERENCES

1. Aghajanian, G. K. (1972): LSD and CNS transmission. *Annu. Rev. Pharmacol.,* 12:157–168.
2. Anlezark, G. M. (1977): The role of cerebral monoamines in reflex epilepsy. Ph.D. thesis, University of London.
3. Anlezark, G. M., Pycock, C., and Meldrum, B. S. (1976): Ergot alkaloids as dopamine agonists: Comparison in two rodent models. *Eur. J. Pharmacol.,* 37: 295–302.
4. Boggan, W. O., and Seiden, L. S. (1971): Dopa reversal of reserpine enhancement of audiogenic seizure susceptibility in mice. *Physiol. Behav.,* 6:215–217.
5. Corrodi, H., Farnebo, L.-O., Fuxe, K., and Hamberger, B. (1975): Effect of ergot drugs on central 5-hydroxytryptamine neurons: Evidence for 5-hydroxytryptamine release or 5-hydroxytryptamine receptor stimulation. *Eur. J. Pharmacol.,* 30: 172–181.
6. Costall, B., and Naylor, R. J. (1975): The role of the raphé and extrapyramidal nuclei in the stereotyped and circling responses to quipazine. *J. Pharm. Pharmacol.,* 27:368–371.
7. Da Prada, M., Saner, A., Burkard, W. P., Bartholini, G., and Pletscher, A. (1975): Lysergic acid diethylamide: Evidence for stimulation of cerebral dopamine receptors. *Brain Res.,* 94:67–73.
8. Fuxe, K., Corrodi, H., Hokfelt, T., Lidbrink, P., and Ungerstedt, U. (1974): Ergocornine and 2-Br-α-ergocryptine. Evidence for prolonged dopamine receptor stimulation. *Med. Biol.,* 52:121–132.
9. Haigler, H. J., and Aghajanian, G. K. (1974): Lysergic acid diethylamide and serotonin: A comparison of effects on serotoninergic neurons and neurons receiving a serotoninergic input. *J. Pharmacol. Exp. Ther.,* 188:688–699.
10. Horton, R. W., Anlezark, G. M., Sawaya, M. C. B., and Meldrum, B. S. (1977): Monoamine and GABA metabolism and the anticonvulsant action of di-n-propylacetate and ethanolamine-O-sulphate *Eur. J. Pharmacol.,* 41:387–397.
11. Lehmann, A. (1970): Psychopharmacology of the response to noise, with special reference to audiogenic seizures in mice. In: *Physiological Effects of Noise,* edited by B. L. Welch and A. S. Welch, pp. 227–257. Plenum Press, New York.
12. Maynert, E. W., Marczynski, T. J., and Browning, R. A. (1975): The role of the neurotransmitters in the epilepsies. *Adv. Neurol.,* 13:79–147.
13. McKenzie, G. M., and Soroko, F. E. (1972): The effects of apomorphine, (+)-amphetamine and L-dopa on maximal electroshock convulsions—a comparative study in the rat and mouse. *J. Pharm. Pharmacol.,* 24:686–701.
14. Pieri, M., Pieri, L., Saner, A., Da Prada, M., and Haefely, W. (1975): A comparison of drug-induced rotation in rats lesioned in the medial forebrain bundle with 5,6-dihydroxytryptamine or 6-hydroxydopamine. *Arch. Int. Pharmacodyn. Ther.,* 217:118–130.
15. Rodriguez, R., Rojas-Ramirez, J. A., and Drucker-Colin, R. R. (1973): Serotonin-like actions of quipazine on the central nervous system. *Eur. J. Pharmacol.,* 24: 164–171.

16. Vuillon-Cacciuttolo, G., Meldrum, B. S., and Balzamo, E. (1973): Electroretinogram and afferent visual transmission in the epileptic baboon, *Papio papio:* Effects of drugs influencing monoaminergic systems. *Epilepsia,* 14:213–221.
17. Walter, S., Balzamo, E., Vuillon-Cacciuttolo, G., and Naquet, R. (1971): Effets comportementaux et électrographiques du diethylamide de l'acide d'lysergique (LSD 25) sur le *Papio papio* photosensible. *Electroencephalogr. Clin. Neurophysiol.,* 30:294–305.

Advances in Biochemical Psychopharmacology, Vol. 19,
edited by P. J. Roberts et al.
Raven Press, New York © 1978.

Brain Catecholamine Concentrations and Convulsions in El Mice

Mutsutoshi Kohsaka, Midori Hiramatsu, and Akitane Mori

Institute for Neurobiology, Okayama University Medical School, Shikata-cho, Okayama, 700 Japan

The El mouse is an inbred strain with a convulsive disposition discovered in 1954 by Imaizumi et al. (2). Convulsions are produced in adult El mice of both sexes 6 to 7 weeks after birth by postural stimulation, i.e., a violent tonic-clonic convulsion follows after mice are gently thrown up several times.

Recently, we analyzed the brain catecholamine levels of 11 strains of mice and found that the brain dopamine of previously unstimulated El mice was higher and norepinephrine level lower than in other tested strains of mice (1). In this chapter we report on brain catecholamine levels of El mouse before, during, and after convulsions.

El mice were obtained from our laboratory. Rf, AKR, and C₃H/BifB/Ki strains were supplied from the mouse colonies of Okayama University Medical School, and were used as control species.

The mice were divided into two groups: the nonstimulated control animals and "stimulated" animals. Stimulated mice were regularly thrown 10 to 15 cm high until they started the general convulsion or a maximum of 80 times without convulsion, once a week from 7 weeks of age. For determining pre-convulsive catecholamine levels, mice were thrown for two-thirds of the time required for El mice to minifest convulsions. All mice were housed at $25° \pm 2°C$ at 50% humidity and were maintained under controlled lighting, which provided equal periods of light (1 A.M. to 1 P.M.) and darkness (1 P.M. to 1 A.M.). The experiments were performed between 9 A.M. and 1 P.M.

CATECHOLAMINE ANALYSIS

For catecholamine analysis, the mice were fixed in liquid nitrogen, and the whole brain without the cerebellum was rapidly removed. Analysis of brain catecholamines was carried out by our method which is a modification of the Kawai and Tamura method (4).

TABLE 1. Effect of "throwing" stimulation on catecholamine levels of El mouse brain

Groups	N	Catecholamine concentrations (μg/g tissue) M $\pm$ S.D.		
		Dopamine	Norepinephrine	Epinephrine
Non-stimulated control group	7	1.305 $\pm$ 0.187	0.286 $\pm$ 0.050	0.037 $\pm$ 0.003
Stimulated groups				
Resting	6	0.693 $\pm$ 0.056[b]	0.258 $\pm$ 0.009[a]	0.053 $\pm$ 0.021[b]
Preconvulsion	6	0.342 $\pm$ 0.059[d]	0.134 $\pm$ 0.055[d]	0.046 $\pm$ 0.015
During convulsion	6	0.600 $\pm$ 0.194	0.202 $\pm$ 0.058[d]	0.050 $\pm$ 0.010
Hours after convulsion				
1	6	0.758 $\pm$ 0.096[c]	0.327 $\pm$ 0.063[d]	0.032 $\pm$ 0.022
3	6	0.815 $\pm$ 0.086[d]	0.364 $\pm$ 0.055[d]	0.052 $\pm$ 0.022
6	8	0.551 $\pm$ 0.092[d]	0.355 $\pm$ 0.051[d]	0.034 $\pm$ 0.017
24	5	0.634 $\pm$ 0.118	0.291 $\pm$ 0.241	0.035 $\pm$ 0.012

[a] $p < 0.01$, compared to nonstimulated control group.
[b] $p < 0.001$, compared to nonstimulated control group.
[c] $p < 0.01$, compared to resting (stimulated group) state.
[d] $p < 0.001$, compared to resting (stimulated group) state.

El Mouse

At first, we determined catecholamine levels in El mice brain. Table 1 summarizes the catecholamine levels associated with convulsions. In resting stage (stimulated series), the dopamine concentration was 50% of the non-stimulated control level; norepinephrine was slightly lower, and conversely, the epinephrine level was higher. At the preconvulsive stage, dopamine and norepinephrine concentrations decreased further to 50% of the levels at the resting stage. During convulsion, the dopamine level was still high, while the norepinephrine level rose to a level higher than the control level. Three hours after convulsions, the dopamine level was at a peak, and norepinephrine likewise reached its peak level. Then 24 hr after convulsions, the dopamine and norepinephrine concentrations returned almost to the resting levels.

Next we determined brain catecholamine levels in mice of other strains.

Rf Mouse

Rf mice, a normal strain of mice with a nonconvulsive disposition, were exposed to the "throwing" stimulation once a week from 5 weeks of age. In the resting stage, the dopamine level in the stimulated series was 50% of the nonstimulated control level; epinephrine also decreased markedly, but no significant difference was observed in norepinephrine level. Just after 80 "throws," the epinephrine level decreased significantly, although no significant differences were observed in dopamine and norepinephrine levels.

C₃H/BifB/Ki Mouse

The 80 "throws" stimulation produced no significant changes in dopamine and norepinephrine levels during or just after stimulation; however, the epinephrine level was significantly lower. Three hours after the "throwing" stimulation, the brain dopamine level was lower even in this strain of mouse.

AkR Mouse

No significant changes in dopamine, norepinephrine, and epinephrine levels were seen, except for a slight decrease in dopamine 3 hr after the stimulations.

DISCUSSION

Recent investigations have indicated that dopamine and/or norepinephrine is important functionally in the convulsive seizure mechanism. For instance, norepinephrine has been reported to be a modulator of audiogenic convulsions (3); reserpine has been found to induce reduction of the electro-stock seizure threshold and was related to decreased brain catecholamines and 5-hydroxytryptamine; and electroshock seizure threshold was reported to be regulated by the dopamine level. These results show that the convulsive threshold correlated closely with biogenic amines, i.e., the threshold was elevated when the amine level was high and decreased when the amine level was low.

Our experimental results on the El mouse also show that the catecholamine levels at the resting stage of the "stimulated" series were lower than those of the nonstimulated control and the "stimulated" group preconvulsion levels of dopamine and norepinephrine were the lowest of the experimental series.

The decrease in brain catecholamines in the resting stage induced by the "throwing" stimulation was observed not only in the El mouse but also in the Rf mouse, a nonconvulsive strain of mouse. This finding suggests that the decrease in catecholamines is not a specific response of the El mouse and could result from the "throwing" stimulation. On the other hand, the response to stimulation differed by strains, i.e., marked decreases in dopamine and norepinephrine were observed in the El mice just after stimulation, but not in the Rf, C₃H/BifB/Ki, and AKR mice, although some decreases were observed 1 to 3 hr later. Minor catecholamine changes were found in Rf and C₃H/BifB/Ki mice. This suggests that the low brain levels of dopamine and norepinephrine were induced by the "throwing" stimulation. The higher sensitivity of these catecholamines in response to "throwing" stimulation in El mice could be an important mechanism in the induction of convulsive seizures.

REFERENCES

1. Hiramatsu, M., Kobayashi, K., and Mori, A. (1976): Brain catecholamine levels in eleven strains of mice. *I.R.C.S. Med. Sci.,* 4:365.
2. Imaizumi, K., Ito, S., Kuzukake, G., et al. (1959): The epilepsy-like abnormalities in a strain of mouse. *Bull. Exp. Anim.,* 8:6–10.
3. Jobe, P. C., Picchioni, A. L., and Chin, L. (1973): Role of brain norepinephrine in audiogenic seizure in the rat. *J. Pharmacol. Exp. Ther.,* 184:1–10.
4. Kawai, S., and Tamura, Z. (1968): Gas chromatography of catecholamines as their trifluoroacetates. *Chem. Pharm. Bull.,* 16:699–701.

Advances in Biochemical Psychopharmacology, Vol. 19,
edited by P. J. Roberts et al.
Raven Press, New York © 1978.

Lisuride- and D-LSD-Induced Changes of Monoamine Turnover in the Rat Brain

H. H. Keller, W. P. Burkard, L. Pieri, E. P. Bonetti,
and M. Da Prada

*Pharmaceutical Research Department, F. Hoffmann-La Roche & Co., Ltd.,
Basel, Switzerland*

Lisuride (lisuride hydrogen maleate, Lysenyl®, Spofa) is a semisynthetic ergot derivative stereochemically related to isolysergic acid, and carries a substituted amino function in the 8 S position. Like D-lysergic acid diethylamide (LSD) and several other ergot alkaloids, lisuride has been recently shown to stimulate dopamine (DA) receptors in the central nervous system (5,6). Lisuride is said to be nonhallucinogenic and is used as an antimigraine drug. We have studied its biochemical and behavioral effects in rats in comparison with those of LSD.

MATERIALS AND METHODS

Male albino rats (stock Füllinsdorf, SPF, 150 to 250 g) were used. Unless otherwise stated, all drugs, dissolved in 0.9% NaCl, were injected intraperitoneally. The doses of the ergot derivatives refer to the salts, i.e., lisuride hydrogen maleate, lisuride (5R, 8R) HCl H_2O, and LSD tartrate. The monoamines and their metabolites were determined fluorimetrically (7) either in single whole brains or in pools (two each) of dissected brain parts (4); adenylate cyclase activity was measured in striatal homogenates or slices of limbric forebrain (7). Some rats, with or without i.p. pretreatment with methiothepin maleate [a compound blocking brain 5-hydroxytryptamine (5-HT), DA, and norepinephrine (NE) receptors], received, under halothane anesthesia, stereotaxic injections of either lisuride or LSD into the raphe medianus and dorsalis (each 5 μg/2 μl saline on the left and right side of the two nuclei) 55 min before decapitation (8). In other animals, drug-induced rotation was recorded in a rotometer using rats lesioned unilaterally in the medial forebrain bundle with 5,6-dihydroxytryptamine (9).

RESULTS AND DISCUSSION

In the whole brain, lisuride at 1 mg/kg induced within 30 min a minor but significant increase of DA to 113.3% (all results refer to untreated controls = 100%) and 5-HT (to 110.5%) and a considerable decrease of NE (to 71.7%), effects similar to those seen with LSD (1 mg/kg) which, for both drugs, confirms earlier findings (3,5). Lisuride, in the whole brain, caused a decrease of homovanillic acid (HVA) (maximum reduction to 64.2% at 0.05 mg/kg) as well as of 5-hydroxyindolacetic acid (5-HIAA) (to 78.0% at 1 mg/kg) for at least 2 hr.

In contrast, 3-methoxy-4-hydroxyphenylethyleneglycol sulfate (MOPEG-SO$_4$) was markedly elevated (for at least 4 hr) by lisuride, whereas LSD (1 mg/kg) caused only a minor and transient increase. As shown in Table 1, lisuride-induced reduction of HVA was most marked in the striatum but quite distinct also in the limbic forebrain and the frontal cortex, whereas LSD at 0.1 mg/kg had no such effect, and at 1 mg/kg even increased HVA in these three brain regions. Both drugs reduced 5-HIAA in limbic forebrain and striatum to about the same degree. The lisuride-induced elevation of MOPEG-SO$_4$ was marked in the cortex and hypothalamus, less pronounced in the limbic forebrain, and did not occur in the striatum; similar but less pronounced effects were seen with LSD.

The lisuride-induced decrease of HVA and 5-HIAA levels accompanied by a slight increase of DA and 5-HT are interpreted as a reduction of the turnover of DA and 5-HT, respectively. The same is proposed for LSD at low doses, whereas at 1 mg/kg LSD seems to enhance DA turnover. The

TABLE 1. Monoamine metabolite levels in rat brain regions 1 hr after lisuride or D-LSD

	Drug dose mg/kg i.p.	Lisuride			D-LSD		
		MOPEG-SO$_4$	HVA	5-HIAA	MOPEG-SO$_4$	HVA	5-HIAA
Cortex[a]	0.1	—	84.8[b] ±5.3	—	—	115.0 ±7.3	—
	1.0	191.6[d] ±9.4	85.4[b] ±3.5	—	132.2[c] ±9.7	154.4[d] ±8.8	—
Limbic forebrain	0.1	—	68.6[c] ±4.5	97.3 ±4.2	—	110.7 ±11.2	100.2 ±3.9
	1.0	152.0[d] ±11.7	77.5[b] ±8.9	80.1[d] ±2.3	132.5[d] ±5.1	137.0[d] ±8.9	90.8[c] ±2.5
Striatum	0.1	—	59.2[d] ±4.6	93.7 ±3.3	—	102.7 ±7.9	93.1 ±3.3
	1.0	116.9 ±12.1	47.9[d] ±5.6	85.3[c] ±3.8	116.9 ±8.8	130.7[d] ±6.6	91.7 ±3.7
Hypothalamus	1.0	205.1[d] ±6.4	—	—	146.7[d] ±8.3	—	—

Tissue levels are given as % of controls (=100%) and are means ± SEM of 7 to 16 single values. Difference from control (t-test): [b] p < 0.05; [c] p < 0.01; [d] p < 0.001; all others: p > 0.05.

[a] MOPEG-SO$_4$ was determined in the whole cortex without the limbic cortex; HVA was measured in the frontal cortex excluding the limbic part.

elevated MOPEG-SO$_4$ levels concomitant with a reduction in NE indicate that both drugs enhance NE turnover.

A decrease of the DA turnover, probably mediated by DA receptor stimulation, is further suggested by the finding that both lisuride and LSD reduced the DA synthesis rate, as judged by an attenuated accumulation of L-DOPA (after injection of the DOPA decarboxylase inhibitor NSD-1015) in the nucleus caudatus, nucleus accumbens septi, and the retina of reserpine-pretreated rats. Furthermore, lisuride (0.05 mg/kg), like LSD and apomorphine, induced contralateral circling in rats unilaterally lesioned in the medial forebrain bundle with 5,6-dihydroxytryptamine (2) which could be inhibited by haloperidol. *In vitro,* lisuride inhibited the DA-stimulated formation of cAMP in rat striatal homogenates (IC$_{50}$ = 1.2 × 10^{-7} M) suggesting that lisuride interacts with DA receptor sites. However, lisuride *per se* was not able to stimulate cAMP formation (6), as found *in vitro* for other ergot derivatives (10). In limbic slices, the NE-stimulated cAMP formation was inhibited by lisuride (IC$_{50}$ = 8 × 10^{-8} M) and LSD (IC$_{50}$ = 3 × 10^{-6} M), indicating that the increase in MOPEG-SO$_4$ and the reduction in NE levels found for lisuride (and to a lesser extent for LSD) are, at least in part, mediated by blockade of central NE receptors (6). This is further suggested by the finding *in vivo* that the α-receptor-stimulating agent clonidine completely prevented the lisuride-induced elevation of MOPEG-SO$_4$. The reduction of 5-HT turnover by lisuride is assumed to be due to stimulation of 5-HT autoreceptors (somatic and/or dendritic 5-HT receptors). In fact, lisuride (but not LSD) when injected stereotaxically in the vicinity of the 5-HT-containing cell bodies of the raphe nuclei was able to completely prevent the methiothepin-induced increase of 5-HIAA in the telencephalon (8). 5-HT receptor stimulation is further supported by the observation that lisuride, but not LSD, induced homosexual mounting in rats of both sexes, a behavior which has been associated with reduced serotoninergic neurotransmission in the brain (1).

In conclusion, the present biochemical and behavioral findings suggest that in rat brain lisuride potently stimulates dopaminergic and, to a lesser extent, serotoninergic receptors (preferably autoreceptors), and at higher doses blocks noradrenergic receptors.

ACKNOWLEDGMENT

Part of these data were presented at the Spring Meeting of the Union of Swiss Societies of Experimental Biology, Zurich, 1977 (for abstract see ref. 6).

REFERENCES

1. Da Prada, M., Bonetti. E. P., and Keller, H. H. (1977): Induction of mounting behaviour in female and male rats by lisuride. *Neurosci. Lett.,* 6:349–353.

2. Da Prada, M., Pieri, L., Keller, H. H., Pieri, M., and Bonetti, E. P. (1978): Effect of 5,6- and 5,7-dihydroxytryptamine on rat CNS after intraventricular or intracerebral application and on blood platelets in vitro. Conference on Serotonin Neurotoxins. *Ann. N.Y. Acad. Sci. (in press).*

3. Diaz, P. M., Ngai, S. H., and Costa, E. (1968): Factors modulating brain serotonin turnover. *Adv. Pharmacol.,* 6B:75–92.

4. Glowinski, J., and Iversen, L. L. (1966): Regional studies of catecholamines in the rat brain. *J. Neurochem.,* 13:655–669.

5. Kehr, W. (1977): Effect of lisuride and other ergot derivatives on monoaminergic mechanisms in rat brain. *Eur. J. Pharmacol.,* 41:261–273.

6. Keller, H. H., Burkard, W., and Da Prada, M. (1977): Lisuride and D-LSD: Effects on the monoaminergic system in the rat brain. *Experientia,* 33:806.

7. Keller, H. H., Burkard, W. P., Pieri, L., Gerecke, M. and Da Prada, M. (1978): Effects of lisuride and D-LSD on the cerebral monoaminergic system of the rat. *J. Pharmacol. Exp. Ther. (in press).*

8. Pieri, L., Keller, H. H., Burkard, W. P., and Da Prada, M. (1978): Effects of lisuride and LSD on cerebral monamine systems and hallucinosis. *Nature,* 272:278–280.

9. Pieri, M., Schaffner, R., and Haefely, W. (1977): Central dopamine-receptor stimulation by LSD and lisuride. *Experientia,* 33:808.

10. Schmidt, M. J., and Hill, L. E. (1977): Effects of ergots on adenylate cyclase activity in the corpus striatum and pituitary. *Life Sci.,* 20:789–798.

Advances in Biochemical Psychopharmacology, Vol. 19,
edited by P. J. Roberts et al.
Raven Press, New York © 1978.

Complementary Distribution of Dopamine, Substance P, and Acetylcholine in the Rat Prefrontal Cortex and Septum

P. C. Emson

MRC Neurochemical Pharmacology Unit, Department of Pharmacology, Medical School, Cambridge, England

In many brain areas the distributions of substance P and monoamines, especially dopamine, are very similar suggesting the possibility of pharmacological interactions (in particular, feedback interactions) between transmitters (1,13,14). During a study on the origin and distribution of dopaminergic projections to the rat frontal cortex we used a sensitive radioimmunoassay procedure (7) to measure the content of substance P in the same frontal cortex areas we had previously assayed for dopamine content (4). The amount of substance P and the regional distribution of assayable substance P in the frontal cortex were similar to the dopamine content of these same frontal cortex areas (Table 1). Further studies in the medial prefrontal cortex indicate that the substance P and dopamine have an almost identical laminar distribution (Table 1).

The laminar distribution of substance P in the medial frontal area was confirmed when immunohistochemical procedures demonstrated the presence of substance P immunoreactive nerve terminals in the deeper layers of the medial prefrontal cortex (15) (Fig. 1A). These substance P immunoreactive terminals disappeared after hemisections at all levels down to the brainstem

TABLE 1. *Distribution of dopamine and substance P in the frontal cortex of the rat*

A. Cortex area	Dopamine (ng/g)	Substance P (ng/g)	B. Laminar distribution in the medial prefrontal cortex		
				SP (ng/g)	DA (ng/g).
Dorsal prefrontal area	19.6 ± 3.6	27.4 ± 5.0	Layers I–III	34.1 ± 5.4	45.0 ± 63
Lateral prefrontal area	14.3 ± 15.4	26.7 ± 3.1			
Medial prefrontal area	88.8 ± 21.4	83.4 ± 11.5			
			Layers IV–V	54.0 ± 6.0	55.2 ± 10.1
Ventral prefrontal area	26.4 ± 5.7	35.0 ± 4.0			
Piriform cortex	34.0 ± 6.4	53.0 ± 6.0	Layers V–VI	87.8 ± 13.2	71.2 ± 8.7

Units represent means ± SEM of a minimum of 4 separate determinations.

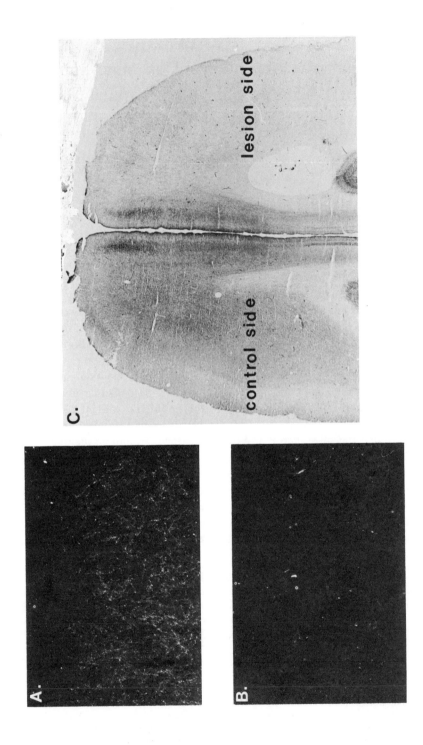

[approximately level A 100 μm according to the atlas of Konig and Klippel (9)] (Fig. 1B). This finding indicated the existence of a long axoned substance P projection from the brainstem (caudal to A 100 μm) projecting to frontal cortex (15). This projection is separate from the dopaminergic projection to the frontal cortex as hemisections caudal to substantia nigra-ventral tegmental area depleted the cortex of substance P fibers, whereas the dopamine terminals remained (2,4,12). The pile-up of immunoreactive substance P within the medial forebrain bundle caudal (15) to the hemisection indicated that, like the dopamine projections to frontal cortex (12), the substance P projection ascends in the medial forebrain bundle.

As a routine histological control we stained alternate sections from the hemisected rat brains for acetylcholinesterase (AChE) activity by the method of Koelle and Friedenwald (8). As has been observed by other authors (10,16), the frontal cortex is only weakly stained for AChE, and the AChE staining is most evident in the deeper layers of the medial prefrontal area (Fig. 1C). Although the AChE and choline acetyltransferase (ChAT) content of this medial area was not affected by knife cuts isolating the globus pallidus from the caudate nucleus and overlying cortex, the dorsal and lateral frontal cortex areas were depleted (Fig. 1C). Presumably this indicates the presence of a cholinergic projection to the dorsal and lateral frontal cortex from the globus pallidus. Additionally, in agreement with other authors (10,11,16) we found that medial prefrontal areas and septum received a cholinergic innervation from the lateral preoptic area and the diagonal band region. Thus, parasagittal cuts between the diagonal band nuclei and the diagonal band tract depleted the septum and prefrontal cortex of AChE, ChAT, dopamine, and substance P.

In our view the coexistence of these three transmitter systems (substance P, dopaminergic, and cholinergic) within the prefrontal cortex is additional evidence to support the inclusion of this neocortical area within the limbic system. Consistent with this idea there is now substantial evidence to show the coexistence of these three transmitters in other limbic areas such as amygdala, nucleus accumbens, and olfactory tubercle (3,5,6).

FIG. 1. A: Substance P innervation of the medial prefrontal cortex in a frontal section at level A 10,300 μm. (Immunohistochemical technique to demonstrate substance P immunoreactive nerve terminals.)

B: The same medial prefrontal area after a hemisection transecting the medial forebrain bundle showing the complete disappearance of substance P-containing fibers.

C: A horizontal longitudinal section to show the distribution of acetylcholinesterase (AChE) in the medial prefrontal cortex. The dorsal and lateral cortex on the right-hand side has been depleted of AChE by a knife cut isolating the globus pallidus from the caudate nucleus and overlying cortex.

ACKNOWLEDGMENTS

I am grateful to my colleagues G. Paxinos, who carried out the initial knife lesions, T. Jessell, who performed the substance P assays, and Mrs. Jenny Reed, who contributed superb technical assistance.

REFERENCES

1. Bartholini, G., Stadler, H., Gadea-Ciria, M., and Lloyd, K. G. (1977): Interaction of dopaminergic and cholinergic neurons in the extra pyramidal and limbic systems. *Adv. Biochem. Psychopharmacol.,* 16:391–396.
2. Dahlström, A., and Fuxe, K. (1964): Evidence for the existence of monoamine-containing neurons in the central nervous system. I. Demonstration of monoamines in the cell bodies of brain stem neurons. *Acta Physiol. Scand. [Suppl. 232]* 62:1–55.
3. Emson, P. C. (1978): Neurotransmitters in the amygdala, a brief review. In: *Amino Acids as Chemical Transmitters,* edited by F. Fonnum. Plenum Press, New York.
4. Emson, P. C., and Koob, G. (1978): The origin and distribution of dopamine-containing afferents to the rat frontal cortex. *Brain Res.,* 142:249–267.
5. Fonnum, F., Walaas, I., and Iversen, E. (1977): Localization of GABAergic, cholinergic and aminergic structures in the mesolimbic system. *J. Neurochem.,* 29:221–230.
6. Hökfelt, T., Johansson, O., Fuxe, K., Elde, R., Goldstein, M., Park, D., Efendic, S., Luft, R., Fraser, H., and Jeffcoate, S. (1977): Hypothalamic dopamine neurons and hypothalamic peptides. *Adv. Biochem. Psychopharmacol.,* 16:99–108.
7. Kanazawa, I., and Jessell, T. (1976): Post mortem changes and regional distribution of substance P in the rat and mouse nervous system. *Brain Res.,* 117:362–367.
8. Koelle, G., and Friedenwald, J. S. (1949): A histochemical method for localizing cholinesterase activity. *Proc. Soc. Exp. Biol. Med.,* 70:617–622.
9. Konig, J. F. R., and Klippel, R. A. (1963): *The Rat Brain.* Williams & Wilkins Co., Baltimore.
10. Krnjevic, K., and Silver, A. (1965): A histochemical study of cholinergic fibres in the cerebral cortex. *J. Anat.,* 99:711–759.
11. Lindvall, O. (1975): Mesencephalic dopaminergic afferents to the lateral septal nucleus of the rat. *Brain Res.,* 87:89–95.
12. Lindvall, O., Björklund, A., Moore, R. Y., and Stenevi, U. (1974): Mesencephalic dopamine neurons projecting to neocortex. *Brain Res.,* 81:325–331.
13. Mantovani, P., Bartolini, A., and Pepeu, G. (1977): Interrelationships between dopaminergic and cholinergic systems in the cerebral cortex. *Adv. Biochem. Psychopharmacol.,* 16:423–427.
14. Nilsson, G., Hökfelt, T., and Pernow, P. (1974): Distribution of substance P-like immunoreactivity in the rat central nervous system as revealed by immunohistochemistry. *Med. Biol.,* 52:424–427.
15. Paxinos, G., Emson, P. C., and Cuello, A. C. (1978): The substance P projections to the frontal cortex and the substantia nigra. *Neurosci. Lett.,* 7:127–132.
16. Shute, C. C. D., and Lewis, P. R. (1967): The ascending cholinergic reticular system: Neocortical, olfactory and subcortical projections. *Brain,* 90:497–520.

Advances in Biochemical Psychopharmacology, Vol. 19,
edited by P. J. Roberts et al.
Raven Press, New York © 1978.

Regulation of GABA Release by Dopamine in the Rat Substantia Nigra

*J.-C. Reubi, L. L. Iversen, and T. M. Jessell

MRC Neurochemical Pharmacology Unit, Department of Pharmacology, Medical School,
Cambridge, England

The dendrites of dopaminergic neurons in the mammalian substantia nigra have been shown to contain relatively high concentrations of dopamine which can be released by a variety of evoking stimuli both *in vitro* and *in vivo* (1). The release of dopamine from dendrites may play a physiological role in regulating the activity of afferent inputs to the substantia nigra (2). A dopamine-sensitive adenylate cyclase has been demonstrated in the substania nigra which appears to be located presynaptically on the axon terminals of neurons originating in the corpus striatum and globus pallidus (3) that use either substance P or GABA as their transmitter. Since the topographic projections of the substance P and GABA-containing striatonigral pathways are similar, it has so far been impossible to determine whether dopamine receptors in the substantia nigra are associated with substance P- or GABA-containing terminals.

In an attempt to localize the site of action of dopamine, we have investigated the effects of dopamine on the release of substance P and GABA from superfused slices of rat substantia nigra *in vitro*. The results show that dopamine stimulated selectively the release of GABA from axon terminals within the substantia nigra.

METHODS

Substantia nigra tissue was dissected from 0.8-mm coronal sections of fresh chilled rat mesencephalon, and 0.2 × 0.2 mm slices were prepared using a McIlwain tissue chopper. Initially, the high-affinity uptake of ^{3}H-GABA was measured, using the method of Iversen and Johnston (4); after 10 min of incubation with 10^{-7} M ^{3}H-GABA at 37°C, a tissue:medium ratio of 72.9 ± 2.1 (mean ± SEM; $N = 4$) was found, indicating that slices of substantia nigra were able to accumulate exogenous GABA from the external medium. Substance P release from superfused slices was measured

---

* Present address: Brain Research Institute, Zurich, Switzerland.

as described previously (5). In experiments to measure GABA release, substantia nigra slices from two rats were incubated for 20 min in Krebs-bicarbonate solution containing 10^{-7} M ^{3}H-GABA, transferred to a super-fusion chamber and superfused at 37°C, with Krebs-bicarbonate containing 30 mg/liter ascorbic acid and 10 mg/liter disodium ethylenediamine-tetra-acetate to inhibit the spontaneous breakdown of dopamine. The tritium content was determined in superfusate samples collected at 2-min intervals, and substantia nigra tissue was recovered at the end of superfusion. In similar experiments more than 90% of the radioactivity was found to represent unchanged ^{3}H-GABA (6).

RESULTS

After a rapid initial efflux rate, the spontaneous release of ^{3}H-GABA remained constant at approximately 0.7% to 0.9% of the total tissue stores released per minute. Addition of 11 mM potassium into the medium for 4 min produced a ^{3}H-GABA release of 3.78 ± 0.56% (mean ± SEM; $N=4$). This release was concentration dependent (over the range of 11 to 47 mM) and was abolished in media with reduced calcium and elevated magnesium.

Addition of dopamine (5 to 500 μM) to the superfusing medium produced a concentration-dependent increase in ^{3}H-GABA release which was abolished in medium containing 0.1 mM calcium and 12 mM magnesium (Fig. 1a and b). The simultaneous application of 50 μM dopamine and 11 mM potassium did not produce a significantly greater release of ^{3}H-GABA than application of 11 mM potassium alone. Addition of the dopamine receptor antagonists α-flupenthixol (1 μM) (Fig. 1c) and fluphenazine (1 μM) to the superfusing medium completely abolished the dopamine-evoked release; haloperidol also partly suppressed this release. The application of the dopamine agonist 4-amino, 6-7-dihydroxy-1,2,3,4-tetrahydronaphthalene (ADTN) (50 μM) given for 4 min also produced a large release of ^{3}H-GABA (Fig. 1d).

D-Amphetamine (50μM), which is thought to release dopamine from intracellular storage sites (1,2), caused a small but significant ($p < 0.05$) release of ^{3}H-GABA when added to the superfusing medium for 4 min (Fig. 1e). The effects of amphetamine could be blocked by addition of α-flupenthixol (1 μM). The stable cyclic AMP analogue dibutyryl cyclic AMP (1.2 mM) administered for 6 min produced a marked increase in the release of ^{3}H-GABA (Fig. 1f) which was calcium dependent.

In control experiments, dopamine (50 μM) did not evoke a significant release of ^{3}H-GABA in the corpus striatum or hippocampus, suggesting that this interaction may be specific to the substantia nigra. It is unlikely that the GABA release measured in the present experiments originated from glial cells since 50 μM dopamine did not affect the spontaneous efflux of ^{3}H-β-alanine, a specific marker for GABA uptake sites into glial cells. The

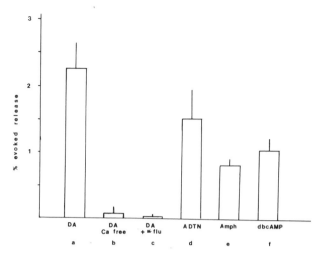

FIG. 1. Release of ³H-GABA from rat substantia nigra. Each column represents the total release of ³H-GABA evoked by drug application, expressed as percentage of the total tissue content.
a: Release of ³H-GABA evoked by addition of 50 μM dopamine (N = 8).
b: Effect of 50 μM dopamine on ³H-GABA release in medium containing 0.1 mM calcium and 12 mM magnesium (N = 4).
c: Effect of 50 μM dopamine on ³H-GABA release after addition of α-flupenthixol (1 μM) (N = 4).
d: Release of ³H-GABA evoked by ADTN (50 μM) (N = 4).
e: Release of ³H-GABA evoked by D-amphetamine (50 μM) (N = 5).
f: Release of ³H-GABA evoked by 1.2 mM dibutyryl-cyclicAMP (N = 4).

spontaneous and potassium-evoked release of substance P was found to be unaffected by addition of 50 μM dopamine.

DISCUSSION

The present results suggest that dopamine produces a selective stimulation of GABA release within the substantia nigra. In addition, the actions of dopamine are likely to be mediated by dopamine receptors with a similar pharmacological specificity to dopamine receptors found in other regions of the central nervous system. The release of GABA appears to originate from striatonigral axon terminals since in other experiments it has been shown that the dopamine-sensitive adenylate cyclase in the substantia nigra is abolished by transection of the striatonigral pathway (3). The lack of effect of dopamine on substance P release indicates that dopamine receptors may be located predominantly on the GABA-containing striatonigral terminals. Amphetamine supposedly acts presynaptically in the caudate nucleus to release dopamine and inhibit its reuptake; stimulation of GABA release by amphetamine in the substantia nigra therefore suggests that a release of endogenous dopamine from the dendrites of the substantia nigra is able to stimulate a local release of ³H-GABA.

The cellular mechanisms responsible for the dopamine-evoked GABA release are unknown; however, an activation of cyclic AMP may be involved, since dibutyryl-cyclic AMP appears to mimick the dopamine-evoked release of GABA.

The selective enhancement of the spontaneous release of GABA without affecting the potassium-evoked release may provide a more subtle mechanism for controlling the firing rate of dopaminergic neurons; thus, during intense striatonigral inhibiting activity, the excitatory effects of dopamine may be abolished.

In conclusion, the present results provide one possible mechanism for the local feedback inhibition of dopaminergic neurons within the substantia nigra.

ACKNOWLEDGMENTS

J. C. R. was supported by the Slack-Gyr Foundation, an ETP grant, and a Swiss NSF grant No. 3.636.75. T. M. J. is an MRC Scholar.

REFERENCES

1. Geffen, L. B., Jessell, T. M., Cuello, A. C., and Iversen, L. L. (1976): Release of dopamine from dendrites in rat substantia nigra. *Nature,* 260:258–260.
2. Groves, P. M., Wilson, C. J., Young, S. J., and Rebec, G. V. (1975): Self-inhibition by dopaminergic neurones. *Science,* 190:522–529.
3. Iversen, L. L. (1977): Catecholamine-sensitive adenylate cyclase in nervous tissues. *J. Neurochem.,* 29:5–12.
4. Iversen, L. L., and Johnston, G. A. R. (1971): GABA uptake in rat central nervous system: Comparison of uptake in slices and homogenates and the effects of some inhibitors. *J. Neurochem.,* 18:1939–1950.
5. Jessell, T. M., Iversen, L. L., and Kanazawa, I. (1976): Release and metabolism of substance P in rat hypothalamus. *Nature,* 264:81–83.
6. Srinivasan, V., Neal, M. J., and Mitchell, J. F. (1969): The effect of electrical stimulation and high potassium concentrations on the efflux of ^{3}H-GABA from brain slices. *J. Neurochem.,* 16:1235–1244.

Advances in Biochemical Psychopharmacology, Vol. 19,
edited by P. J. Roberts et al.
Raven Press, New York © 1978.

In Vitro Uptake of Dopamine in Serotoninergic Nerve Terminals: A Fluorescence Histochemical Study on Vibratome Sections of the Rat Cerebral Cortex

Brigitte Berger

INSERM U134, Laboratoire de Neuropathologie Charles Foix, Hopital Salpêtrière, 75634 Paris, Cedex 13 France

The present study was undertaken to develop an *in vitro* approach allowing the separate visualization of noradrenergic and dopaminergic nerve terminals in rat cerebral tissue sections. We tried to use experimental conditions close to those selected in biochemical studies carried out on synaptosomal preparations for the analysis of the amine uptake processes.

Following the depletion of catecholamine stores by a pharmacological treatment, fluorescence histochemical studies were performed on thin tissue sections from normal or lesioned rats. The sections were incubated in the presence of different exogenous amines and of catecholamine uptake inhibitors, and the minimal concentrations of amines and drugs required were determined.

It was thus observed that in contrast to norepinephrine (NE), dopamine (DA) was taken up not only in catecholaminergic but also in serotoninergic nerve terminals. We report here briefly on the experimental conditions allowing the identification of the three types of aminergic terminals.

METHODS

Endogenous catecholamines were detectable in cerebral tissue sections of normal rats incubated in a physiological medium. Thus, it was necessary to deplete the endogenous stores of these transmitters in order to properly evaluate the accumulation of exogenous amines. All the animals were therefore pretreated with α-methyl-*p*-tyrosine (7) (150 mg/kg) 12 hr and (200 mg/kg) 2 hr before sacrifice. In addition, lesions of the aminergic systems were performed in some cases: bilateral destruction of the ascending noradrenergic pathways; high-frequency electrolytic lesions in the ventral tegmental area (VTA) to destroy the mesocortical dopaminergic neurons; and elimination of the serotoninergic innervation of the cerebral cortex and hippocampus following local microinjections of 5,7-dihydroxytryptamine in the tegmentum. Biochemical analysis had previously confirmed the validity of the lesion models used (8,10; D. Nelson, C. Euvrard, A. Herbert, and J. Glowinski, *personal communication*).

In all these cases, coronal sections 30 μm thick were prepared with a vibratome from the entire frontal lobe or from the parietal, hippocampal, or cerebellar cortices and incubated according to the technique of Hamberger (3). Pargyline 10^{-4} M as a MAO inhibitor and amine uptake inhibitors were introduced at the beginning of the 10-min preincubation period. Exogenous amines were introduced during the 10-min incubation period. The glyoxylic acid method (5) was then applied, modified as previously described (1).

RESULTS

Identification of Dopaminergic Fibers

The best procedure to selectively visualize the dopaminergic fibers was to incubate cerebral tissue sections with DA (10^{-6} M) in the presence of desmethylimipramine (DMI) (5×10^{-6} M). At this concentration this inhibitor blocked the amine uptake in noradrenergic and also in serotoninergic fibers, without affecting the transport of DA in dopaminergic fibers in agreement with biochemical findings.

The morphological aspect and the distribution of the fluorescent fibers were similar to those of the dopaminergic arborizations previously identified (1,5). They were easily detected in the medial frontal and the rhinal cortex but not in the hippocampal and cerebellar cortex known to be devoid of DA innervation. They were not observed when benztropine (10^{-5} M), a potent blocker of the active transport in DA fibers (2,9), was used instead of DMI. They disappeared following lesions in the VTA but were not affected by the destruction of the ascending noradrenergic pathways.

Identification of Serotoninergic Fibers

When inhibitors of DA uptake were not added during the preincubation, DA (10^{-6} M) was also found to be taken up in fibers exhibiting morphological characteristics distinct from those of dopaminergic and noradrenergic fibers. These fibers were thinner and less sinuous than the dopaminergic arborizations with small and irregularly spaced varicosities. They were also seen in areas lacking dopaminergic innervation, such as the parietal cerebral cortex, the gyrus dentatus, and the cerebellar cortex.

Several facts suggested that this third type of fluorescent fiber could represent serotoninergic nerve terminals:

1. They appeared located in areas known to be innervated by serotoninergic neurons.
2. They were not seen in tissue sections of the hippocampus and the

cerebral cortex of rats lesioned with 5,7-dihydroxytryptamine, although NA and DA arborizations could still be visualized.

3. They were present in the cerebral and hippocampal cortices of rats lesioned with 6-hydroxydopamine to selectively destroy the ascending noradrenergic pathways. They could also be observed in some rats lesioned in the VTA when the electrolytic lesion spared the serotoninergic axons passing close to this mesencephalic zone.

4. They could not be observed in the presence of fluoxetine (10^{-6} M), a selective inhibitor of 5-HT uptake (11). Indeed, this drug did not influence the transport of exogenous amines in catecholaminergic fibers under our experimental conditions.

5. Furthermore, in the presence of 5-HT (10^{-6} to 10^{-5} M) added to compete with DA (10^{-6} M) for the membrane 5-HT carrier, the third type of fluorescent fibers was no longer seen.

Benztropine (10^{-5} M) at a concentration which blocked the transport of DA in dopaminergic fibers, slightly reduced the visualization of this third type of fluorescent fiber. Nevertheless, they could be identified easily. Maprotiline, at a concentration (10^{-5} M) which completely inhibited DA uptake in noradrenergic fibers, also affected, but to a lesser extent, the transport of DA in the serotoninergic arborization. At a lower concentration of the inhibitor (10^{-6} M), the serotoninergic innervation was easily detectable but the typical noradrenergic fibers were less fluorescent and slightly less numerous. In contrast, the inhibiting effect of DMI on the amine transport in the two types of terminals was observed not only at the concentration of 5×10^{-6} M necessary to completely block the amine uptake in NA fibers, but was observed also at a lower concentration (10^{-6} M).

Several concentrations of DA were tested in order to visualize the serotoninergic fibers (10^{-7} M, 5×10^{-7} M, and 10^{-6} M). The optimal concentration was 10^{-6} M since fewer fluorescent axonal terminals were seen with lower concentrations. In contrast to that observed with DA, the serotoninergic fibers could not be seen when NE or α-methylnorepinephrine was used as exogenous amine regardless of the concentration tested (10^{-6}, 10^{-5} M).

Identification of Noradrenergic Axons

Fluorescent axons, exhibiting the morphological aspect of typical NE terminals (1), were observed in tissue sections incubated with exogenous NE (10^{-6} M) in the presence of benztropine (10^{-5} M). Under these conditions, the noradrenergic fibers are the only ones seen, since at this concentration benztropine is completely effective in blocking NE transport into dopaminergic neurons. Furthermore, in contrast to DA, NE is not accumulated in serotoninergic fibers.

These axons were not detectable when DMI 5×10^{-6} or maprotiline 10^{-5} M was present in the incubation medium instead of benztropine; nor were they seen after the destruction of the ascending noradrenergic pathways. In contrast, they did persist after destruction of the DA neurons in the VTA.

REFERENCES

1. Berger, B., Thierry, A. M., Tassin, J. P., and Moyne, M. A. (1976): Dopaminergic innervation of the rat prefrontal cortex: A fluorescence histochemical study. *Brain Res.*, 106:133–145.
2. Coyle, S. T., and Snyder, S. H. (1969): Antiparkinsonian drugs: Inhibition of dopamine uptake in the corpus striatum as a possible mechanism of action. *Science,* 166:899–901.
3. Hamberger, B. (1967): Reserpine resistant uptake of catecholamines in isolated tissues of the rat. *Acta Physiol. Scand. [Suppl.]*, 295:1–56.
4. Lidbrink, P., Jonsson, G., and Fuxe, K. (1971): The effect of imipramine-like drugs and antihistamine drugs on uptake mechanism in the central noradrenaline and 5-hydroxytryptamine neurons. *Neuropharmacology*, 10:521–536.
5. Lindvall, O., and Björklund, A. (1974): The glyoxylic acid fluorescence histochemical method: A detailed account of the methodology for the visualization of the central catecholamine neurons. *Histochemistry, 39*:97–127.
6. Shaskan, E., and Snyder, S. H. (1970): Kinetics of serotonin accumulation into slices from rat brain: Relationship to catecholamine uptake. *J. Pharmacol. Exp. Ther.,* 175:404–418.
7. Spector, S., Sjoerdsma, A., Udenfried, S. (1965): Blockade of endogenous norepinephrine synthesis by α-methyl-tyrosine, an inhibitor of tyrosine hydroxylase. *J. Pharmacol. Exp. Ther.*, 147:86–95.
8. Tassin, J. P., Stinus, L., Simon, H., Blanc, G., Thierry, A. M., Le Moal, M., Cardo, B., and Glowinski, J. (1978): Relationship between the locomotor hyperactivity induced by A_{10} lesions and the destruction of the fronto-cortical dopaminergic innervation in the rat. *Brain Res.*, 141:267–281.
9. Tassin, J. P., Thierry, A. M., Blanc, G., and Glowinski, J. (1974): Evidence for a specific uptake of dopamine by dopaminergic terminals of the rat cerebral cortex. *Naunyn-Schmiedberg's Arch. Pharmacol.*, 282:239–244.
10. Thierry, A. M., Stinus, L., Blanc, G., and Glowinski, J. (1973): Some evidence for the existence of dopaminergic neurons in the rat cortex. *Brain Res.*, 50:230–234.
11. Wong, D. T., Bymaster, F. P., Horng, J. S., and Molloy, B. B. (1975): A new selective inhibitor for uptake of serotonin into synaptosomes of rat brain: 3-(p-trifluoromethylphenoxy)-N-Methyl-6,3-phenylpropylamine. *J. Pharmacol. Exp. Ther.,* 193:804–811.

Subject Index